ACSM's
CLINICAL
CERTIFICATION
REVIEW

ACSM Exercise Specialist®
ACSM Program Director$_{SM}$

SENIOR EDITORS
Michael S. Wegner, PhD, FACSM
Professional Services
Medical Liaison
KOS Pharmaceuticals, Inc.
Miami Lakes, Florida

Jeanne E. Ruff, MS, FAACVPR
Director of Cardiac/Pulmonary Rehabilitation and Health Promotion
Peninsula Regional Medical Center
Salisbury, Maryland

ASSOCIATE EDITOR
Walter R. Thompson, PhD, FACSM, FAACVPR
Professor of Kinesiology and Health (College of Education)
Professor of Nutrition (College of Health and Human Sciences)
Georgia State University
Atlanta, Georgia

ACSM's CLINICAL CERTIFICATION REVIEW

ACSM EXERCISE SPECIALIST®
ACSM PROGRAM DIRECTOR$_{SM}$

AMERICAN COLLEGE OF SPORTS MEDICINE

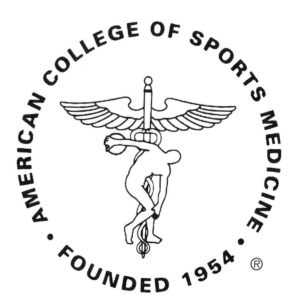

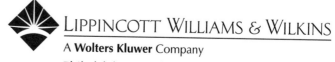

LIPPINCOTT WILLIAMS & WILKINS
A **Wolters Kluwer** Company

Philadelphia • Baltimore • New York • London
Buenos Aires • Hong Kong • Sydney • Tokyo

Editor: Peter Darcy
Editorial Director: Julie P. Scardiglia
Development Editors: Rosanne Hallowell and Kevin Law
Managing Editor: Amy G. Dinkel
Marketing Manager: Christen DeMarco
ACSM Publications Committee Chair: W. Larry Kenney, PhD, FACSM
ACSM Group Publisher: D. Mark Robertson

Lippincott Williams & Wilkins
351 West Camden Street
Baltimore, Maryland 21201-2436 USA

530 Walnut Street
Philadelphia, Pennsylvania 19106 USA

The publisher is not responsible (as a matter of product liability, negligence, or otherwise) for any injury resulting from any material contained herein. This publication contains information relating to general principles of medical care which should not be construed as specific instructions for individual patients. Manufacturers' product information and package inserts should be reviewed for current information, including contraindications, dosages, and precautions.

Printed in the United States of America

The publishers have made every effort to trace the copyright holders for borrowed material. If they have inadvertently overlooked any, they will be pleased to make the necessary arrangements at the first opportunity.

We'd like to hear from you! If you have comments or suggestions regarding this Lippincott Williams & Wilkins title, please contact us at the appropri-ate customer service number listed below, or send correspondence to **book_comments@lww.com.** If possible, please remember to include your mail-ing address, phone number, and a reference to the book title and author in your message. To purchase additional copies of this book call our cus-tomer service department at **(800) 638-3030** or fax orders to **(301) 824-7390.** International customers should call **(301) 714-2324.**

01 02 03
1 2 3 4 5 6 7 8 9 10

CONTRIBUTORS

THEODORE J. ANGELOPOULOS, PhD, MPH, FACSM
Professor and Director
Exercise Physiology Laboratory
University of Central Florida
Department of Human Services and Wellness
College of Education
Orlando, Florida
Chapter 12, Electrocardiography

KHALID W. BIBI, PhD
Associate Professor, Sports Medicine, Health & Human
Performance
Director, Health and Human Performance Center
Canisius College
Buffalo, New York
Chapter 11, Metabolic Calculations

KIMBERLY A. BONZHEIM, MSA, FACSM
Assistant Director
Cardiac Rehabilitation and Exercise Laboratories
William Beaumont Hospital
Birmingham, Michigan
Chapter 9, Nutrition and Weight Management

KATHLEEN M. CAHILL, MS, ATC, RCEP
President
Health Enhancements
Germantown, Tennessee
Chapter 8, Exercise Programming

FREDERICK S. DANIELS, MS, HFD
President
CPTE Health Group, Inc.
Nashua, New Hampshire
Chapter 7, Safety, Injury Prevention, and Emergency Care

PATRICK J. DUNN, MS, MBA
Executive Director
New Heart Cardiovascular Disease Management
Program
Albuquerque, New Mexico
Chapter 2, Exercise Physiology

GREGORY B. DWYER, PhD, FACSM, ETT, ES, PD, RCEP
Assistant Professor
Department of Movement Studies and Exercise Science
East Stroudsburg University
East Stroudsburg, Pennsylvania
Chapter 10, Program Administration / Management

KELLY M. EBERLEIN, RD
Diabetes and Endocrinology Associates, PC
Decatur, Georgia
Chapter 9, Nutrition and Weight Management

STEPHEN C. GLASS, PhD, FACSM
Division Head / Dean
Wayne State College
Division of Human Performance and Leisure Studies
Wayne, Nebraska
Chapter 6, Health Appraisal and Fitness Testing

CHAD HARRIS, PhD
Associate Professor
Department of Kinesiology
Boise State University
Boise, Idaho
Chapter 1, Functional Anatomy and Biomechanics

MARK J. KASPER, EdD
Associate Professor
Valdosta State University
Department of Kinesiology and Physical Education
Valdosta, Georgia
Chapter 4, Pathophysiology / Risk Factors

ROBERT S. MAZZEO, PhD, FACSM
University of Colorado
Department of Kinesiology and Applied Physiology
Boulder, Colorado
Chapter 3, Human Development and Aging

EILEEN UDRY, PhD
Department of Physical Education
Indiana University Purdue University Indianapolis
Indianapolis, Indiana
Chapter 5, Human Behavior and Psychology

Contents

FOREWORD

Advances in modern medicine have contributed immensely to the detection and treatment of chronic diseases. Moreover, exercise testing and training are now widely accepted as part of our diagnostic and therapeutic armamentarium. As a result, mortality and recurrence rates have declined, and the patients' symptomatology and quality of life have improved.

The emergence of this new clinical specialty, preventive and rehabilitative medicine—including multifactorial lifestyle alterations, behavior change, and contemporary pharmacotherapies aimed at the primary and secondary prevention of disease—has created the need for educating and training physicians and allied health professionals to deliver these services. Although numerous organizations have responded to this void through their sponsorship of conferences, establishment of committees, and publication of educational materials, none have done it with the fervor of the American College of Sports Medicine (ACSM). Since 1975, the ACSM has uniquely promulgated quality control and knowledge and proficiency standards for program personnel through their Guidelines, workshops, and certification examinations, which are now held in 13 countries worldwide!

It is an honor and a privilege for me to introduce you to this text, *ACSM's Clinical Certification Review*, which was written to cover the critical knowledge, skills, and abilities (KSAs) for Clinical Track certifications as delineated in the sixth edition of *ACSM's Guidelines for Exercise Testing and Prescription*—a virtual pharmacopoeia of scientifically based exercise recommendations for a broad spectrum of persons with and without chronic disease.

This clinical review text includes KSAs presented in outline form; a plethora of tables and figures to highlight key or salient points; 12 clinically germane chapters with end-of-chapter Review Test questions; and Comprehensive Examination questions at the end of the book. It provides an overview of the fundamental competencies that must be mastered by candidates applying for the ACSM's Program Director$_{SM}$ and Exercise Specialist® certifications. Accordingly, the editors have recruited a prestigious group of scientists, clinicians, researchers and, most importantly, outstanding teachers who have painstakingly worked to summarize, in a clear and concise manner, pertinent information relative to the KSAs.

For nearly 20,000 exercise professionals, ACSM certification has served as a springboard to launching a satisfying and rewarding career—an investment in helping others "help themselves" to achieve the health and fitness dividends that result from a physically active lifestyle. This book serves as a compass to navigate the reader on his or her journey toward accomplishing this objective, by providing an invaluable study guide in preparing for clinical certifications.

The challenge is yours!

Barry A. Franklin, PhD, FACSM
Director, Cardiac Rehabilitation
and Exercise Laboratories
William Beaumont Hospital
Royal Oak, Michigan

PREFACE

The *ACSM's Clinical Certification Review* is one of two review books for ACSM certification; the other book is the *ACSM's Health & Fitness Certification Review*. Along with the *ACSM's Resource Manual for Guidelines for Exercise Testing and Prescription, 4th edition*, these review books present materials relevant to ACSM certification in an organized and user-friendly fashion.

The information in the *ACSM's Clinical Certification Review* covers almost all of the knowledge, skills and abilities (KSAs) for the clinical track, both for the ACSM Program Director$_{SM}$ (PD) and the ACSM Exercise Specialist$_{SM}$ (ES) certifications.

Features. The chapters in the *ACSM's Clinical Certification Review* coincide with the major categories of the KSAs and are presented in **outline form** to allow quick, topical review of each area. This type of presentation is possible because of the new organization of the KSAs. **Tables and figures** supplement the outline text and allow for easy access to supporting information. At the conclusion of each chapter there is a **Review Test** consisting of multiple-choice study questions written in the same format and at about the same difficulty level as the examination questions in the ACSM's Clinical Track certification exam. A **Comprehensive Examination** is presented at the end of the book for additional practice. It too has been formulated using the same "blueprint" as the certification examination so that candidates get a taste of the true written examination process. **Answers with explanations** are provided for each Review Test and Comprehensive Examination question. In the Review Tests and Comprehensive Examination, the candidate will find questions that are representative of the KSAs and applicable to each level of certification. A listing of **Recommended Readings** pertaining to each chapter can also be found at the end of the book, preceding the Comprehensive Examination; these references can be consulted for more-detailed information about the topics outlined in this study guide.

How to Use This Book. The *ACSM's Clinical Certification Review* is meant to be used by ACSM Clinical Track certification candidates who are ready (or nearly ready) for the certification examination and want to review the KSAs. Those candidates who are just beginning the study process may want to use this study guide to identify their "weak areas" where more intense study may be necessary. This book is *not* meant to be a primary resource; it is really a "skeletal" outline of the critical KSAs for the Clinical Track certification. The reader is further advised that the two basic study books for all ACSM Certification candidates are the *ACSM's Guidelines for Exercise Testing and Prescription*, 6th edition (© 2000) and the *ACSM's Resource Manual for Guidelines for Exercise Testing and Prescription*, 4th edition (© 2001). These are invaluable and primary resources for all certification candidates and professionals who need supplemental information about the ACSM's Guidelines and their derivation.

Summary. The features contained in the *ACSM's Clinical Certification Review*—the outline format, the tables and illustrations, the practice questions for each chapter, and the comprehensive examination at the end of the book—should make this study guide a great aid to those preparing for certification. It is our hope that this type of presentation will assist all candidates for these certifications to increase their level of knowledge and preparation for the examination and certification process.

Acknowledgments. We would like to acknowledge the support and participation of our loved ones (Joanie, Caroline and Sarah), and thank them for their patience with our participation in this project and the hours we spent away from them. Additionally, we would like to acknowledge the individuals we work with everyday. Their support towards our efforts in contributing to our profession and ACSM is greatly appreciated. And finally, we would like to thank the following manuscript reviewers:

Charles Emory, PhD
Reed Humphrey, PhD, FACSM
Doug Post, MS, PT
F. Stuart Sanders, MD, FACSM
Renee Wall, MS, RDLD, CDE
Rose Mary Wasielewski, MSN, RN, C
Robert Wester, MPH
Mitchell Whaley, PhD, FACSM
Mark Williams, PhD, FACSM

KNOWLEDGE, SKILLS, AND ABILITIES (KSAS) FOR ACSM EXERCISE SPECIALIST® AND ACSM PROGRAM DIRECTOR_{SM} CERTIFICATIONS

KSA Numbering System. The first number in the sequence denotes the certification level of the KSA. KSAs numbered "1.—" are specific to Group Exercise Leader; KSAs numbered "2.—" are specific to Health/Fitness Instructor; and so on. The first numbers denote level of certification as follows:

1.— Exercise Leader
2.— Health/Fitness Instructor
3.— Health/Fitness Director
4.— Exercise Specialist
5.— Program Director

The second number in the sequence denotes the content matter of the KSA. For example, KSAs numbered "—.1" are related to Anatomy and Biomechanics; KSAs numbered "—.2" are related to Exercise Physiology. The second numbers denote content matter as follows:

—.1 Anatomy and Biomechanics
—.2 Exercise Physiology
—.3 Human Development and Aging
—.4 Pathophysiology and Risk Factors
—.5 Human Behavior and Psychology
—.6 Health Appraisal and Fitness Testing
—.7 Safety and Injury Prevention
—.8 Exercise Programming
—.9 Nutrition and Weight Management
—.10 Program and Administration/Management
—.11 Electrocardiography

Example. A KSA numbered "1.3.—" is a KSA for an Exercise Leader that relates to Human Development and Aging. A KSA numbered "4.4.—" is for an Exercise Specialist that relates to Pathophysiology and Risk Factors.

This numbering system allows exact determination of KSAs specific to the level of certification and the content matter.

ANATOMY AND BIOMECHANICS

1.1.0	Knowledge of anatomy as it relates to exercise and health.
1.1.0.1	Knowledge of the basic structures of bone, skeletal muscle, and connective tissues.
1.1.0.2	Knowledge of the basic anatomy of the cardiovascular system and respiratory system.
1.1.0.3	Ability to identify the major bones and muscles. Major muscles include, but are not limited to, the following: trapezius, pectoralis major, latissimus dorsi, biceps, triceps, *rectus abdominis,* internal and external obliques, erector spinae, gluteus maximus, quadriceps, hamstrings, adductors, abductors, and gastrocnemius.
1.1.0.4	Knowledge of the definition of the following terms: supination, pronation, flexion, extension, adduction, abduction, hyperextension, rotation, circumduction, agonist, antagonist, and stabilizer.
1.1.0.5	Ability to identify the joints of the body.
1.1.1	Knowledge of biomechanical aspects of exercise participation.
1.1.1.1	Knowledge to identify the plane in which each muscle action occurs.
1.1.1.2	Knowledge of the interrelationships among center of gravity, base of support, balance, stability, and proper spinal alignment.
1.1.1.3	Ability to describe the following curvatures of the spine: lordosis, scoliosis, and kyphosis.
1.1.1.4	Knowledge of and skill to demonstrate exercises designed to enhance muscular strength and/or endurance of specific major muscle groups.
1.1.1.5	Knowledge of and skill to demonstrate exercises for enhancing musculoskeletal flexibility.
1.1.1.6	Knowledge to describe the myotatic stretch reflex.
1.1.1.7	Knowledge to identify the primary action and joint range of motion for each major muscle group.

2.1.0   Knowledge of functional anatomy and biomechanics.

2.1.0.1   Knowledge of the structure and ability to describe movements for the major joints of the body.

2.1.0.2   Ability to locate the anatomic landmarks for palpation of peripheral pulses.

2.1.0.3   Ability to locate the brachial artery and correctly place the cuff and stethoscope in position for blood pressure measurement.

2.1.0.4   Ability to locate common sites for measurement of skinfold thicknesses and circumferences (for determination of body composition and waist-hip ratio).

2.1.1   Knowledge of biomechanical principles that underlie performance of the following activities: walking, jogging, running, swimming, cycling, weight lifting, and carrying or moving objects.

3.1.0   Ability to describe modifications in exercise prescription for individuals with functional disabilities and musculoskeletal injuries.

3.1.1   Ability to describe the relationship between biomechanical efficiency, oxygen cost of activity (economy), and performance of physical activity.

4.1.0   Knowledge of anatomy as it relates to exercise testing and programming.

4.1.0.1   Ability to locate anatomic landmarks for palpitation of radial, brachial, carotid, femoral, popliteal, and tibialis arteries.

4.1.0.2   Ability to locate the appropriate sites for the limb and chest leads for resting, standard, and exercise (Mason Likar) electrocardiograms (ECGs), as well as commonly used bipolar systems (e.g., CM-5).

4.1.0.3   Knowledge of coronary anatomy.

4.1.0.4   Knowledge of basic joint movements, muscle actions, and points of insertions as it relates to exercise programming.

4.1.1   Knowledge of the biomechanical factors associated with various disease states, neuromuscular disorders, and orthopedic limitations.

4.1.1.1   Knowledge of common gait abnormalities as they relate to exercise testing and programming.

4.1.1.2   Knowledge of neuromuscular disorders (e.g., Parkinson's disease, multiple sclerosis) as they relate to modifications of exercise testing and programming.

4.1.1.3   Knowledge of orthopedic limitations (e.g., gout, foot drop, specific joint problems) as they relate to modifications of exercise testing and programming.

5.1.1   Knowledge of standard auscultatory regions in the chest for listening to heart sounds, murmurs, and lung sounds.

5.1.1.1   Ability to list regions of auscultatory interest (e.g., aortic, pulmonic, tricuspid, mitral areas).

5.1.1.2   Knowledge of heart sounds and murmurs (e.g., first heart sound, second heart sound, gallop sounds, midsystolic clicks, systolic ejection murmurs, diastolic murmurs).

5.1.1.3   Knowledge of lung sounds (e.g., rales, crackles).

EXERCISE PHYSIOLOGY

1.2.0   Basic knowledge of exercise physiology as it relates to exercise prescription.

1.2.1   Ability to define aerobic and anaerobic metabolism.

1.2.2   Knowledge of the role of aerobic and anaerobic energy systems in the performance of various activities.

1.2.3 Knowledge of the following terms: ischemia, angina pectoris, tachycardia, bradycardia, arrhythmia, myocardial infarction, cardiac output, stroke volume, lactic acid, oxygen consumption, hyperventilation, systolic blood pressure, diastolic blood pressure, and anaerobic threshold.

1.2.4 Knowledge of the role of carbohydrates, fats, and proteins as fuels for aerobic and anaerobic metabolism.

1.2.5 Knowledge of the components of fitness: cardiorespiratory fitness, muscular strength, muscular endurance, flexibility, and body composition.

1.2.6 Knowledge to describe normal cardiorespiratory responses to static and dynamic exercise in terms of heart rate, blood pressure, and oxygen consumption.

1.2.7 Knowledge of how heart rate, blood pressure, and oxygen consumption responses change with adaptation to chronic exercise training.

1.2.8 Knowledge of the physiological adaptations associated with strength training.

1.2.9 Ability to identify and apply to both groups and individuals methods used to monitor exercise intensity, including heart rate and rating of perceived exertion.

1.2.10 Knowledge of the physiological principles related to warm-up and cool-down.

1.2.11 Knowledge of the common theories of muscle fatigue and delayed onset muscle soreness (DOMS).

2.2.0 Knowledge of exercise physiology including the role of aerobic and anaerobic metabolism, muscle physiology, cardiovascular physiology, and respiratory physiology at rest and during exercise. In addition, demonstrate an understanding of the components of physical fitness, the effects of aerobic and strength and/or resistance training on the fitness components and the effects of chronic disease.

2.2.1 Knowledge of the physiological adaptations that occur at rest and during submaximal and maximal exercise following chronic aerobic and anaerobic exercise training.

2.2.2 Knowledge of the differences in cardiorespiratory response to acute graded exercise between conditioned and unconditioned individuals.

2.2.3 Knowledge of the structure of the skeletal muscle fiber and the basic mechanism of contraction.

2.2.4 Knowledge of the characteristics of fast and slow twitch fibers.

2.2.5 Knowledge of the sliding filament theory of muscle contraction.

2.2.6 Knowledge of twitch, summation, and tetanus with respect to muscle contraction.

2.2.7 Ability to discuss the physiological principles involved in promoting gains in muscular strength and endurance.

2.2.8 Ability to define muscular fatigue as it relates to task, intensity, duration, and the accumulative effects of exercise.

2.2.9 Knowledge of the relationship between the number of repetitions, intensity, number of sets, and rest with regard to strength training.

2.2.10 Knowledge of the basic properties of cardiac muscle and the normal pathways of conduction in the heart.

2.2.11 Knowledge of the response of the following variables to acute exercise: heart rate, stroke volume, cardiac output, pulmonary ventilation, tidal volume, respiratory rate, and arteriovenous oxygen difference.

2.2.12 Knowledge of the differences in the cardiorespiratory responses to static exercise compared with dynamic exercise, including possible hazards and contraindications.

2.2.13 Ability to describe how each of the following differs from the normal condition: premature atrial contractions and premature ventricular contractions.

2.2.14 Knowledge of blood pressure responses associated with acute exercise, including changes in body position.

2.2.15 Knowledge of and ability to describe the implications of ventilatory threshold (anaerobic threshold) as it relates to exercise training and cardiorespiratory assessment.

2.2.16 Knowledge of and ability to describe the physiological adaptations of the respiratory system that occur at rest and during submaximal and maximal exercise following chronic aerobic and anaerobic training.

2.2.17 Ability to describe how each of the following differs from the normal condition: dyspnea, hypoxia, and hypoventilation.

2.2.18 Knowledge of and ability to discuss the physiological basis of the major components of physical fitness: flexibility, cardiovascular fitness, muscular strength, muscular endurance, and body composition.

2.2.19 Ability to explain how the principle of specificity relates to the components of fitness.

2.2.20 Ability to explain the concept of detraining or reversibility of conditioning and its implications in fitness programs.

2.2.21 Ability to discuss the physical and psychological signs of overtraining and to provide recommendations for these problems.

2.2.22 Ability to describe the physiological and metabolic responses to exercise associated with chronic disease (heart disease, hypertension, diabetes mellitus, and pulmonary disease).

3.2.0   Knowledge of the muscular, cardiorespiratory, and metabolic responses to decreased exercise intensity.

4.2.0   Knowledge of exercise physiology as it relates to exercise testing and training.

4.2.0.1   Ability to describe the physiological effects of bed rest and discuss the appropriate physical activities that might be used to counteract these changes.

4.2.0.2   Ability to describe the normal and abnormal cardiorespiratory responses at rest and exercise.

4.2.0.3   Ability to describe the principle of specificity of training as it relates to the mode of exercise testing and training.

4.2.0.4   Ability to list the cardiorespiratory responses associated with postural changes.

4.2.0.5   Knowledge of acute and chronic adaptations to exercise for apparently healthy individuals (low risk) and for those with cardiovascular, pulmonary, and metabolic diseases.

4.2.0.6   Ability to describe normal and abnormal chronotropic and inotropic responses to exercise testing and training.

4.2.1   Knowledge of activities that are primarily aerobic and anaerobic.

4.2.1.1   Ability to describe the aerobic and anaerobic metabolic demands of exercise for individuals with cardiovascular, pulmonary, and/or metabolic diseases undergoing exercise testing or training and the implications of such exercise.

4.2.1.2   Ability to identify the metabolic equivalent (MET) requirements of various occupational, household, sport/exercise, and leisure time activities.

4.2.2   Knowledge of the unique hemodynamic responses of arm versus leg exercise and of static versus dynamic exercise.

4.2.2.1   Ability to describe the differences in the physiological responses to various modes of ergometry (e.g., treadmill, cycle and arm ergometers) as they relate to exercise testing and training.

4.2.2.2   Ability to discuss the effects of isometric exercise in individuals with cardiovascular, pulmonary, and/or metabolic diseases or with low functional capacity.

4.2.3   Knowledge of the determinants of myocardial oxygen consumption and the effects of exercise training on those determinants.

4.2.3.1   Ability to explain maximal oxygen (O_2) consumption and how it is measured.

4.2.3.2   Ability to list and explain the variables measured during cardiopulmonary exercise testing (e.g., heart rate, blood pressure, rate of perceived exertion, ventilation, oxygen consumption, ventilatory threshold, pulmonary circulation) and their potential relationship to cardiovascular, pulmonary, and metabolic disease.

4.2.3.3   Ability to list and plot the normal resting and exercise values associated with increasing exercise intensity (and how they may differ for diseased population) for the following: heart rate, stroke volume, cardiac output, double product, arteriovenous O_2 difference, O_2 consumption, systolic and diastolic blood pressure, minute ventilation, tidal volume, breathing frequency, Vd/Vt, VE/VCO$_2$.

5.2.0   Ability to discuss the mechanisms by which functional capacity and cardiovascular, pulmonary, metabolic, endocrine, and neuromuscular adaptations occur in response to exercise testing and training in healthy and various diseased states.

HUMAN DEVELOPMENT AND AGING

1.3.0   Knowledge of the benefits and risks associated with exercise training in prepubescent and postpubescent youth.

1.3.1   Knowledge of the benefits and precautions associated with resistance and endurance training in older adults.

1.3.2   Ability to describe specific leadership techniques appropriate for working with participants of all ages.

2.3.0   Knowledge of the changes that occur during growth and development from childhood to old age.

2.3.0.1   Ability to modify cardiovascular and resistance exercises based on age and physical condition.

2.3.0.2   Knowledge of and ability to describe the changes that occur in maturation from childhood to adulthood for the following: skeletal muscle, bone structure, reaction time, coordination, heat and cold tolerance, maximal oxygen consumption, strength, flexibility, body composition, resting and maximal heart rate, and resting and maximal blood pressure.

2.3.0.3   Knowledge of the effect of the aging process on the musculoskeletal and cardiovascular structure and function at rest, during exercise, and during recovery.

2.3.0.4   Ability to characterize the differences in the development of an exercise prescription for children, adolescents, and older participants.

2.3.0.5   Knowledge of and ability to describe the unique adaptations to exercise training in children, adolescents, and older participants with regard to strength, functional capacity, and motor skills.

2.3.0.6   Knowledge of common orthopedic and cardiovascular considerations for older participants and the ability to describe modifications in exercise prescription that are indicated.

4.3.0   Knowledge of selecting appropriate testing and training modalities according to the age and functional capacity of the individual.

4.3.0.1   Ability to select an appropriate test protocol according to the age and functional capacity of the individual.

4.3.1   Ability to describe the importance of and appropriate methods for resistance training in older individuals.

5.3.0   Ability to explain differences in overall policy and procedures for the inclusion of different age groups in an exercise program.

5.3.1   Ability to discuss facility and equipment adaptations necessary for different age groups.

PATHOPHYSIOLOGY/RISK FACTORS

1.4.0   Knowledge of cardiovascular, respiratory, metabolic, and musculoskeletal risk factors that may require further evaluation by medical or allied health professionals before participation in physical activity.

1.4.0.1   Ability to determine those risk factors that may be favorably modified by physical activity habits.

1.4.0.2   Knowledge to define the following terms: total cholesterol (TC), high-density lipoprotein cholesterol (HDL-C), TC/HDL-C ratio, low-density lipoprotein cholesterol (LDL-C), triglycerides, hypertension, and atherosclerosis.

1.4.0.3   Knowledge of plasma cholesterol levels for adults as recommended by the National Cholesterol Education Program (NCEP II).

2.4.0   Knowledge of the pathophysiology of atherosclerosis and how this process is influenced by physical activity.

2.4.1   Knowledge of the risk factor concept of CAD and the influence of heredity and lifestyle on the development of CAD.

2.4.2   Knowledge of the atherosclerotic process, the factors involved in its genesis and progression, and the potential role of exercise training in treatment.

2.4.3   Ability to discuss in detail how lifestyle factors, including nutrition, physical activity, and heredity, influence lipid and lipoprotein profiles.

2.4.4 Knowledge of cardiovascular risk factors or conditions that may require consultation with medical personnel before testing or training, including inappropriate changes in resting or exercise heart rate and blood pressure, new onset discomfort in chest, neck, shoulder, or arm, changes in the pattern of discomfort during rest or exercise, fainting or dizzy spells, and claudication.

2.4.5 Knowledge of respiratory risk factors or conditions that may require consultation with medical personnel before testing or training, including asthma, exercise-induced bronchospasm, extreme breathlessness at rest or during exercise, bronchitis, and emphysema.

2.4.6 Knowledge of metabolic risk factors or conditions that may require consultation with medical personnel before testing or training, including body weight more than 20% above optimal, BMI 1 30, thyroid disease, diabetes or glucose intolerance, and hypoglycemia.

2.4.7 Knowledge of musculoskeletal risk factors or conditions that may require consultation with medical personnel before testing or training, including acute or chronic back pain, osteoarthritis, rheumatoid arthritis, osteoporosis, tendonitis, and low back pain.

3.4.0 Ability to define atherosclerosis, the factors causing it, and the interventions that may potentially delay or reverse the atherosclerotic process.

3.4.1 Ability to describe the causes of myocardial ischemia and infarction.

3.4.2 Ability to describe the pathophysiology of hypertension, obesity, hyperlipidemia, diabetes, chronic obstructive pulmonary diseases, arthritis, osteoporosis, chronic diseases, and immunosuppressive disease.

3.4.3 Ability to describe the effects of the above diseases and conditions on cardiorespiratory and metabolic function at rest and during exercise.

4.4.0 Ability to risk stratify individuals with cardiovascular, pulmonary, and metabolic diseases, using appropriate materials and understanding the prognostic indicators for high-risk individuals.

4.4.1 Ability to list the effects of cardiovascular, pulmonary, and metabolic diseases on performance and safety during exercise testing and training.

4.4.2 Knowledge of the common procedures used for radionuclide imaging (e.g., thallium, technetium, sestamibi, single photon emission computed tomography (SPECT), planar).

4.4.3 Ability to define myocardial ischemia and ability to identify the methods used to measure ischemic response.

4.4.4 Ability to describe the cardiorespiratory and metabolic responses in myocardial dysfunction and ischemia at rest and during exercise.

4.4.5 Knowledge of the differences between typical, atypical, and vasospastic angina.

4.4.6 Knowledge of the pathophysiology of the healing myocardium and the potential complications after acute myocardial infarction (MI) (extension, expansion, rupture).

4.4.7 Knowledge of the purpose of coronary angiography.

4.4.8 Knowledge of the indications for use of streptokinase, tissue plasminogen activase, and other thrombolytic agents.

4.4.9 Ability to describe PTCA and other catheter revascularization techniques (e.g., atherectomy, stent placement) as an alternative to medical management or coronary artery bypass surgery (CABS).

4.4.10 Ability to demonstrate an understanding of the indications and limitations for medical management and interventional techniques in different subsets of individuals with CAD and CABS.

4.4.11 Ability to describe the cardiorespiratory and metabolic responses that accompany or result from pulmonary diseases at rest and during exercise.

4.4.12 Ability to describe reversible airway (obstructive) and restrictive lung diseases and their effect on exercise testing and training.

4.4.13 Ability to describe the signs and symptoms of peripheral vascular diseases and their effect on exercise.

4.4.14 Ability to describe the metabolic responses at rest and during exercise and potential complications in individuals with type 1 or type 2 diabetes.

4.4.15 Ability to describe the influence of exercise on weight reduction, hyperlipidemia, hypertension, and diabetes.

4.4.16 Knowledge of the effects of variation in ambient temperature, humidity, carbon dioxide, ozone, and altitude on functional capacity for normal individuals and those with cardiovascular, pulmonary, and metabolic diseases.

4.4.17   Skill in adapting the exercise prescription appropriately in environmental extremes for normal individuals and those with cardiovascular, pulmonary, and metabolic diseases.

5.4.0   Knowledge of the atherosclerotic process, including current hypotheses regarding onset and rate of progression and/or regression.

5.4.1   Knowledge of the lipoprotein classifications and their relationship to atherosclerosis or other diseases.

5.4.2   Ability to identify and explain the mechanisms by which exercise may contribute to preventing or rehabilitating individuals with cardiovascular, pulmonary, and metabolic diseases.

5.4.3   Knowledge and ability to describe coronary angiography, radionuclide imaging, echocardiography imaging, and pharmacologic studies, including the type of information obtained, sensitivity, specificity, predictive value, and associated risks and indications for use.

HUMAN BEHAVIOR AND PSYCHOLOGY

1.5.0   Ability to identify and define at least five behavioral strategies to enhance exercise and health behavior change (i.e., reinforcement, goal setting, social support).

1.5.1   Ability to list and define the five important elements that should be included in each counseling session.

1.5.2   Knowledge of specific techniques to enhance motivation (e.g., posters, recognition, bulletin boards, games, competitions). Define extrinsic and intrinsic reinforcement and give examples of each.

1.5.3   Knowledge of the stages of motivational readiness.

1.5.4   Ability to list and describe three counseling approaches that may assist less motivated clients to increase their physical activity.

2.5.0   Ability to list and describe the specific strategies aimed at encouraging the initiation, adherence, and return to participation in an exercise program.

2.5.1   Knowledge of symptoms of anxiety and depression that may necessitate referral.

2.5.2   Knowledge of the potential symptoms and causal factors of test anxiety (i.e., performance, appraisal threat during exercise testing) and how it may affect physiological responses to testing.

3.5.0   Knowledge of and ability to apply basic cognitive-behavioral intervention such as shaping, goal setting, motivation, cueing, problem solving, reinforcement strategies, and self-monitoring.

3.5.1   Knowledge of the selection of an appropriate behavioral goal and the suggested method to evaluate goal achievement for each stage of change.

4.5.0   Ability to identify and explain five behavioral strategies as they apply to lifestyle modifications, such as exercise, diet, stress, and medication management.

4.5.1   Ability to describe signs and symptoms of maladjustment and/or failure to cope during an illness crisis and/or personal adjustment crisis (e.g., job loss) that might prompt a psychological consult or referral to other professional services.

4.5.2   Ability to describe the general principles of crisis management and factors influencing coping and learning in illness states.

4.5.3   Ability to describe the psychological issues to be confronted by the patient and by family members of patients who have cardiorespiratory disease and/or who have had an acute MI or cardiac surgery.

4.5.4   Knowledge of the psychological issues associated with an acute cardiac event versus those associated with chronic cardiac conditions.

4.5.5   Knowledge of the psychological stages involved with the acceptance of death and dying and ability to recognize when it is necessary for a psychological consult or referral to a professional resource.

5.5.0   Ability to demonstrate an understanding of the need for psychosocial consultation and referral of individuals who exhibit signs of psychological distress.

5.5.1   Knowledge of community resources for psychosocial support and behavior modification and outline an example of a referral system.

5.5.2   Knowledge of the observable signs and symptoms of anxiety or depressive symptoms secondary to cardiopulmonary disorders.

HEALTH APPRAISAL AND FITNESS TESTING

1.6.1   Knowledge of the importance of a health/medical history.

1.6.2   Knowledge of the value of a medical clearance prior to exercise participation.

1.6.3   Skill to measure pulse rate accurately both at rest and during exercise.

2.6.0   Knowledge, skills, and abilities to assess the health status of individuals and the ability to conduct fitness testing.

2.6.0.1   Ability to obtain a health history and risk appraisal that includes past and current medical history, family history of cardiac disease, orthopedic limitations, prescribed medications, activity patterns, nutritional habits, stress and anxiety levels, and smoking and alcohol use.

2.6.0.2   Ability to describe the categories of participants who should receive medical clearance prior to administration of an exercise test or participation in an exercise program.

2.6.0.3   Ability to identify relative and absolute contraindications to exercise testing or participation.

2.6.0.4   Ability to discuss the limitations of informed consent and medical clearance prior to exercise testing.

2.6.0.5   Ability to obtain informed consent.

2.6.0.6   Ability to explain the purpose and procedures for monitoring clients prior to, during, and after cardiorespiratory fitness testing.

2.6.0.7   Skill in instructing participants in the use of equipment and test procedures.

2.6.0.8   Ability to describe the purpose of testing, select an appropriate submaximal or maximal protocol, and conduct an assessment of cardiovascular fitness on the cycle ergometer or the treadmill.

2.6.0.9   Skill in accurately measuring heart rate, blood pressure, and obtaining rating of perceived exertion (RPE) at rest and during exercise according to established guidelines.

2.6.0.10   Ability to locate and measure skinfold sites, skeletal diameters, and girth measurements used for estimating body composition.

2.6.0.11   Ability to describe the purpose of testing, select appropriate protocols, and conduct assessments of muscular strength, muscular endurance, and flexibility.

2.6.0.12   Skill in various techniques of assessing body composition.

2.6.0.13   Knowledge of the advantages/disadvantages and limitations of the various body composition techniques.

2.6.0.14   Ability to interpret information obtained from the cardiorespiratory fitness test and the muscular strength and endurance, flexibility, and body composition assessments for apparently healthy individuals and those with stable disease.

2.6.0.15   Ability to identify appropriate criteria for terminating a fitness evaluation and demonstrate proper procedures to be followed after discontinuing such a test.

2.6.0.16   Ability to modify protocols and procedures for cardiorespiratory fitness tests in children, adolescents, and older adults.

2.6.0.17   Knowledge of common drugs from each of the following classes of medications and ability to describe the principal action and the effects on exercise testing and prescription:

2.6.0.17.1   Antianginals
2.6.0.17.2   Antihypertensives
2.6.0.17.3   Antiarrhythmics
2.6.0.17.4   Bronchodilators
2.6.0.17.5   Hypoglycemics
2.6.0.17.6   Psychotropics
2.6.0.17.7   Vasodilators
2.6.0.18   Ability to identify the effects of the following substances on exercise response: antihistamines, tranquilizers, alcohol, diet pills, cold tablets, caffeine, and nicotine.
2.6.0.19   Skill in techniques for calibration of a cycle ergometer and a motor-driven treadmill.

3.6.0   Knowledge of the use and value of the results of the fitness evaluation and exercise test for various populations.
3.6.1   Ability to design and implement a fitness testing/health appraisal program that includes, but is not limited to, staffing needs, physician interaction, documentation, equipment, marketing, and program evaluation.
3.6.2   Ability to recruit, train, and evaluate appropriate staff personnel for performing exercise tests, fitness evaluations, and health appraisals.
3.6.3   Ability to identify and describe the principal action, mechanisms of action, and major side effects from each of the following classes of medications:
3.6.3.1   Antianginals
3.6.3.2   Antihypertensives
3.6.3.3   Antiarrhythmics
3.6.3.4   Bronchodilators
3.6.3.5   Hypoglycemics
3.6.3.6   Psychotropics
3.6.3.7   Vasodilators

4.6.0   Knowledge and skills necessary for interpreting medical history and physical examination findings as they relate to health appraisal and exercise testing.
4.6.0.1   Ability to obtain a routine medical history prior to health appraisal and exercise testing.
4.6.0.2   Ability to identify individuals for whom physician supervision is recommended during maximal and submaximal exercise testing.
4.6.0.3   Ability to identify appropriate individuals who require exercise testing prior to exercise training.
4.6.1   Knowledge and skills necessary to conduct pretest procedures.
4.6.1.1   Knowledge of basic equipment and facility requirements for exercise testing.
4.6.1.2   Ability to obtain a standard and modified (Mason-Likar) 12-lead ECG on a participant in different body positions.
4.6.1.3   Ability to minimize resting ECG artifact.
4.6.1.4   Ability to accurately record a right and left arm blood pressure in different body positions.
4.6.1.5   Ability to instruct the test participant in the use of the RPE scale and other appropriate subjective scales, such as the dyspnea and angina scales.
4.6.1.6   Ability to gain informed consent.
4.6.1.7   Knowledge of the absolute and relative contraindications to an exercise test.
4.6.2   Knowledge and skills necessary for administering an exercise test.
4.6.2.1   Ability to calibrate testing equipment and explain procedures for calibration (e.g., a motor-driven treadmill, mechanical cycle ergometer, arm ergometer, electrocardiograph, and aneroid and mercury sphygmomanometers).
4.6.2.2   Knowledge of procedures and protocols for the exercise test, including the selection of the exercise test protocol in terms of modes of exercise, starting levels, increments of work, ramping versus standard protocols, length of stages, and frequency of measures.
4.6.2.3   Knowledge of appropriate techniques of measurement of physiological and subjective responses (e.g., symptoms, ECG, blood pressure, heart rate, RPE and other scales, oxygen saturation, and oxygen consumption measures) at appropriate intervals during the test.

4.6.2.4   Knowledge of how age, weight, level of fitness, and health status are considered in the selection of an exercise test protocol.

4.6.2.5   Knowledge of the technical factors that may indicate test termination (e.g., loss of ECG signal, loss of power).

4.6.2.6   Knowledge of the clinical factors that may indicate test termination (e.g., termination criteria).

4.6.2.7   Knowledge of immediate postexercise procedures and ability to list various approaches to cool-down.

4.6.2.8   Ability to record, organize, and perform necessary calculations of test data for summary presentation.

4.6.3   Knowledge and skills necessary to interpret the exercise test.

4.6.3.1   Knowledge of the prognostic implications of the exercise ECG and hemodynamic responses in light of the current medication status of the participant as well as any comorbidities.

4.6.3.2   Ability to provide objective recommendations to an individual regarding such factors as physical conditioning, return to work, and performance of selected activities for daily living (such as driving, stair climbing, sexual activity) based on exercise test results and clinical status.

4.6.4   Knowledge and skills necessary for administering an exercise test with special populations or test considerations.

4.6.4.1   Knowledge of exercise testing procedures for various clinical populations including those individuals with cardiovascular, pulmonary, and metabolic diseases in terms of exercise modality, protocol, physiological measurements, and expected outcomes.

4.6.4.2   Knowledge of the appropriate end points for exercise testing for various clinical populations.

4.6.4.3   Ability to describe silent ischemia and its implications for exercise testing and training.

4.6.4.4   Knowledge of techniques for measurement of oxygen consumption at appropriate intervals during an exercise test for special populations (e.g., congestive heart failure, valvular heart disease, coronary artery disease).

4.6.4.5   Ability to explain indications for combining exercise testing with radionuclide imaging.

4.6.4.6   Knowledge of the differences in test protocol and procedures when the exercise test involves the addition of various methodologies to increase the sensitivity and/or specificity of the test, such as radionuclide imaging or echocardiography.

4.6.4.7   Knowledge of testing procedures and protocol for children and the elderly with or without various clinical conditions.

4.6.5   Knowledge in recognizing medications commonly encountered during exercise testing and training and knowledge of the indications and effects on the ECG, heart rate, and blood pressure at rest and during exercise.

4.6.5.1   Antianginals

4.6.5.2   Antihypertensives

4.6.5.3   Antiarrhythmics

4.6.5.4   Bronchodilators

4.6.5.5   Hypoglycemics

4.6.5.6   Psychotropics

4.6.5.7   Vasodilators

4.6.5.8   Anticoagulant and antiplatelet drugs (warfarin, aspirin, ticlopidine, clopidogrel, etc.)

4.6.5.9   Lipid-lowering agents

4.6.6   Knowledge and ability to administer and interpret basic resting spirometric tests and measures including forced expiratory volume in 1 second ($FEV_{1.0}$), FVC, and MVV.

5.6.0   Knowledge of the various diagnostic and treatment modalities currently used in the management of cardiovascular disease.

5.6.1   Knowledge of the diagnostic and prognostic value of the results of the graded exercise test for various populations.

SAFETY, INJURY PREVENTION, AND EMERGENCY CARE

1.7.0   Knowledge of and skill in obtaining basic life support and cardiopulmonary resuscitation certification.

1.7.1   Knowledge of appropriate emergency procedures (i.e., telephone procedures, written emergency procedures, personnel responsibilities) in the group exercise setting.

1.7.2   Knowledge of basic first aid procedures for exercise-related injuries, such as bleeding, strains/sprains, fractures, and exercise intolerance (dizziness, syncope, heat injury).

1.7.3   Knowledge of basic precautions taken in a group exercise setting to ensure participant safety.

1.7.4   Ability to identify the physical and physiological signs and symptoms of overtraining.

1.7.5   Ability to list the effects of temperature, humidity, altitude, and pollution on the physiological response to exercise.

1.7.6   Knowledge of the following terms: shin splints, sprain, strain, tennis elbow, bursitis, stress fracture, tendonitis, patellar femoral pain syndrome, low back pain, plantar fasciitis, and rotator cuff tendonitis.

1.7.7   Skill to demonstrate exercises used for people with low back pain.

1.7.8   Knowledge of hypothetical concerns and potential risks that may be associated with the use of exercises such as straight leg sit-ups, double leg raises, full squats, hurdlers stretch, yoga plough, forceful back hyperextension, and standing bent-over toe touch.

2.7.0   Skill in demonstrating appropriate emergency procedures during exercise testing and/or training.

2.7.1   Knowledge of safety plans, emergency procedures, and first aid techniques needed during fitness evaluations, exercise testing, and exercise training.

2.7.2   Ability to identify the components that contribute to the maintenance of a safe environment.

2.7.3   Knowledge of the health/fitness instructor's responsibilities, limitations, and the legal implications of carrying out emergency procedures.

2.7.4   Ability to describe potential musculoskeletal injuries (e.g., contusions, sprains, strains, fractures), cardiovascular/pulmonary complications (e.g., tachycardia, bradycardia, hypotension/hypertension, tachypnea) and metabolic abnormalities (e.g., fainting/syncope, hypoglycemia/hyperglycemia, hypothermia/hyperthermia).

2.7.5   Knowledge of the initial management and first aid techniques associated with open wounds, musculoskeletal injuries, cardiovascular/pulmonary complications, and metabolic disorders.

2.7.6   Knowledge of the components of an equipment maintenance/repair program and how it may be used to evaluate the condition of exercise equipment to reduce the potential risk of injury.

3.7.0   Ability to identify the process to train the exercise staff in cardiopulmonary resuscitation.

3.7.1   Ability to design and evaluate emergency procedures for a preventive exercise program and an exercise testing facility.

3.7.2   Ability to train staff in safety procedures, risk reduction strategies, and injury care techniques.

3.7.3   Knowledge of the legal implications of documented safety procedures, the use of incident documents, and ongoing safety training.

4.7.0   Knowledge in responding with appropriate emergency procedures to situations which might arise before, during, and after administration of an exercise test and/or exercise session.

4.7.1   Ability to list and describe the use of emergency equipment and personnel that should be present in an exercise testing laboratory and rehabilitative exercise training setting.

4.7.2   Knowledge of verifying operating status of and maintaining emergency equipment.

4.7.3   Ability to describe emergency procedures that may arise during exercise testing or training, including (but not limited to):

4.7.3.1   Cardiac arrest

4.7.3.2   Hypoglycemia and hyperglycemia

4.7.3.3   Bronchospasm

4.7.3.4   Sudden onset hypotension

4.7.3.5   Serious (including possibly life-threatening) arrhythmias (VT, Vfib, etc.)

4.7.3.6   ICD discharge

4.7.3.7   TIA

4.7.3.8   MI

4.7.3.9   Coronary thrombosis

4.7.4 Ability to identify the emergency drugs that should be available in exercise testing sessions and training sessions and to describe the mechanisms of action.

4.7.5 Ability to possess necessary emergency skills similar to or associated with current Advanced Cardiac Life Support (ACLS) policies and procedures.

5.7.0 Ability to diagram an emergency response system and discuss minimum standards for equipment and personnel required in settings for rehabilitative exercise programs.

5.7.1 Ability and knowledge to discuss the concepts of informed consent, risk management, negligence, and standards of care as they relate to exercise testing and training.

5.7.2 Ability and knowledge to discuss procedures for training and drilling staff on emergency response.

EXERCISE PROGRAMMING

1.8.0 Knowledge of the recommended intensity, duration, frequency, and type of physical activity necessary for development of cardiorespiratory fitness in an apparently healthy population.

1.8.1 Ability to differentiate between the amount of physical activity required for health benefits and the amount of exercise required for fitness development.

1.8.2 Ability to describe exercises designed to enhance muscular strength and/or endurance of specific major muscle groups.

1.8.3 Knowledge of the principles of overload, specificity, and progression and how they relate to exercise programming.

1.8.4 Skill to teach and demonstrate appropriate exercises used in the warm-up and cool-down of a variety of group exercise classes.

1.8.5 Ability to teach the components of an exercise session (i.e., warm-up, aerobic stimulus phase, cool-down, muscular strength/endurance, flexibility).

1.8.6 Knowledge of the following terms: progressive resistance, isotonic/isometric, concentric, eccentric, atrophy, hypertrophy, sets, repetitions, plyometrics, Valsalva maneuver.

1.8.7 Skill to teach class participants how to monitor intensity of exercise using heart rate and rating of perceived exertion.

1.8.8 Skill to teach participants how to use RPE and heart rate to adjust the intensity of the exercise session.

1.8.9 Ability to calculate training heart rates using two methods: percent of age-predicted maximum heart rate and heart rate reserve (Karvonen).

1.8.10 Skill to teach and demonstrate appropriate modifications in specific exercises for the following groups: older adults, pregnant and postnatal women, obese persons, and persons with low back pain.

1.8.11 Ability to recognize proper and improper technique in the use of resistive equipment such as stability balls, weights, bands, resistance bars, and water exercise equipment.

1.8.12 Ability to recognize proper and improper technique in the use of cardiovascular conditioning equipment (e.g., steps, cycles, slides).

1.8.13 Skill to teach and demonstrate appropriate exercises for improving range of motion of all major joints.

1.8.14 Ability to modify exercises in the group setting for apparently healthy persons of various fitness levels.

1.8.15 Ability to teach a progression of exercises for all major muscle groups to improve muscular strength and endurance.

1.8.16 Knowledge to describe the various types of interval, continuous, and circuit training programs.

1.8.17 Knowledge to describe various ways a leader can take a position relative to the group to enhance visibility, participant interactions, and communication.

1.8.18 Ability to communicate effectively with exercise participants in the group exercise session.

1.8.19 Knowledge to describe partner resistance exercises that can be used in a group class setting.

1.8.20 Ability to demonstrate techniques for accommodating various fitness levels within the same class.

1.8.21 Knowledge of the properties of water that affect the design of a water exercise session.

1.8.22 Knowledge of basic music fundamentals, including downbeat, 8 count, and 32 count.

1.8.23 Skill to effectively use verbal and nonverbal cues in the group exercise setting, including anticipatory, motivational, safety, and educational.

1.8.24 Skill to demonstrate the proper form, alignment, and technique in typical exercises used in the warm-up, stimulus, muscle conditioning and cool-down phases of the group session.

1.8.25 Ability to evaluate specific exercises in terms of safety and effectiveness for various participants.

1.8.26 Ability to demonstrate a familiarity with a variety of group exercise formats (e.g., traditional, step, slide, muscle conditioning, flexibility, indoor cycling, water fitness, walking).

2.8.0 Knowledge, skills, and abilities to prescribe and administer exercise programs for apparently healthy individuals, individuals at higher risk, and individuals with known disease.

2.8.0.1 Ability to design, implement, and evaluate individualized and group exercise programs based on health history and physical fitness assessments.

2.8.0.2 Ability to modify exercises based on age and physical condition.

2.8.0.3 Knowledge, skills, and abilities to calculate energy cost, $\dot{V}O_2$, METs, and target heart rates and apply the information to an exercise prescription.

2.8.0.4 Ability to convert weights from pounds (lb) to kilograms (kg) and speed from miles per hour (mph) to meters per minute (m.min^{-1}).

2.8.0.5 Ability to convert METs to $\dot{V}O_2$ expressed as mL.kg^{-1}.min^{-1}, L.min^{-1}, and/or mL.kg FFW^{-1}.min^{-1}.

2.8.0.6 Ability to calculate the energy cost in METs and kilocalories for given exercise intensities in stepping exercise, cycle ergometry, and during horizontal and graded walking and running.

2.8.0.7 Knowledge of approximate METs for various sport, recreational, and work tasks.

2.8.0.8 Ability to prescribe exercise intensity based on $\dot{V}O_2$ data for different modes of exercise, including graded and horizontal running and walking, cycling, and stepping exercise.

2.8.0.9 Ability to explain and implement exercise prescription guidelines for apparently healthy clients, increased risk clients, and clients with controlled disease.

2.8.0.10 Ability to adapt frequency, intensity, duration, mode, progression, level of supervision, and monitoring techniques in exercise programs for patients with controlled chronic disease (heart disease, diabetes mellitus, obesity, hypertension), musculoskeletal problems, pregnancy and/or postpartum, and exercise-induced asthma.

2.8.0.11 Ability to understand the components incorporated into an exercise session and the proper sequence (i.e., pre-exercise evaluation, warm-up, aerobic stimulus phase, cool-down, muscular strength and/or endurance, and flexibility).

2.8.0.12 Skill in the use of various methods for establishing and monitoring levels of exercise intensity, including heart rate, RPE, and METs.

2.8.0.13 Knowledge of special precautions and modifications of exercise programming for participation at altitude, different ambient temperatures, humidity, and environmental pollution.

2.8.0.14 Ability to design resistive exercise programs to increase or maintain muscular strength and/or endurance.

2.8.0.15 Ability to evaluate flexibility and prescribe appropriate flexibility exercises for all major muscle groups.

2.8.0.16 Knowledge of the importance of recording exercise sessions and performing periodic evaluations to assess changes in fitness status.

2.8.0.17 Knowledge of the advantages and disadvantages of implementation of interval, continuous, and circuit training programs.

2.8.0.18 Ability to design training programs using interval, continuous, and circuit training programs.

2.8.0.19 Ability to discuss the advantages and disadvantages of various commercial exercise equipment in developing cardiorespiratory fitness, muscular strength, and muscular endurance.

2.8.0.20 Knowledge of the types of exercise programs available in the community and how these programs are appropriate for various populations.

4.8.0 Knowledge of the implications (benefits versus risks) of exercise for individuals with CAD risk factors and for individuals with established stable cardiovascular, pulmonary, metabolic, and/or orthopedic disorders.

4.8.1 Knowledge, skills, and abilities necessary to establish and supervise individualized exercise prescriptions based on medical information and exercise test data, including intensity, duration, frequency, progression, precautions, and type of physical activity for a variety of chronic disease and disability conditions, including, but not limited to:

4.8.1.1 CAD/MI

4.8.1.2 PTCA/stent

4.8.1.3   CHF
4.8.1.4   Heart transplantation
4.8.1.5   COPD
4.8.1.6   Asthma
4.8.1.7   Bronchitis
4.8.1.8   Stroke/TIA
4.8.1.9   Diabetes
4.8.1.10   Hypertension
4.8.1.11   Obesity
4.8.1.12   Renal disease/transplantation
4.8.1.13   Common orthopedic and neuromuscular conditions
4.8.2   Ability to modify exercise (type of physical activity, intensity, duration, progression) according to the current health status.
4.8.3   Knowledge of basic mechanisms of action of medications that may affect exercise testing and the exercise prescription, including:
4.8.3.1   b-Adrenergic blockers
4.8.3.2   Diuretics
4.8.3.3   Calcium channel blockers
4.8.3.4   Antihypertensives
4.8.3.5   Antihistamines
4.8.3.6   Antihyperglycemics
4.8.3.7   Psychotropics
4.8.3.8   Alcohol
4.8.3.9   Diet pills
4.8.3.10   Cold tablets
4.8.3.11   Caffeine
4.8.3.12   Nicotine
4.8.4   Ability to discuss warm-up and cool-down phenomena with *specific reference* to angina and ischemic ECG changes, arrhythmias, and blood pressure changes, and with *general reference* to cardiovascular, pulmonary, and metabolic diseases.
4.8.5   Ability to discuss the appropriate use of static and dynamic exercise for individuals with cardiovascular, pulmonary, and metabolic disease.
4.8.6   Knowledge in the design of a strength and flexibility program for the following individuals or groups:
4.8.6.1   Cardiovascular disease, pulmonary disease, metabolic disease, or musculoskeletal disorders
4.8.6.2   Elderly
4.8.6.3   Children
4.8.7   Ability to discuss modifications in monitoring of exercise intensity for various disease groups (cardiovascular, pulmonary, and metabolic diseases).
4.8.8   Ability to discuss possible adverse responses to exercise in various patient groups (cardiovascular, pulmonary, and metabolic diseases) and what precautions may be taken to prevent them.
4.8.9   Knowledge of the relative and absolute contraindications to exercise training as related to the current health status of the patient.
4.8.10   Ability to devise a supervised exercise program for the first 6 weeks after hospitalization and for the following 3 months for the following conditions:
4.8.10.1   MI
4.8.10.2   Angina
4.8.10.3   Congestive heart failure
4.8.10.4   PTCA
4.8.10.5   CABG
4.8.10.6   Stents and other catheter revascularization techniques
4.8.10.7   Chronic pulmonary disease
4.8.10.8   Transplants
4.8.11   Ability to identify characteristics that correlate or predict poor compliance to exercise programs, and strategies to increase exercise adherence.
4.8.12   Ability to identify and describe the role of various allied health professionals and the indications and procedures for referral necessary in a multidisciplinary rehabilitation program.
4.8.13   Knowledge of the concept of "Activities of Daily Living" (ADLs) and its importance in the overall rehabilitation of the individual.

4.8.14   Knowledge prescribing exercise using nontraditional exercise modalities (e.g., bench stepping, elastic bands, isodynamic exercise, water aerobics) for individuals with cardiovascular, pulmonary, or metabolic diseases, or those with orthopedic limitations.

5.8.0   Ability to discuss the level of supervision and level of monitoring recommended for various chronic disease conditions during exercise testing and training using risk stratification.

NUTRITION AND WEIGHT MANAGEMENT

1.9.0   Knowledge to define the following terms: obesity, overweight, percent fat, lean body mass, anorexia nervosa, bulimia, and body fat distribution.

1.9.1   Knowledge of the relationship between body composition and health.

1.9.2   Knowledge of the effects of diet plus exercise, diet alone, and exercise alone as methods for modifying body composition.

1.9.3   Knowledge of the importance of an adequate daily energy intake for healthy weight management.

1.9.4   Ability to differentiate between fat-soluble and water-soluble vitamins.

1.9.5   Ability to describe the importance of maintaining normal hydration before, during, and after exercise.

1.9.6   Knowledge of the USDA Food Pyramid.

1.9.7   Knowledge of the importance of calcium and iron in women's health.

1.9.8   Ability to describe the myths and consequences associated with inappropriate weight loss methods (e.g., saunas, vibrating belts, body wraps, electric simulators, sweat suits, fad diets).

1.9.9   Knowledge of the number of kilocalories in one gram of carbohydrate, fat, protein, and alcohol.

1.9.10   Knowledge of the number of kilocalories equivalent to losing 1 pound of body fat.

2.9.0   Knowledge, skills, and abilities to provide information concerning nutrition and the role of diet and exercise on body composition and weight control.

2.9.0.1   Ability to describe the health implications of variation in body fat distribution patterns and the significance of the waist to hip ratio.

2.9.0.2   Knowledge of the guidelines for caloric intake for an individual desiring to lose or gain weight.

2.9.0.3   Knowledge of common nutritional ergogenic aids, the purported mechanism of action, and any risk and/or benefits (e.g., carbohydrates, protein/amino acids, vitamins, minerals, sodium bicarbonate, creatine, bee pollen).

2.9.0.4   Knowledge of nutritional factors related to the female athlete triad syndrome (i.e., eating disorders, menstrual cycle abnormalities, and osteoporosis).

2.9.0.5   Knowledge of the NIH Consensus statement regarding health risks of obesity, Nutrition for Physical Fitness Position Paper of the American Dietetic Association, and the ACSM Position Stand on proper and improper weight loss programs.

2.9.0.6   Knowledge of NCEP II guidelines for lipid management.

PROGRAM AND ADMINISTRATION/MANAGEMENT

2.10.0   Knowledge, skills, and ability to administer and deliver health/fitness programs.

2.10.0.1   Knowledge of the health/fitness instructor's supportive role in administration and program management within a health/fitness facility.

2.10.0.2   Ability to administer fitness-related programs within established budgetary guidelines.

2.10.0.3   Ability to develop marketing materials for the purpose of promoting fitness-related programs.
2.10.0.4   Ability to use various sales techniques for prospective program clients/participants.
2.10.0.5   Ability to describe and use the documentation required when a client shows signs or symptoms during an exercise session and should be referred to a physician.
2.10.0.6   Ability to create and maintain records pertaining to participant exercise adherence, retention, and goal setting.
2.10.0.7   Ability to develop and administer educational programs (e.g., lectures, workshops) and educational materials.
2.10.0.8   Knowledge of management of a fitness department (e.g., working within a budget, training exercise leaders, scheduling, running staff meetings).
2.10.0.9   Knowledge of the importance of tracking and evaluating member retention.

3.10.0   Ability to manage personnel effectively.
3.10.0.1   Ability to describe a management plan for the development of staff, continuing education, marketing and promotion, documentation, billing, facility management, and financial planning.
3.10.0.2   Ability to describe the decision-making process related to budgets, market analysis, program evaluation, facility management, staff allocation, and community development.
3.10.0.3   Ability to describe the development, evaluation, and revision of policies and procedures for programming and facility management.
3.10.0.4   Ability to describe how the computer can assist in data analysis, spreadsheet report development, and daily tracking of customer utilization.
3.10.0.5   Ability to define and describe the total quality management (TQM) and continuous quality improvement (CQI) approaches to management.
3.10.0.6   Ability to interpret applied research in the areas of exercise testing, exercise programming, and educational programs to maintain a comprehensive and current state-of-the-art program.
3.10.0.7   Ability to develop a risk factor screening program, including procedures, staff training, feedback, and follow-up.
3.10.1   Knowledge of administration, management and supervision of personnel.
3.10.1.1   Ability to describe effective interviewing, hiring, and employee termination procedures.
3.10.1.2   Ability to describe and diagram an organizational chart and show the relationships between a health/fitness director, owner, medical advisor, and staff.
3.10.1.3   Knowledge of and ability to describe various staff training techniques.
3.10.1.4   Knowledge of and ability to describe performance reviews and their role in evaluating staff.
3.10.1.5   Knowledge of the legal obligations and problems involved in personnel management.
3.10.1.6   Knowledge of compensation, including wages, bonuses, incentive programs, and benefits.
3.10.1.7   Knowledge of methods for implementing a sales commission system.
3.10.1.8   Ability to describe the significance of a benefits program for staff and demonstrate an understanding in researching and selecting benefits.
3.10.1.9   Ability to write and implement thorough and legal job descriptions.
3.10.1.10 Knowledge of personnel time management techniques.
3.10.2   Knowledge of administration, management, and development of a budget and of the financial aspects of a fitness center.
3.10.2.1   Knowledge of the principles of financial management.
3.10.2.2   Knowledge of basic accounting principles such as accounts payable, accounts receivable, accrual, cash flow, assets, liabilities, and return on investment.
3.10.2.3   Ability to identify the various forms of a business enterprise such as sole proprietorship, partnership, corporation, and S-corporation.
3.10.2.4   Knowledge of the procedures involved with developing, evaluating, revising, and updating capital and operating budgets.
3.10.2.5   Ability to manage expenses with the objective of maintaining a positive cash flow.
3.10.2.6   Ability to understand and analyze financial statements, including income statements, balance sheets, cash flows, budgets, and pro forma projections.
3.10.2.7   Knowledge of program-related break-even and cost/benefit analysis.
3.10.2.8   Knowledge of the importance of short-term and long-term planning.
3.10.3   Knowledge of the principles of marketing and sales.
3.10.3.1   Ability to identify the steps in the development, implementation, and evaluation of a marketing plan.
3.10.3.2   Knowledge of the components of a needs assessment/market analysis.
3.10.3.3   Knowledge of various sales techniques for prospective members.

3.10.3.4   Knowledge of techniques for advertising, marketing, promotion, and public relations.

3.10.3.5   Ability to describe the principles of developing and evaluating products and services, and establishing pricing.

3.10.4   Knowledge of the principles of day-to-day operation of a fitness center.

3.10.4.1   Knowledge of the principles of pricing and purchasing equipment and supplies.

3.10.4.2   Knowledge of facility layout and design.

3.10.4.3   Ability to establish and evaluate an equipment preventive maintenance and repair program.

3.10.4.4   Ability to describe a plan for implementing a housekeeping program.

3.10.4.5   Ability to identify and explain the operating policies for preventive exercise programs, including data analysis and reporting, confidentiality of records, relationships with health care providers, accident and injury reporting, and continuing education of participants.

3.10.4.6   Knowledge of the legal concepts of tort, negligence, liability, indemnification, standards of care, health regulations, consent, contract, confidentiality, malpractice, and the legal concerns regarding emergency procedures and informed consent.

3.10.4.7   Ability to implement capital improvements with minimal disruption of client or business needs.

3.10.4.8   Ability to coordinate the operations of various departments, including, but not limited to, the front desk, fitness, rehabilitation, maintenance and repair, day care, housekeeping, pool, and management.

3.10.5   Knowledge of management and principles of member service and communication.

3.10.5.1   Skills in effective techniques for communicating with staff, management, members, health care providers, potential customers, and vendors.

3.10.5.2   Knowledge of and ability to provide strong customer service.

3.10.5.3   Ability to develop and implement customer surveys.

3.10.5.4   Knowledge of the strategies for management conflict.

3.10.6   Knowledge of the principles of health promotion and ability to administer health promotion programs.

3.10.6.1   Knowledge of health promotion programs (e.g., nutrition and weight management, smoking cessation, stress management, back care, body mechanics, and substance abuse).

3.10.6.2   Knowledge of the specific and appropriate content and methods for creating a health promotion program.

3.10.6.3   Knowledge of and ability to access resources for various programs and delivery systems.

3.10.6.4   Knowledge of the concepts of cost-effectiveness and cost-benefit as they relate to the evaluation of health promotion programming.

3.10.6.5   Ability to describe the means and amounts by which health promotion programs might increase productivity, reduce employee loss time, reduce health care costs, and improve profitability in the workplace.

5.10.0   Knowledge and ability to administer a clinical exercise program, including personnel, finance, risk management, program development, outcomes measurement, and continuous quality improvement.

5.10.1   Knowledge of general human resource policy and procedures, including job descriptions, leave policies, disabilities, discipline, and job performance evaluations.

5.10.2   Ability to diagram and explain an organizational chart and show staff relationships between an exercise program director, governing body, exercise leader, exercise specialist, registered nurse, physical therapist, medical director or advisor, and a participant's personal physician.

5.10.3   Ability to identify and explain operating policies for preventive and rehabilitative exercise programs.

5.10.4   Ability to describe the role of the medical director and referring physician in the program design and implementation, and to describe the responsibility of the program director to these individuals.

5.10.5   Ability to describe and explain strategies for enhancing the understanding of the role of rehabilitation on the part of the public, health care policy makers, health care providers, and the medical community.

5.10.6   Ability to discuss the role of the rehabilitative staff in the development and implementation of the comprehensive patient care plan.

5.10.7   Ability to justify the inclusion of a comprehensive rehabilitation program in the health care setting.

5.10.8   Ability to describe the concept of risk stratification and its application to program administration.

5.10.9   Ability to identify and explain operating policies and procedures for clinical exercise programs including data analysis and reporting, reimbursement of service fees, confidentiality of records, relationships between program and referring physicians, continuing education of participants and family, legal liability, and accident or injury reporting.

5.10.10   Ability to assume fiscal (financial) responsibility for clinical programs.

5.10.11   Knowledge and ability to implement and monitor a comprehensive continuous quality improvement process.

5.10.12   Knowledge of the relationship between insurance reimbursement and services fees.

5.10.13   Knowledge of awareness of health care reform and the potential impact upon preventive and rehabilitative exercise programs.

5.10.14   Knowledge of marketing and public relation functions for a rehabilitative exercise program.

5.10.15   Ability to identify ways to increase physician and nonphysician referrals into a comprehensive rehabilitative exercise program.

Electrocardiography

4.11.0   Knowledge and skills necessary to identify resting and exercise ECG changes associated with the following abnormalities:

4.11.0.1   Bundle branch blocks and bifascicular blocks

4.11.0.2   Atrioventricular blocks

4.11.0.3   Sinus bradycardia and tachycardia

4.11.0.4   Sinus arrest

4.11.0.5   Supraventricular premature contractions and tachycardia

4.11.0.6   Ventricular premature contractions (including frequency, form, couplets, salvos, tachycardia)

4.11.0.7   Atrial flutter and fibrillation

4.11.0.8   Ventricular fibrillation

4.11.0.9   Myocardial ischemia, injury, and infarction

4.11.1   Knowledge and skills necessary to define the limits or considerations for initiating and terminating exercise testing or training based on the ECG abnormalities listed above.

4.11.2   Knowledge and skills necessary to identify myocardial ischemia, injury, and infarction.

4.11.2.1   Ability to identify ECG changes that correspond to ischemia in various myocardial regions (e.g., inferior, posterior, anteroseptal, anterior, anterolateral, lateral).

4.11.2.2   Ability to differentiate between Q-wave and non-Q-wave infarction.

4.11.2.3   Ability to identify ECG changes that typically occur due to hyperventilation, electrolyte abnormalities, and drug therapy.

4.11.3   Knowledge and skills necessary to identify cardiac arrhythmias and conduction defects during exercise.

4.11.3.1   Knowledge of the potential causes of various cardiac arrhythmias.

4.11.3.2   Knowledge of the significance of arrhythmia occurrence during rest, exercise, and recovery.

4.11.3.3   Ability to identify potentially hazardous arrhythmias or conduction defects observed on the ECG at rest, during exercise, and recovery.

4.11.3.4   Knowledge of appropriate procedures in the event of such arrhythmias or conduction defects.

4.11.4   Knowledge of the important ECG patterns at rest and during exercise in healthy persons and in patients with cardiovascular, pulmonary, and metabolic diseases.

4.11.4.0   Ability to identify resting ECG changes associated with diseases other than coronary artery disease (such as hypertensive heart disease, cardiac chamber enlargement, pericarditis, pulmonary disease, metabolic disorders).

4.11.4.1   Ability to identify the significance of important ECG abnormalities in the designation of the exercise prescription and in activity selection.

4.11.5   Knowledge of the indications and methods for ECG monitoring during exercise testing and during exercise sessions.

4.11.6   Knowledge of the causes and means of reducing false positive and false negative exercise ECG responses.

4.11.7   Knowledge of ECG patterns and responses of pacemakers and programmable cardioverter defibrillators.

5.11.0   Knowledge of the implications of various ECG patterns for exercise testing, exercise programming, prognosis, and risk stratification.

5.11.1   Knowledge of the diagnostic and prognostic significance of ischemic ECG responses and arrhythmias at rest, during exercise, or recovery.

5.11.2   Knowledge of Baye's theorem as it relates to pretest likelihood of CAD and the predictive value of positive or negative diagnostic exercise ECG results.

5.11.3   Knowledge of the role of the ECG during exercise testing as it relates to radionuclide imaging and echocardiography imaging.

1

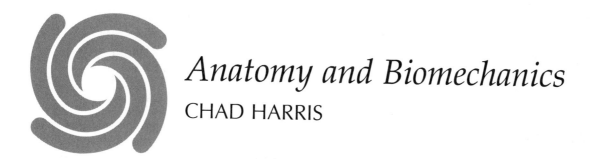

Anatomy and Biomechanics
CHAD HARRIS

I. ANATOMICAL LOCATIONS

A. ORIENTATION (Figure 1-1)

1. **Proximal:** nearest to the body center, joint center, or reference point.

2. **Distal:** away from the body center, joint center, or reference point.

3. **Superior** (cranial): above, toward the head.

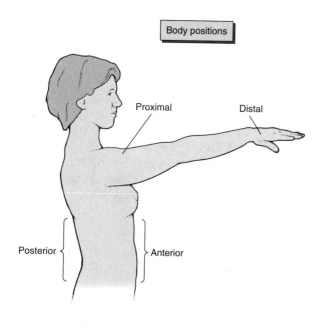

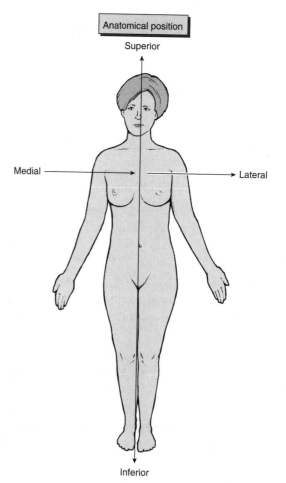

FIGURE 1-1 Anatomical orientations. (From *ACSM's Resource Manual for Guidelines for Exercise Testing and Prescription,* 3rd ed. Baltimore, Williams & Wilkins, 1998, p 90.)

4. **Inferior** (caudal): lower than, toward the feet.
5. **Anterior** (ventral): toward the front.
6. **Posterior** (dorsal): toward the back.
7. **Medial:** near the midline.
8. **Lateral:** away from the midline.

B. **PLANES AND AXES**

1. **Planes** are three perpendicular spatial dimensions in which whole body and segmental movement occurs (**Figure 1-2**).

   a. The **sagittal plane** divides the body into symmetrical right and left halves.

   b. The **frontal plane** divides the body into front and back halves.

   c. The **transverse plane** divides the body in half superiorly and inferiorly.

2. **Axes**

   –Segmental movements occur around an axis and in a plane. Each plane has an associated axis lying perpendicular to it:

   a. The **mediolateral axis** lies perpendicular to the sagittal plane.

   b. The **anteroposterior axis** lies perpendicular to the frontal plane.

   c. The **longitudinal axis** lies perpendicular to the transverse plane.

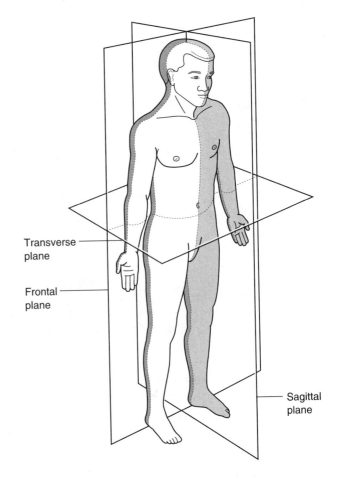

FIGURE 1-2 Planes and axes of the human body.

II. MOVEMENT

–Depending on the type of articulation between adjacent segments, one or more movements are possible at a joint (**Figure 1-3**).

A. **FLEXION** is movement that decreases the joint angle; occurs in a sagittal plane around a mediolateral axis.

B. **EXTENSION** is movement opposite to flexion, increasing the joint angle; occurs in a sagittal plane around a mediolateral axis.

C. **ADDUCTION** is movement toward the midline of the body in a frontal plane around an anteroposterior axis.

D. **ABDUCTION** is movement away from the midline of the body in a frontal plane around an anteroposterior axis.

E. **ROTATION** is movement around a longitudinal axis and in the transverse plane, either toward the midline (internal) or away from the midline (external).

F. **CIRCUMDUCTION** is a combination of flexion, extension, abduction, and adduction. The segment moving in circumduction describes a cone.

G. **PRONATION** is rotational movement at the radioulnar joint in a transverse plane about a longitudinal axis that results in the palm facing downward.

H. **SUPINATION** is rotational movement at the radioulnar joint in a transverse plane around a longitudinal axis that results in the palm facing upward.

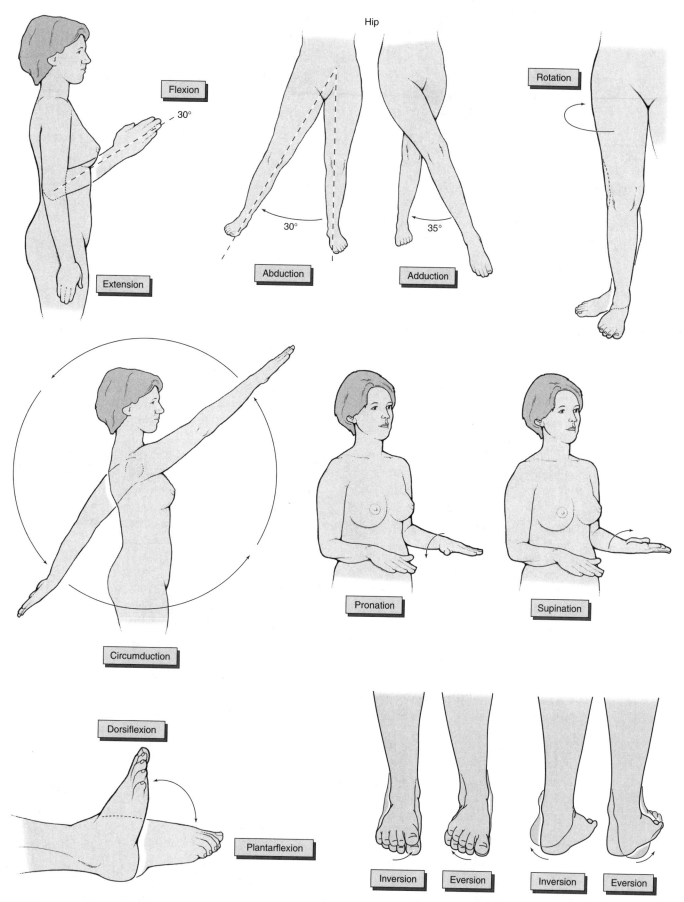

FIGURE 1-3 Body movements at joints. (Adapted in part from *ACSM's Resource Manual for Guidelines for Exercise Testing and Prescription,* 3rd ed. Baltimore, Williams & Wilkins, 1998, pp 83, 90, 91.)

I. PLANTARFLEXION is extension at the ankle joint.

J. DORSIFLEXION is flexion at the ankle joint.

K. EVERSION is turning the sole of the foot outward.

L. INVERSION is turning the sole of the foot inward.

III. FUNCTIONAL ANATOMY

A. UPPER BODY

1. The **axial skeleton** comprises the skull, vertebral column, ribs, and sternum (**Figure 1-4**).

    a. **Skull**

    –Of the 29 bones of the skull, the most significant in terms of exercise testing is the **mandible,** which serves as an orienting landmark for palpating the carotid artery when assessing pulse.

    b. **Vertebral column**

    –comprises **33 vertebrae** in 5 regions: 7 cervical, 12 thoracic, 5 lumbar, 5 fused sacral, and 4 fused coccygeal.

    –**Intervertebral discs** are fibrocartilaginous pads separating the vertebrae.

    –**Normal spinal curves** are present in the major regions of the vertebral column when viewed sagittally.

    (1) The **thoracic curve** and **sacral curve** are posteriorly directed and termed primary curves, because they retain the same directional curvature as the spine in the fetus.

    (2) The **cervical curve** and **lumbar curve** are anteriorly directed curves, called secondary curves, which develop after birth as the infant progresses in weight bearing.

    c. **Ribs**

    –There are **12 pairs of ribs: 7 pairs of true ribs,** in which the costal cartilage articulates directly with the sternum, and five pairs that do not articulate directly with the sternum.

    –The costal cartilage of **ribs 8, 9, and 10** articulates with the costal cartilage of the adjacent superior rib. The cartilaginous ends of **ribs 11 and 12** are free from articulation.

    –The spaces between the ribs are called **intercostal spaces.** Palpation of the intercostal spaces of the true ribs is **important for correct placement of electrocardiography (ECG) electrodes** (in the fourth and fifth intercostal spaces).

    d. **Sternum**

    –lies in the midline of the chest and comprises three parts: the **manubrium** (superior), the **body** (middle), and the **xyphoid process** (inferior).

    (1) The **sternal angle** is a slightly raised surface landmark where the manubrium meets the body of the sternum.

    (2) The **xiphoid process** is also a surface landmark, situated at the bottom of the sternum and in the middle of the inferior border of the rib cage. **Palpation of the xiphoid** is necessary for cardiopulmonary resuscitation (CPR).

    (3) Palpation of the manubrium helps determine proper paddle placement in defibrillation.

2. The **appendicular skeleton** of the upper body comprises the bones of the pectoral girdle (clavicles and scapulae), upper arm, forearm, and hand.

    a. **Clavicles** articulate with the sternal manubrium proximally and the scapulae distally and are positioned just superior to the first rib. Palpation of the clavicles helps determine electrode placement for defibrillation.

    b. **Scapulae** are situated on the posterior side of the body in the region of the first seven ribs. Each scapula has two important landmarks:

    (1) The **inferior angle** (used for skinfold site location) at the bottom of the scapulae forming the junction between the medial and lateral borders.

    (2) The **acromion process** (used for shoulder breadth measurement), the bony process at the most lateral part of the shoulder.

    c. **Upper arm**

    (1) The **humerus** proximally articulates with the glenoid fossa of the scapula and distally articulates with the ulna and radius.

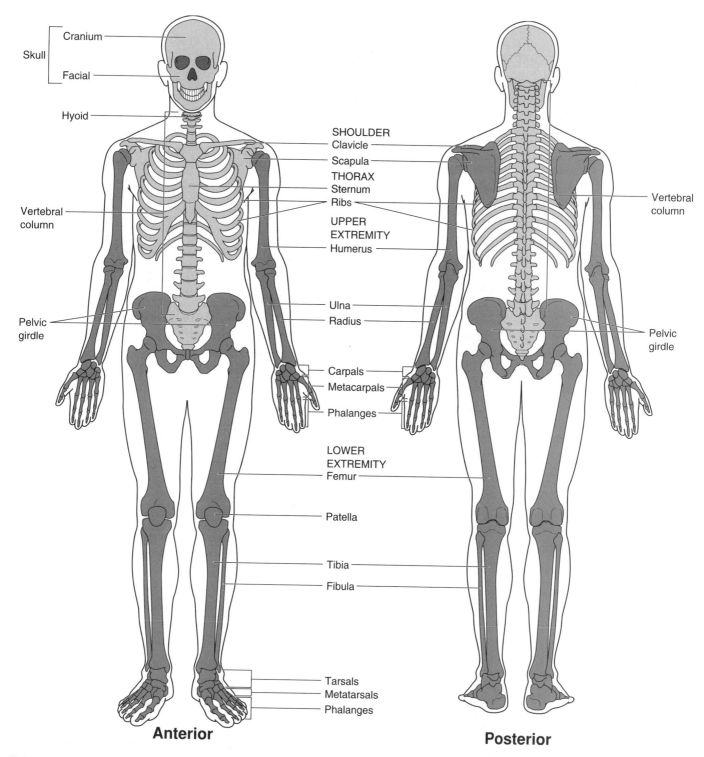

FIGURE 1-4 Major bones of the human body. (With permission from Tortora G, Anagnostakos N: *Principles of Anatomy and Physiology,* 6th ed. New York, Harper & Row, 1992, p 163.)

(2) The most easily palpable aspects of the humerus are the **medial and lateral epicondyles** at its distal end. The epicondyles are located for elbow width measurement in estimating frame size.

  d. Forearm

    –includes two bones: the **ulna** and the **radius.**

(1) The most prominent bony landmark of the proximal forearm is the **olecranon process** on the posterior ulna.

(2) At the distal end of the forearm are the **radial styloid process** laterally and the **ulnar styloid process** medially. These areas help identify the proper location for assessing radial pulse.

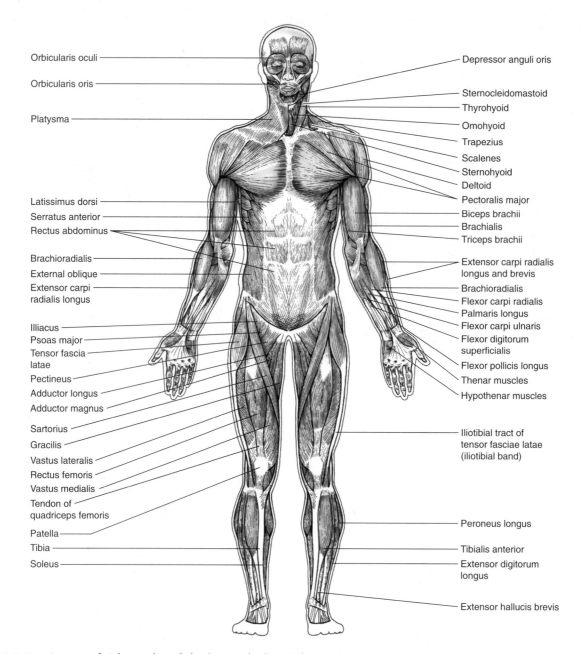

Orbicularis oculi
Orbicularis oris
Platysma
Latissimus dorsi
Serratus anterior
Rectus abdominus
Brachioradialis
External oblique
Extensor carpi radialis longus
Illiacus
Psoas major
Tensor fascia latae
Pectineus
Adductor longus
Adductor magnus
Sartorius
Gracilis
Vastus lateralis
Rectus femoris
Vastus medialis
Tendon of quadriceps femoris
Patella
Tibia
Soleus

Depressor anguli oris
Sternocleidomastoid
Thyrohyoid
Omohyoid
Trapezius
Scalenes
Sternohyoid
Deltoid
Pectoralis major
Biceps brachii
Brachialis
Triceps brachii
Extensor carpi radialis longus and brevis
Brachioradialis
Flexor carpi radialis
Palmaris longus
Flexor carpi ulnaris
Flexor digitorum superficialis
Flexor pollicis longus
Thenar muscles
Hypothenar muscles
Iliotibial tract of tensor fasciae latae (iliotibial band)
Peroneus longus
Tibialis anterior
Extensor digitorum longus
Extensor hallucis brevis

FIGURE 1-5 Anterior superficial muscles of the human body. (With permission from Tortora G, Anagnostakos N: *Principles of Anatomy and Physiology,* 6th ed. New York, Harper & Row, 1992, p 266.)

3. **Musculature**

   a. The superficial anterior and posterior muscles of the upper body are shown in **Figures 1-5** and **1-6**.

   b. Of particular importance to exercise testing are identification and palpation of the **sternocleidomastoid, pectoralis major, biceps brachii,** and **triceps brachii.**

4. **Arteries**

   a. Arteries carry blood away from the heart, either to the lungs (pulmonary arteries) or to other organs and the skeletal muscles (systemic arteries).

   b. For exercise testing and evaluation, identification and palpation of the **carotid, brachial,** and **radial arteries** are important (see III C 1 below).

B. **LOWER BODY**

1. The **appendicular skeleton** comprises the bones of the pelvic girdle, thigh, leg, and foot.

   a. **Pelvic girdle**

      –comprises the hip bones (**ilium, ischium,** and **pubis**), **sacrum,** and **coccyx.**

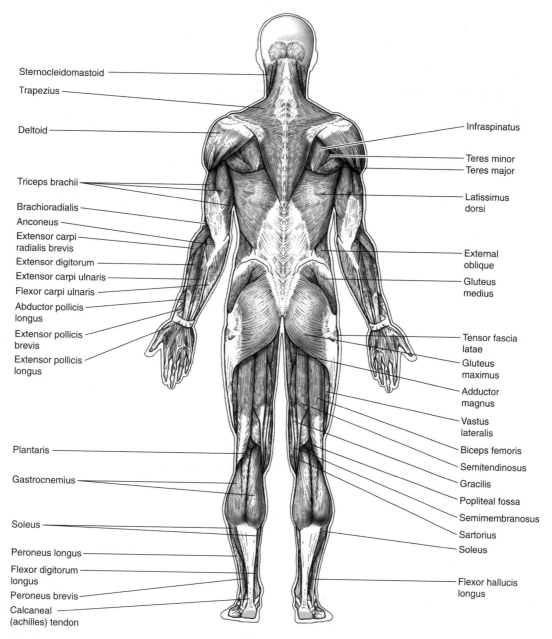

FIGURE 1-6 Posterior superficial muscles of the human body. (With permission from Tortora G, Anagnostakos N: *Principles of Anatomy and Physiology*, 6th ed. New York, Harper & Row, 1992, p 265.)

–Of the hip bones, the **ilium** is the most noteworthy in terms of exercise testing. Its superiormost structure **(iliac crest)** and anteriormost structure **(anterior superior iliac spine)** are easily palpated and serve as landmarks for skinfold measurements.

b. Thigh

–Skeletally, the thigh is formed by the **femur.** Its most easily palpable landmark is the **greater trochanter** on the proximal lateral side.

–Distally, the **patella** is located anterior to the knee joint. It serves as a landmark for locating the thigh skinfold.

2. Musculature

a. Of particular importance to exercise testing are identification and palpation of the **gluteus maximus, quadriceps femoris,** and **gastrocnemius.**

b. An important landmark for skinfold measurement is the **inguinal crease,** a natural diagonal crease in the skin formed where the musculature of the thigh meets the pelvic girdle.

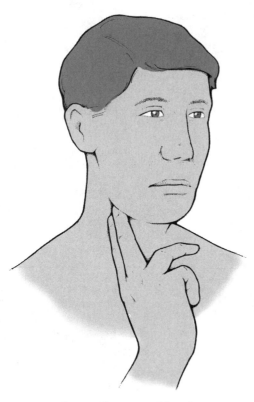

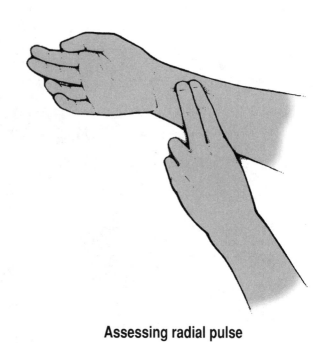

Assessing radial pulse

Assessing carotid pulse

FIGURE 1-7 The carotid pulse is palpated by placing the first two fingers in the groove between the trachea and the sternocleidomastoid muscle and pressing gently inward. The radial pulse is palpated by placing the first two fingers as shown and pressing gently. (Adapted from *ACSM's Resource Manual for Guidelines for Exercise Testing and Prescription,* 3rd ed. Baltimore, Williams & Wilkins, 1998, p 94.)

C. SURFACE ANATOMY

–Knowledge of basic surface anatomy is essential to assessing pulses and blood pressure, obtaining anthropometric measurements, determining ECG lead placements, and performing CPR and emergency defibrillation.

1. **Pulse** is assessed at a palpable artery, most commonly the brachial, carotid, or radial artery (**Figure 1-7**).

   a. The **carotid artery** runs along the trachea as the **common carotid.** Approximately at the level of the mandible, the common carotid bifurcates to the **external and internal carotid arteries.** The carotid artery can be palpated inferior to the mandible and lateral to the larynx in the groove between the trachea and the sternocleidomastoid muscle.

   b. The **brachial artery** runs along the medial side of the upper arm between the biceps brachii and triceps brachii muscles to a point just distal of the elbow joint. The artery can be palpated in the groove between the biceps and triceps or, more commonly, at the medial antecubital space, located on the frontal aspect of the elbow.

   c. The **radial artery** divides from the brachial artery and continues down the forearm on the radial(thumb) side. The radial artery is easily palpable at the distal lateral forearm.

2. In **blood pressure measurement,** the arterial reference indicator on the cuff is placed over the brachial artery. The bottom of the cuff is located approximately 1 inch above the antecubital space, and the stethoscope is positioned in the medial antecubital space (**Figure 1-8**).

3. **Anthropometric measurements**

   a. **Skinfold measurements**

   –Because of the assumed relationship between subcutaneous fat and total body fat, skinfold measurements are a common method of **estimating body fat percentage.** Various skinfold sites may be measured (**Figure 1-9**):

   (1) Chest/pectoral: diagonal fold, one-half the distance between the anterior axillary line and the nipple in men, or one-third of this distance in women.

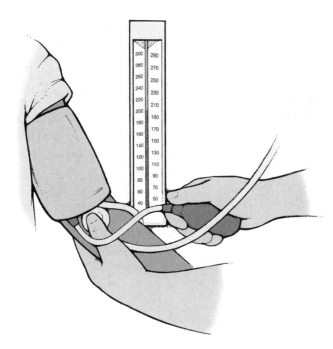

FIGURE 1-8 When measuring blood pressure, the stethoscope is placed over the brachial artery as shown. (From *ACSM's Resource Manual for Guidelines for Exercise Testing and Prescription,* 3rd ed. Baltimore, Williams & Wilkins, 1998, p 93.)

(2) Midaxillary: vertical fold, on the midaxillary line at the level of the xiphoid process.

(3) Subscapular: diagonal fold (45-degree angle), 1-2 cm inferior to and along the line of the inferior angle of the scapula.

(4) Triceps brachii: vertical fold, on the posterior midline of the upper arm midway between the acromion and olecranon processes.

(5) Biceps brachii: vertical fold, on the anterior arm over the belly of the muscle, 1 cm above the triceps brachii site.

(6) Abdominal: vertical fold, 2 cm to the right of the umbilicus.

(7) Suprailiac: diagonal fold, on the anterior axillary line, immediately superior to the natural line of the iliac crest.

(8) Thigh: vertical fold, on the anterior midline of the thigh, midway between the inguinal crease and superior patellar border.

(9) Calf: vertical fold, at the midline of the medial border of calf at the greatest circumference.

b. Body circumferences

–Circumference, or girth, is measured at selected sites to estimate body fat

percentage or for comparative purposes in weight loss/management programs. Common sites include the following (**Figure 1-10**):

(1) Arm: midway between the acromion and olecranon processes.

(2) Forearm: at the maximum forearm circumference.

(3) Abdomen: at the level of the umbilicus.

(4) Waist: at the narrowest part of the torso, inferior to the xiphoid process and superior to the umbilicus.

(5) Hip: at the greatest circumference of the hips/buttocks, above the gluteal fold.

(6) Thigh: at the greatest circumference of the thigh, below the gluteal fold.

(7) Calf: at the maximum circumference between the knee and ankle joint.

c. Body widths

–Skeletal widths may be used for estimating body frame size; two sites are measured:

(1) Elbow: the distance between the lateral and medial epicondyles, with the elbow flexed to 90 degrees.

(2) Bisacromial: the distance between the acromion processes.

4. Electrocardiography lead placement (Figure 1-11)

a. The **standard or Mason-Likar 12-lead system** uses 10 electrodes: four limb electrodes and six precordial electrodes.

(1) Limb electrodes

(a) Right arm (RA) and left arm (LA) electrodes are positioned just inferior to the distal ends of the right and left clavicle, respectively.

(b) Right leg (RL) and left leg (LL) electrodes are positioned just superior to the iliac crest along the midclavicular line.

(2) Precordial (or "V") electrodes

(a) V1 and V2 are positioned at the fourth intercostal space on the right and left sternal border, respectively.

(b) V4 is located on the midclavicular line at the fifth intercostal space.

(c) V3 is positioned at the midpoint between V2 and V4.

(d) V5 and V6 are positioned on the anterior axillary line and midaxillary line, respectively, both at the level of V4.

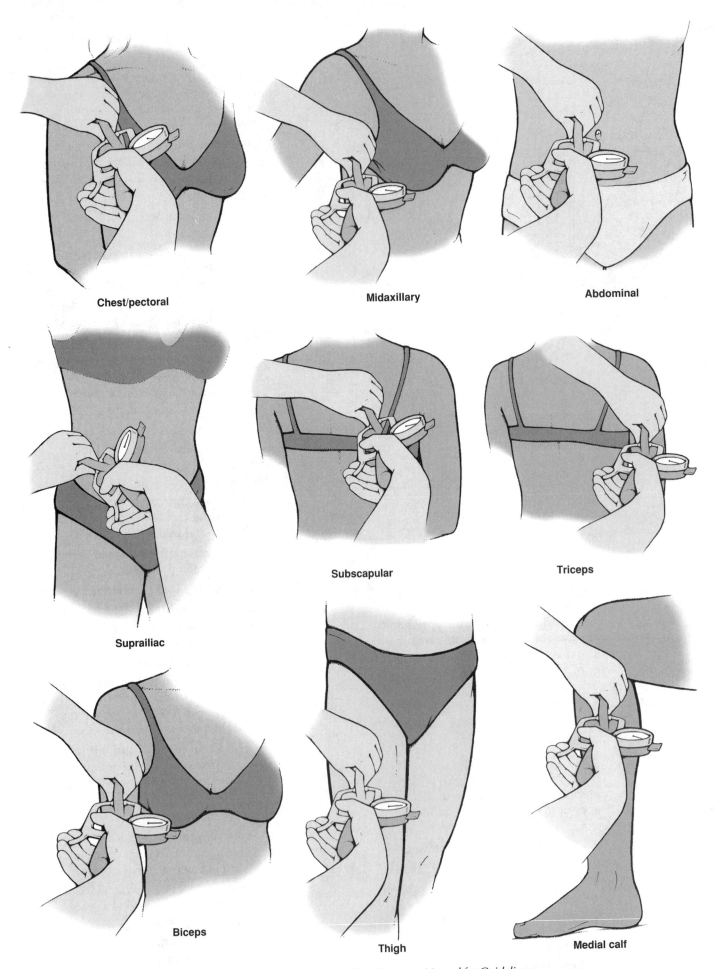

Chest/pectoral

Midaxillary

Abdominal

Suprailiac

Subscapular

Triceps

Biceps

Thigh

Medial calf

FIGURE 1-9 Obtaining skinfold measurements. (Adapted from *ACSM's Resource Manual for Guidelines for Exercise Testing and Prescription,* 3rd ed. Baltimore, Williams & Wilkins, 1998, pp 95–97.)

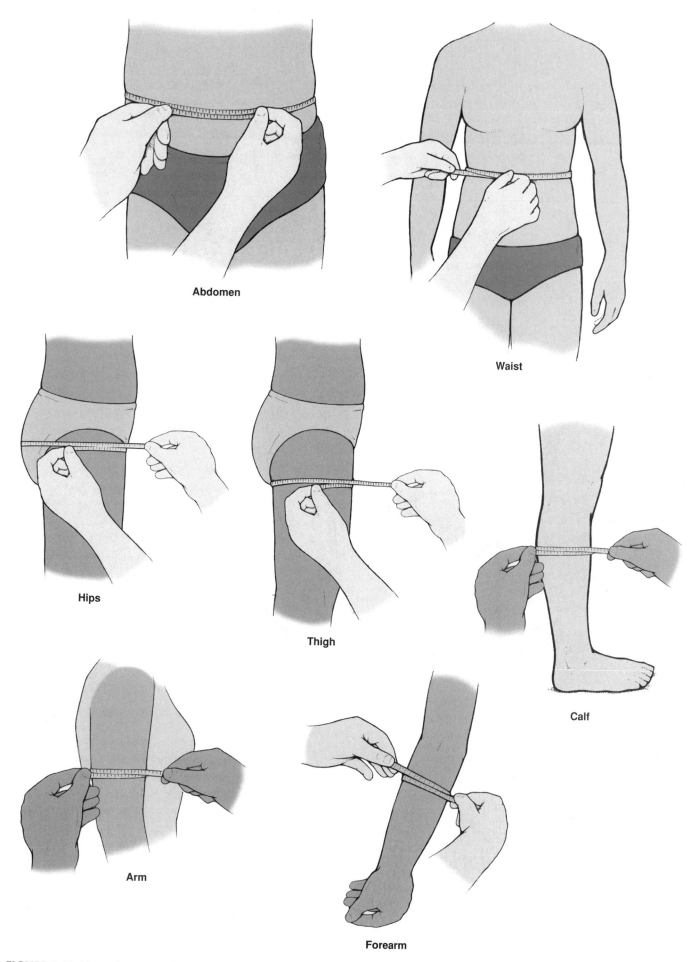

FIGURE 1-10 Measuring circumferences. (Adapted from *ACSM's Resource Manual for Guidelines for Exercise Testing and Prescription,* 3rd ed. Baltimore, Williams & Wilkins, 1998, pp 97–99.)

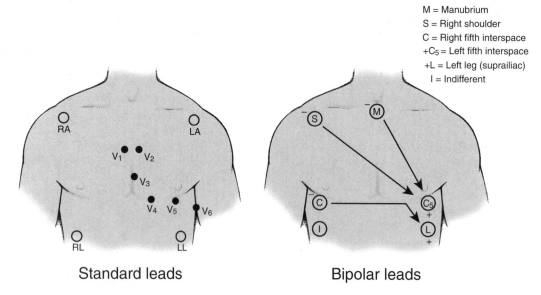

M = Manubrium
S = Right shoulder
C = Right fifth interspace
+C₅ = Left fifth interspace
+L = Left leg (suprailiac)
I = Indifferent

Standard leads

Bipolar leads

FIGURE 1-11 ECG lead placement. (From *ACSM's Resource Manual for Guidelines for Exercise Testing and Prescription,* 3rd ed. Baltimore, Williams & Wilkins, 1998, p 92.)

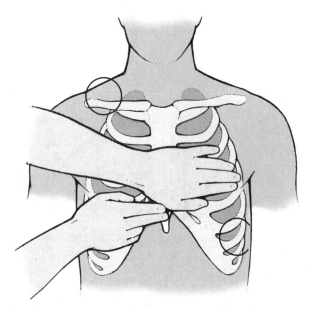

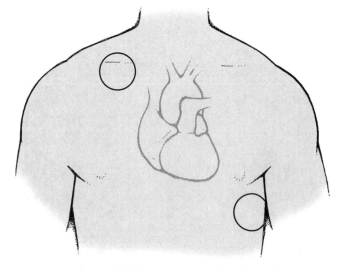

FIGURE 1-13 Standard placement for defibrillation electrodes. (From *ACSM's Resource Manual for Guidelines for Exercise Testing and Prescription,* 3rd ed. Baltimore, Williams & Wilkins, 1998, p 100.)

FIGURE 1-12 Correct hand position for cardiac compressions in CPR. (From *ACSM's Resource Manual for Guidelines for Exercise Testing and Prescription,* 3rd ed. Baltimore, Williams & Wilkins, 1998, p 99.)

b. **Bipolar electrodes**

–Electrode placement for the bipolar leads can take various configurations. Electrodes may be placed at the manubrium, the right fifth intercostal space at the anterior axillary line, and at the standard electrode placements of RA, RL, LL, and V5.

5. **CPR and defibrillation**

a. In **CPR,** chest compressions are done with the hand on the sternal body, at the xyphoid. The middle finger is placed on the xyphoid notch with the index finger next to it. The heel of the opposite hand is then placed superior to the index finger (**Figure 1-12**).

b. The upper electrode for **defibrillation** is placed just inferior to the clavicle and to the right of the sternum. The lower electrode is located at the midaxillary line just lateral to the left nipple (**Figure 1-13**).

IV. BIOMECHANICAL PRINCIPLES

–For movement to occur, a net force must be present. **Biomechanics** is the study of the forces and torques affecting movement and the description of the resulting movement.

A. FORCES

–A **force** can be thought of as a push or a pull that produces or has the capacity to produce a change in motion of a body.

–Multiple forces from multiple directions may act on a body. The sum of these forces, or the **net force,** determines the resulting change in motion.

B. TORQUE

–**Torque** is the product of a force and the perpendicular distance from the line of action of the force and the axis of rotation.

–When a force is applied and rotational movement results, the force must be eccentric to the axis of rotation.

C. NEWTON'S LAWS

–The relationships between forces, torques and the resulting movements were described by Sir Isaac Newton (1642-1727). Three laws describe the interactions:

1. The **law of inertia** states that a body will maintain its state of rest or uniform motion in a straight line unless acted on by an external force.

2. The **law of acceleration** states that the acceleration of a body resulting from an applied force will be proportional to the magnitude of the force, in the direction of the applied force, and inversely proportional to the mass of the body.

3. The **law of reaction** states that when two bodies interact, the force exerted by the first body on the second is met by an equal and opposite force by the second body on the first. In other words, **for every action, there is an equal and opposite reaction.**

D. FORCES AFFECTING MOVEMENT

–The forces influencing movement can be classified as reaction, friction, and muscular.

1. **Ground reaction force**

   a. In accordance with **Newton's law of reaction,** as a body applies a force to the ground, the ground applies an equal and opposite force to the body.

   b. Ground reaction forces are measured with a force plate in **three directions:** vertical, anteroposterior, and mediolateral. The net effect of the three-dimensional forces determines the resulting movement.

   c. **Typical patterns** of ground reaction force are seen in **walking** and **running** (**Figure 1-14**).

   d. **Abnormalities in gait** can be assessed by evaluating ground reaction force patterns.

2. **Frictional force**

   a. When two objects interact, **friction** acts at the surface contact of the objects in a direction opposite the motion or impending motion (**Figure 1-15**).

   b. **Frictional force** (Ff) is influenced by the nature and interaction of the contacting surfaces (the coefficient of friction, m) and the force pressing the surfaces together (normal force, N). The formula for frictional force is:

   $$Ff = m\ N$$

3. **Muscular force**

   a. To move body segments, muscular forces must be present. Muscles provide a **pulling force on bone.** Across any joint, the net effect of individual muscle forces acting across the joint determines the joint movement.

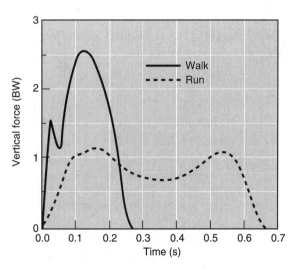

FIGURE 1-14 Vertical ground reaction force component during heel-toe running and walking.

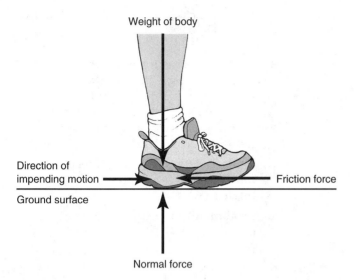

Weight of body

Direction of
impending motion

Ground surface

Friction force

Normal force

FIGURE 1-15 Friction force during foot contact of a running stride. (From *ACSM's Resource Manual for Guidelines for Exercise Testing and Prescription,* 3rd ed. Baltimore, Williams & Wilkins, 1998, p 105.)

b. Because all segmental movement is rotational, not only the net muscular force, but also **the distance the force acts from the rotational axis of the joint,** influence movement.

c. Also affecting movement are the **length of the muscle at the time of contraction** and the **velocity of muscle shortening.**

d. **Normal movement patterns** result from the coordinated actions of the muscles acting across a joint.

e. **Abnormal movement patterns** result from disruptions in the coordinated muscular actions due to application of inappropriate force, co-contraction of musculature, muscular weakness, or neurologic disorders affecting muscular recruitment.

E. APPLICATION TO HUMAN MOVEMENT

1. **Abnormal spinal curvature (Figure 1-16)**

   a. **Kyphosis** is a condition of abnormal posterior curvature. In the lumbar region, it may be associated with posterior pelvic tilt, shortened hip extensors and stretched hip flexors.

   b. **Lordosis** is a condition of abnormal anterior curvature. In lumbar region, it may be associated with anterior pelvic tilt, stretched hip extensors, and shortened hip flexors and trunk extensors.

   c. **Scoliosis** is an abnormal lateral curvature of the spine. Scoliosis may affect the spine's load-bearing capability and, in severe cases, crowd normal organ space.

2. **Gait**

   a. **Normal walking gait**

      (1) Locomotion occurs from repetition of the **gait cycle,** the time between successive ground contacts of the same foot (**Figure 1-17**).

      (a) A **stride** is the time between ground contacts of the right heel.

      (b) One-half of a stride is a **step,** defined as the time from ground contact of one heel to ground contact of the other heel.

      (c) Normally, 60% of the gait cycle is in **stance** (foot in contact with the ground) and 40% is in **swing** (foot not in contact with the ground).

      (2) Typical **walking speed** in adults is approximately 1.5 m/s. Decreases occur with aging, injury, and disease.

      (3) A typical length of stride, or **cycle length (CL),** is approximately 1.5 m, and a typical rate of stride, or **cycle rate (CR),** is about 1 cycle/s. With increasing gait speed, CL and CR increase.

      (4) In the frontal plane, **pelvic movement** during walking is approximately 5 cm on each side, alternating as each leg assumes a support role. In the tranverse plane, the pelvis rotates a total of 8 degrees, half of it anteriorly and half posteriorly.

      (5) In a normal walking gait, the vertical **ground reaction force** pattern is bimodal in shape and of maximum magnitude on the order of 1–1.2 times body weight. The two peaks represent heel contact to midstance and midstance to push-off.

   b. **Abnormal walking gait**

      –Deviations from a normal walking gait occur for various reasons (e.g., pain from injury, decreased flexibility or range of motion) and take many different forms. **Common causes of gait abnormalities** include muscular weakness and neurologic disorders.

      (1) Muscular weakness

      (a) Weakness in the gluteus maximus may contribute to an anterior lean of the upper body at heel strike.

      (b) Weakness in the gluteus medius and minimus decreases their stabilizing function during the stance phase of gait, possibly

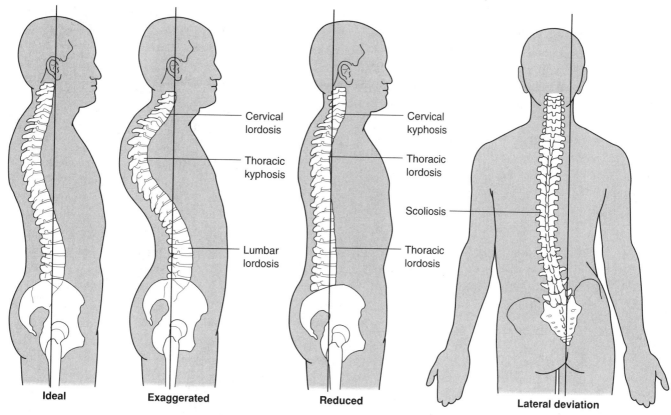

FIGURE 1-16 Ideal and abnormal spinal curvatures.

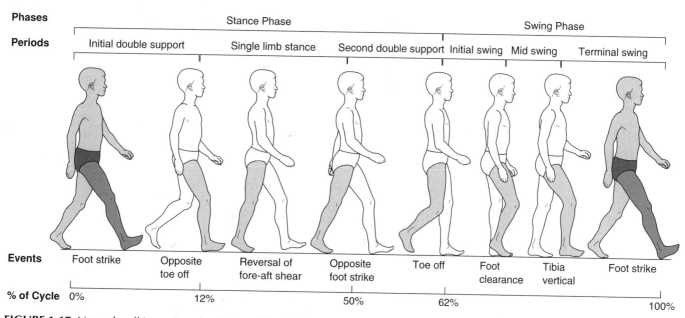

FIGURE 1-17 Normal walking gait cycle. (Adapted from Rose J, Gamble JG [eds]: *Human Walking,* 2nd ed. Baltimore, Williams & Wilkins, 1994, p 26.)

leading to an increased lateral shift in the pelvis (increased frontal plane movement) and side-to-side movement during gait.

(c) Severe **weakness in the plantarflexors** reduces push-off and thus step length on the affected side.

(d) Dorsiflexor insufficiency results in slapping of the foot during heel contact (foot drop) and increased knee and hip flexion during the swing phase.

(e) Due to the inability to adequately support loads or control knee extension, **weakness of the quadriceps femoris** may lead to forward lean of the trunk or hyperextension of the knee joint (genu recurvatum).

(2) Neurologic disorders

(a) In **hemiplegia,** the affected leg is often circumducted during the swing phase, and the affected arm is held across the upper body with flexion in the elbow, wrist, and hand.

(b) Parkinsonism may produce a characteristic gait pattern of increased hip and knee flexion, forward trunk lean, and shuffling step.

c. Normal Running Gait

(1) The normal running gait is similar to the walking gait but with the addition of a **flight phase,** during which both feet are off the ground.

(2) Cycle length and **cycle rate** are related to running speed:

$$velocity = CL \times CR$$

(3) Up to about 5 m/s, CL increases with speed and CR stays relatively constant or increases slightly. Increases in speed beyond 5 m/s generally result from increased CR.

(4) At running speeds up to 6 m/s, vertical **ground reaction forces** are between two and three times body weight. These forces are realized at heel strike as an impact peak and during push-off as an active peak.

d. Abnormal Running Gait

–As with walking, running gait disorders are difficult to generalize due to their complexity and varying manifestations. However, the most common problems associated with running involve rear foot motion during heel strike and push-off.

(1) Pronation

(a) A combination of abduction, eversion, and dorsiflexion, **pronation** is greatest at midstance and may be affected by running speed and shoe hardness and design.

(b) Some degree of pronation is helpful in reducing impact forces. Excessive and very rapid pronation is undesirable. Shoe wear patterns in overpronators show medial wear.

(2) Supination is a combination of adduction, inversion, and plantarflexion. Excessive supination (marked by excessive shoe wear on the lateral side) at take-off may impair running performance due to misdirection of propulsive forces.

REVIEW TEST

DIRECTIONS: Carefully read all questions and select the BEST single answer.

1. For exercise testing, where are the upper extremity limb leads placed?
   (A) On the distal anterior forearm
   (B) Just inferior to the distal clavicle
   (C) At the second intercostal space, along the midclavicular line
   (D) At the fourth intercostal space, at the right and left sternal border

2. In a 12-lead ECG, where are precordial leads V5 and V6 positioned?
   (A) At the fifth intercostal space on the distal clavicular and anterior axillary lines
   (B) On the midaxillary line in the fifth and sixth intercostal spaces
   (C) On the left midaxillary and postaxillary lines of the fifth intercostal space
   (D) On the left anterior and midaxillary lines at the level of the V4 electrode

3. For a bipolar lead arrangement, differences in electrode placement from a 12-lead setup include the
   (A) manubrium of the sternum.
   (B) right third intercostal space, midclavicular line.
   (C) right fourth intercostal space, sternal border.
   (D) xiphoid process.

4. Palpation of the brachial artery is possible
   (A) along the anterior aspect of the biceps brachii.
   (B) in the medial side of the upper arm in the groove between the biceps brachii and triceps brachii.
   (C) 2 cm distal to the antecubital space on the lateral side of the forearm.
   (D) at the level of the antecubital space at the medial condyle of the humerus.

5. The radial pulse is easily palpated at the
   (A) proximal lateral forearm where it divides from the brachial artery.
   (B) medial antecubital space.
   (C) posterior forearm, between the zyloid processes.
   (D) distal lateral forearm.

6. Identifying the proper site for chest compressions in cardiopulmonary resuscitation is best accomplished by
   (A) locating the sternoclavicular joint and placing the compressing hand 2 cm inferior to it.
   (B) locating the sternal angle and placing the hand over it.
   (C) locating the xiphoid process and placing the compressing hand superior to the xiphoid notch.
   (D) placing the hand anywhere along the midline of the sternum.

7. What is the proper orientation and location for obtaining the suprailiac skinfold measurement?
   (A) A diagonal fold at the anterior axillary line along the natural line of the iliac crest
   (B) A diagonal fold at the anterior superior iliac spine
   (C) A vertical fold at the iliac crest, midaxillary line
   (D) A vertical fold just superior to the anterior superior iliac spine

8. What is the orientation and location of the subscapular skinfold?
   (A) 1 inch below the medial border of the scapula as a vertical fold
   (B) As a vertical fold at the inferior angle of the scapula
   (C) Diagonally along the external border at the level of the xiphoid process
   (D) As a diagonal fold 2 cm below and along the line of the inferior angle of the scapula

9. When taking circumference measurements, the abdomen and the waist are
   (A) the same measurement
   (B) different in that the waist is inferior to the abdomen
   (C) the same only if the narrowest part of the torso is at the level of the umbilicus
   (D) different in that the abdomen will be less than the waist

10. Elbow width is used to measure frame size. Where is this width measured?
    (A) At the lateral epicondyles with the elbow and shoulder flexed 90 degrees
    (B) Across the olecranon process with the elbow flexed 90 degrees
    (C) Between the antecubital space and the olecranon process with the elbow fully extended
    (D) Posteriorly at the lateral epicondyles with the elbow fully extended

11. When assessing blood pressure, the diaphragm of the stethoscope is positioned
    (A) on the lateral portion of the antecubital space.
    (B) distal to the antecubital space on the radial artery.
    (C) on the medial side of the upper arm, 2 cm superior to the antecubital space.
    (D) on the medial portion of the antecubital space.

12. The relative change in the velocity of two bodies due to equal external forces occurs in accordance with
    (A) the law of reaction.
    (B) the law of acceleration.
    (C) the law of friction.
    (D) the law of inertia.

13. In a normal healthy adult with an average walking gait, which of the following would be expected?
    (A) A speed of 1.5 m/s and a cycle length of 1.5 m
    (B) A speed of 3.0 m/s and a cycle length of 1.5 m
    (C) A speed of 1.5 m/s and a cycle rate of 1.5 cycles/s
    (D) A speed of 2.5 m/s and a cycle rate of 1 cycle/s

14. When comparing vertical ground reaction forces between walking and running, which of the following is true?
    (A) Impact peaks are higher in running, but active peaks are similar in magnitude between walking and running.
    (B) They are speed dependent in walking but not in running, due to the flight phase of the gait.
    (C) In running, impact peaks are more prominent and active peaks are of greater magnitude.
    (D) Impact peaks are smaller and active peaks are greater in running.

15. An adult with greater than average hip and knee flexion and a short stride length may be suspected of having
    (A) weak quadriceps femoris muscles.
    (B) weak plantarflexors and dorsiflexors.
    (C) hemiplegia.
    (D) weak gluteals.

16. Circumduction of the leg during the swing phase of the walking gait is indicative of
    (A) hemiplegia.
    (B) gluteal weakness.
    (C) Parkinson's disease.
    (D) quadriceps femoris weakness.

17. Across the range of typical distance running speeds, increases in velocity are due to what factors?
    (A) Primarily an increase in cycle time
    (B) Primarily an increase in cycle rate
    (C) Equal increases in cycle rate and cycle length
    (D) Primarily an increase in cycle length

18. With lordosis in the lumbar region, which of the following is NOT uncommon?
    (A) The hip flexors and abdominals are shortened.
    (B) The hip extensors and trunk extensors are stretched.
    (C) The trunk extensors are shortened and the hip extensors are stretched.
    (D) The abdominals are stretched and the hamstrings are shortened.

19. In which of the following conditions would the lumbar curve be attenuated and the thoracic curve be accentuated?
    (A) Thoracic lordosis and lumbar kyphosis
    (B) Thorcic kyphosis and lumbar kyphosis
    (C) Thoracic lordosis and lumbar lordosis
    (D) Thoracic kyphosis and lumbar lordosis

20. A running shoe showing excessive wear on the medial sole may be indicative of
    (A) excessive pronation.
    (B) excessive supination.
    (C) excessive impact force.
    (D) excessive stance time.

ANSWERS AND EXPLANATIONS

1–B. Left arm and right arm electrodes are positioned just inferior to the distal clavicle. Traditional standard resting 12-lead setups place the electrodes on the distal anterior forearm. This is impractical for exercise testing. No limb leads are placed in intercostal spaces.

2–D. Precordial electrodes V5 and V6 are positioned at the same level as V4. Because the ribs curve in a superior direction, following the fifth intercostal space will not allow for correct lead placement. All precordial electrodes are placed on the left side of the body in accordance with the position of the heart.

3–A. The manubrium of the sternum is a common bipolar electrode site. No electrodes are placed at the third intercostal space on the right side or at the xiphoid process.

4–B. The brachial artery is located superficially in the groove between the biceps brachii and triceps brachii on the medial side of the arm. Being superficial, it can be palpated easily. At the level of the antecubital space, it moves anteriorly between the condyles. Approximately ½ inch below the antecubital space, it divides into the radial and ulnar arteries.

5–D. The radial artery divides from the brachial artery just below the bend in the arm. It extends to the distal lateral forearm being covered proximally by the supinator longus muscle. It is superficial and easily palpated at the distal lateral forearm.

6–C. The hand is placed just above the xiphoid notch on the sternum. This positions the hand on the sternal body and helps to ensure that compressions are not performed on the xiphoid, which could damage internal organs. The xiphoid is located by tracing the inferior border of the ribs up to the midline of the body where the xiphoid is located.

7–A. The suprailiac skinfold is a diagonal fold that follows the normal curvature of the iliac crest.

8–D. Subscapular skinfold is taken diagonally just below the inferior angle of the scapula following the line of the inferior. The inferior angle of the scapula is the landmark to palpate for measurement.

9–C. The waist is measured at the level of the narrowest part of the torso. Normally, this places it superior to the abdominal circumference, which is measured at the level of the umbilicus.

10–A. The appropriate measurement is at the lateral and medial epicondyles taken with the elbow and shoulder flexed at 90 degrees.

11–D. The brachial artery is palpated for pulse where it enters the antecubital space on the medial side. This is also where the stethoscope is placed when measuring blood pressure.

12–B. The law of acceleration states that the acceleration of a body is proportional to the net force and inversely proportional to the mass of the body. Therefore, given that an equal force is acting on the unequal masses, the less massive body will experience a greater change in velocity.

13–A. While normal preferred walking speed will vary somewhat, the average speed is 1.5 m/s. Speed is equal to cycle length x cycle rate, with average cycle lengths of about 1.5 m and average cycle rates of about 1.0 Hz.

14–C. The vertical ground reaction force for running shows a sharper impact peak and an active peak of greater magnitude than with walking. In general, the vertical ground reaction forces are approximately 2–3 times body weight in running gait and about 1–1.2 times body weight in walking.

15–B. Plantarflexors are critical in the push-off phase of the walking gait. Weakness in these muscles will reduce stride length. Weakness in the dorsiflexors will result in difficulties in clearing the ground with the feet during the swing phase unless stride adaptations are made. Often, to overcome dorsiflexion insufficiency, hip and knee flexion are increased during the swing phase.

16–A. Neurologic disorders such as paralysis are associated with the gait circumduction of the affected leg during the swing phase as coordinated normal muscular action is impaired. Parkinson's disease is characterized by a shuffling gait and flexion in the hips, knees, and trunk.

17–D. For common distance running speeds, the increase in speed is mainly due to lengthening of the stride, with little change in the rate of stride. As speed approaches maximum, cycle rate becomes the predominant factor as cycle length reaches a maximum and stays relatively consistent.

18–C. Lumbar lordosis involves an accentuated anterior curve in the lumbar region and often a forward tilting of the pelvis, placing the anterior superior iliac spine in front of the symphasis pubis. In this position, the hip flexors are shortened, as are the trunk extensors. The hip extensors are stretched, as are the abdominals.

19–B. In kyphosis, there is abnormal posterior curvature. The thoracic curve is a posterior curve; therefore, an increase of the curve would be abnormal. The lumbar curve is an anterior curve. Reducing the lumbar curve causes abnormal posterior curvature in the lumbar region. A flattened anterior curve or increased posterior curve is a sign of kyphosis.

20–A. Pronation is a combination of abduction, eversion, and dorsiflexion. While this is helpful to absorb shock in running, excessive pronation can lead to injury. Because an overpronator will rapidly evert the foot, wear to the shoe will be seen on the medial side. A supinator, however, will tend to show wear on the lateral side of the shoe, because more time is spent in inversion.

CHAPTER 2

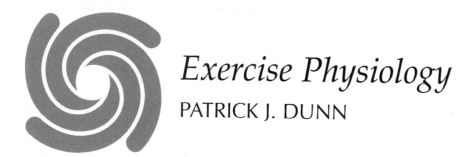

Exercise Physiology
PATRICK J. DUNN

I. ENERGY METABOLISM

–The energy to perform physical work comes from the **breakdown of adenosine triphosphate (ATP).** The amount of directly available ATP is small and lasts only 5–10 seconds; for ATP to continue to work, it must be resynthesized.

–**ATP resynthesis** occurs through a combination of **aerobic and anaerobic processes** via three pathways: the adenosine triphosphate–creatine phosphate (ATP–CP) system (anaerobic), rapid glycolysis (anaerobic), and oxidation (aerobic). See **Figure 2-1.**

–At rest, oxygen (aerobic) is the primary energy source. Increasing intensity of exercise causes a progressive shift to anaerobic sources.

–Clinical exercise physiologists must distinguish between aerobic and anaerobic energy sources in interpreting exercise test results and prescribing an exercise regimen.

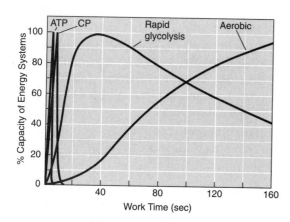

FIGURE 2-1 Interaction between anaerobic and aerobic energy sources during exercise, including ATP, creatine phosphate, rapid glycolysis, and aerobic (oxidative phosphorylation). (From *ACSM's Resource Manual for Guidelines for Exercise Testing and Prescription,* 3rd ed. Baltimore, Williams & Wilkins, 1998, p 132.)

A. ATP-CP SYSTEM

–This is an anaerobic process that lasts 1–30 seconds.

–The ATP–CP process generates rapid energy by transferring high-energy phosphate from creatine phosphate to rephosphorylate ATP.

–**Weight lifting** and **sprinting** are examples of physical activities that use the ATP–CP process.

B. RAPID (ANAEROBIC) GLYCOLYSIS AND LACTIC ACID FORMATION

–This anaerobic process lasts from 30 seconds to 3 minutes.

–The process involves anaerobic degradation of carbohydrate (glucose or glycogen) to either lactate or pyruvate.

–**Lactic acid formation** allows glycolysis to continue.

–Because **pyruvate** can participate in the aerobic production of ATP, glycolysis can also be considered the first step in the aerobic production of ATP.

–Anaerobic production of ATP results in accumulation of lactic acid in the blood. Lactic acid contributes to fatigue, but can also be used as a fuel during and following exercise.

–A **400-meter sprint** is an example of physical activity requiring anaerobic glycolysis to produce energy in the form of ATP.

C. OXIDATION

–This aerobic process is the primary energy source when a person is **at rest,** as well as **when exercise lasts longer than 3 minutes.**

–Oxidation combines two metabolic processes: the **Krebs cycle** and **electron transport.**

–**Oxidative phosphorylation uses oxygen** as the final hydrogen acceptor to form ATP and water. Byproducts are carbon dioxide (CO_2) and water.

–**Oxidation uses fat, carbohydrate, or protein** as an energy source. Fat is broken down aerobically through beta-oxidation; 5 kcal/L of oxygen are consumed.

–**Jogging, walking, swimming, and cycling** are examples of physical activities using oxidation.

II. PHYSIOLOGICAL MEASUREMENTS USED IN EXERCISE TESTING (Table 2-1)

A. HEART RATE

1. **Normal exercise response**

   –**Heart rate increases in a linear fashion** with work rate and oxygen uptake during dynamic exercise.

   –Response is related to age, body position, fitness, type of activity, the presence of heart disease, medications, blood volume, and environment.

   –The increase in heart rate occurring at any fixed submaximal work rate is proportionally greater in untrained persons than in trained persons.

2. **Abnormal exercise responses**

   –**No increase in heart rate** occurs with increased work rate.

   –**Cardiac arrhythmias,** such as atrial fibrillation, supraventricular tachycardia, or ventricular arrhythmias, are present.

3. **Adaptation to training**

   –**Resting heart rate and the heart rate at submaximal exercise intensity** are decreased.

   –**Maximal heart rate** is unchanged or slightly decreased.

B. STROKE VOLUME

–**Stroke volume is a function of preload (diastolic filling), afterload (ventricular outflow), and myocardial contractility.** It is the difference between end-diastolic volume (EDV) and end-systolic volume (ESV).

–**Ejection fraction** is the percentage of the EDV that is ejected from the left ventricle into the aorta with each heart beat (EF = stroke volume/EDV × 100%). The range of normal values is 57%–73%.

–**Normal resting stroke volume** is 60–100 ml/beat.

–**Normal maximal stroke volume** is 100-200 ml/beat.

1. **Normal exercise response**

   –During exercise, **stroke volume increases curvilinearly** with work rate until it reaches near maximum at a level equivalent to approximately 50% of aerobic capacity, then increases only slightly thereafter.

   –According to the **Frank-Starling law,** the left ventricle can contract with greater force during exercise, because of increased EDV and enhanced mechanical ability of muscle fibers to produce force.

2. **Adaptation to training**

   –**Stroke volume increases with endurance training.**

   a. Long-term endurance training increases the force of left ventricular contraction during exercise, resulting in increased ejection fraction.

   b. Long-term endurance training also leads to increased central blood volume and total hemoglobin concentration,

 Table 2-1. Physiological Responses to Aerobic Conditioning in Untrained Individuals

Variable[1]	Unit of Measure	Response
$\dot{V}O_2$max	ml/kg/min	↑
Resting heart rate	beats/min	↓
Exercise heart rate (submax)	beats/min	↓
Maximum heart rate	beats/min	↔ (or slight ↓)
a-VO_2difference	ml O_2/100 ml blood	↑
Maximum minute ventilation	liters/min	↑
Stroke volume	ml/beat	↑
Cardiac output	liters/min	↑
Blood volume (resting)	liters	↑
Systolic blood pressure	mm Hg	↔ (or slight ↑)
Blood lactate	ml/100 ml blood	↑
Oxidative capacity skeletal muscle	multiple variables[2]	↑

[1] at maximum exercise unless otherwise specified.
[2] represents increases in skeletal muscle mitochondrial number and size, capillary density, and/or oxidative enzymes.
↑ = increase
↓ = decrease
↔ = no change
(From *ACSM's Resource Manual for Guidelines for Exercise Testing and Prescription,* 3rd ed. Baltimore, Williams & Wilkins, 1998, p 157.)

which contribute to increased EDV and stroke volume.

 c. Therefore, stroke volume is higher in conditioned persons at any fixed or relative submaximal workload. This allows conditioned persons to exercise at lower heart rates, thus decreasing myocardial oxygen demand.

 d. Normal ventricular wall thickness and elevated EDV result from endurance training, allowing for greater resting and exercise stroke volumes.

C. CARDIAC OUTPUT

–is the volume of blood pumped into the systemic circulation per minute.

–is related to heart rate, preload, afterload, and contractility.

–The formula for determining cardiac output is:

heart rate × stroke volume

–**Normal resting cardiac output** is approximately 5 L/min.

–**Normal cardiac output after maximal exercise** is approximately 20 L/min.

 1. **Normal exercise response**

  –**Cardiac output increases linearly** with increased work rate.

   a. At exercise intensity up to 50% of oxygen capacity (see II F), the cardiac output increase results from increased heart rate and stroke volume.

   b. Thereafter, the increase results almost solely from the continued rise in heart rate.

  –In **untrained persons,** heart rate plays a more significant role in the ability to increase cardiac output.

  –Cardiac output increases with both the concentric and eccentric phases of a muscular contraction.

 2. **Adaptation to training**

  –**Maximal cardiac output increases with increased conditioning,** primarily because of increased stroke volume.

  –Cardiac output remains essentially unchanged at any fixed submaximal workload before and after training and does not differ substantially between conditioned and unconditioned persons.

D. RATE–PRESSURE PRODUCT

–Also called **double product,** rate–pressure product provides an indirect measure of myocardial oxygen consumption.

–It is determined by the following formula:

heart rate × systolic blood pressure

–**Normal resting rate–pressure product** is 5,400–14,000.

–**Normal range of values at maximal physical exertion** is 25,000–40,000.

 1. **Normal exercise response**

  –An adequate rate–pressure product during maximal exercise is > 25,000.

  –Rate–pressure product may be influenced by age, clinical status, and medications (e.g, beta blockers).

 2. **Adaptation to training**

  –Rate–pressure product at rest and at submaximal exercise intensity is decreased, and the maximal rate–pressure product is unchanged.

E. ARTERIOVENOUS OXYGEN (a-vO$_2$) DIFFERENCE

–is the difference between oxygen content of arterial blood and venous blood.

–measures the ability of skeletal muscle tissue to extract oxygen.

–**Normal resting value** is 5 ml O$_2$/100 ml/dl; normal arterial oxygen concentration of 20 ml O$_2$/100 ml/dl minus normal venous oxygen concentration of 15 ml O$_2$/100 ml/dl.

–**Typical maximal value** is 15 ml O$_2$/100 ml/dl; a-vO$_2$ difference is greater at maximal exercise in conditioned persons than in unconditioned persons.

 1. **Normal exercise response**

  –Oxygen extraction by the tissues typically increases from 5 ml O$_2$/100 ml/dl to 15 ml O$_2$/100 ml/dl at exhaustion.

 2. **Adaptation to training**

  –a-vO$_2$ difference increases with training. Long- term training enhances the ability to extract oxygen from the blood, to deliver oxygen to the working muscles, and to remove and use it for generating energy.

F. MAXIMUM OXYGEN CONSUMPTION

–The most widely recognized measure of cardiopulmonary fitness is **aerobic capacity,** or $\dot{V}O_{2max}$, which can be expressed in absolute (L/min) or relative (ml/kg/min) terms.

–**Oxygen consumption** is calculated using the following formula:

cardiac output × a-vO$_2$ difference

–Oxygen consumption can be measured through direct or indirect calorimetry or, more commonly, estimated from workload or the heart rate at a submaximal workload.

–**Normal resting oxygen consumption** is approximately 3.5 ml/kg/min.

–$\dot{V}O_{2max}$ is defined as the highest rate of oxygen transport and use that can be achieved at maximal physical exertion. **Normal $\dot{V}O_{2max}$** ranges from approximately 35 ml/kg/min (10 metabolic equivalents [METs]) for a healthy unconditioned person to 80 ml/kg/min (23 METs) for a world-class endurance athlete.

1. **Normal exercise response**

   –**Oxygen consumption increases** with increasing work rate. Oxygen uptake rises rapidly during the first minutes of exercise; between the third and fourth minutes, when work rate stabilizes, a plateau is reached, and oxygen uptake remains relatively constant throughout the exercise period.

   a. **Steady-state exercise** reflects a balance between the energy required by working muscles and the rate of ATP production through aerobic metabolism.

   b. **Oxygen deficit** is the difference between total oxygen actually consumed and the amount that would have been consumed in a steady state.

   c. **Oxygen debt** is the increased oxygen consumption in excess of the resting oxygen consumption at the end of an exercise session.

2. **Abnormal exercise response**

   –Assessment of oxygen consumption can be used to classify functional impairment (Table 2-2).

3. **Adaptation to training**

   –**Oxygen consumption increases with training.** Healthy persons can increase maximal oxygen consumption by 10%–30%, with the greatest relative improvements occurring in the most unconditioned persons.

G. **MYOCARDIAL OXYGEN CONSUMPTION (MVO₂)(Figure 2-2)**

   –is an indicator of the heart's workload.

   –depends on heart rate, myocardial contractility, and the tension or stress developed in the

Table 2-2. Weber's Classification of Functional Impairment in Aerobic Capacity and Anaerobic Threshold

Class	Severity	$\dot{V}O_2$max (ml/kg/min)	AT ($\dot{V}O_2$max, ml/kg/min)
A	Mild to none	> 20	> 14
B	Mild to moderate	16–20	11–14
C	Moderate to severe	10–16	8–11
D	Severe	6–10	5–8
E	Very severe	< 6	< 4

(Adapted from Weber KT, Janicki JS. Cardiopulmonary exercise testing for evaluation of chronic cardiac failure. *AM J Cardiol* 55(Suppl A):22A–31A, 1985.)

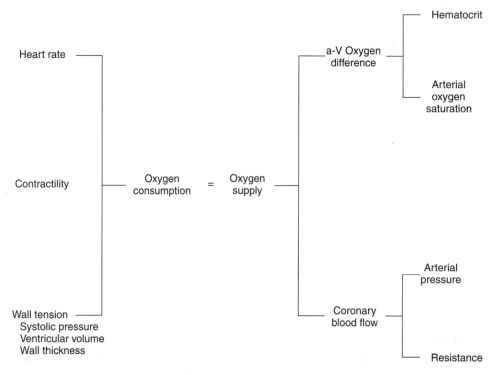

FIGURE 2-2 Determinants of myocardial oxygen demand and supply. (From *ACSM's Resource Manual for Guidelines for Exercise Testing and Prescription,* 3rd ed. Baltimore, Williams & Wilkins, 1998, p 144.)

ventricular wall. Ventricular wall tension is directly related to systolic BP and ventricular volume and inversely related to myocardial wall thickness.

–is best reflected by the rate–pressure product.

–**Normal resting MV̇O₂** is 7.7 ml O₂/100 mg LV/min. At rest, myocardial oxygen use is high in relation to its blood flow. About 70%–80% of oxygen is extracted from the blood.

–**Normal maximal MV̇O₂** is 30 ml O₂/100 mg LV/min.

1. **Normal exercise response**

    –During exercise, increased heart rate is the major contributor to increased MV̇O₂.

    –Oxygen supply is facilitated by increased coronary blood flow and a modest increase in a-vO₂ difference.

2. **Abnormal exercise response**

    –Exercise-induced angina and significant ST segment depression usually occur at the same rate–pressure product in an individual with ischemic heart disease.

3. **Adaptation to training**

    –Long-term exercise training reduces MV̇O₂ during rest and submaximal exercise.

H. BLOOD PRESSURE (Table 2-3)

–Blood pressure (BP) reflects intra-arterial pressure during systole (**systolic BP**) and diastole (**diastolic BP**).

BP = cardiac output × total peripheral resistance.

–**Normal resting BP** values are 90-140 mm Hg systolic and 60-90 mm Hg diastolic.

–**Normal maximal BP** values are 190-220 mm Hg systolic and < 115 mm Hg diastolic.

1. **Normal exercise response**

    a. A linear **increase in systolic BP** occurs with increasing exercise intensity, due to increased cardiac output.

        –The normal incremental rise in systolic BP in response to exercise is 10 mm Hg/MET.

        –BP can increase significantly during resistance training with or without Valsalva's maneuver.

    b. **Diastolic BP may decrease slightly or remain unchanged,** owing to the decreased total peripheral resistance caused by vasodilation.

    c. The **normal postexercise response is a progressive decline in systolic BP.**

        –During passive recovery in an upright posture, systolic BP may decrease

abruptly due to peripheral pooling; it usually normalizes with resumption of the supine position.

    –Systolic BP may remain below pretest resting values for several hours after the test.

    d. **Diastolic BP may also drop** during the postexercise period.

    e. In clients taking vasodilators, calcium channel blockers, angiotensin (ACE) inhibitors, or alpha or beta blockers, the BP response to exercise is variable and cannot be accurately predicted in the absence of clinical test data.

2. **Abnormal exercise response**

    –A **drop in systolic BP or failure of systolic BP to increase with increased exercise intensity (exercise-induced hypotension)** is considered an abnormal response that may reflect coronary artery disease, valvular heart disease, cardiomyopathies, and various arrhythmias.

    –Occasionally, clients without clinically significant heart disease will exhibit exercise-induced hypotension due to antihypertensive therapy, prolonged strenuous exercise, or vasovagal responses.

Table 2-3. Classification of Blood Pressure (BP) for Adults Aged 18 Years and Older*†‡

Category	Systolic BP (mm Hg)		Diastolic BP (mm Hg)
Optimal	<120	and	<80
Normal	120–129	and	80–84
High normal	130–139	or	85–59
Hypertension			
Stage 1	140–159	or	90–99
Stage 2	160–179	or	100–109
Stage 3	≥180	or	≥110

(Reprinted from Sixth Report of the Joint Committee on Prevention, Detection, Evaluation, and Treatment of High Blood Pressure (JNCVI), U.S. Public Health Service, National Institutes of Health, National Heart, Lung and Blood Institute, NIH Publication No. 98-4080, November 1997.)
*Not taking antihypertensive medication and not acutely ill. When systolic and diastolic BPs fall into different categories, the higher category should be selected to classify the individual's BP status. For example, 160/92 mm Hg should be classified as stage 2 hypertension and 174/120 mm Hg should be classified as stage 3 hypertension. Isolated systolic hypertension is defined as systolic BP ≥ 140 mm Hg and diastolic BP < 90 mm Hg and staged appropriately (e.g., 170/82 mm Hg is defined as stage 2 isolated systolic hypertension). In addition to classifying stages of hypertension on the basis of average BP levels, clinicians should specify presence or absence of target organ disease and additional risk factors. This specificity is important for risk classification and treatment.
†Optimal BP with respect to cardiovascular risk is below 120/80 mm Hg. However, unusually low readings should be evaluated for clinical significance.
‡Based on the average of two or more readings taken at each of two or more visits after an initial screening.

–Although the prognosis of exercise-induced hypotension in post-MI patients has not been quantified, **an abnormal systolic BP response to exercise is associated with subsequent cardiac events** in this population.

3. **Adaptation to training**

–In persons who participate in long-term exercise training, **systolic and diastolic BP are lower at rest and at submaximal exercise intensities, and maximal BP remains unchanged.** This is because of reductions in resting and submaximal heart rate and reductions in total peripheral resistance, and because of the effects of exercise on body composition.

–At any fixed submaximal workload, conditioned persons exhibit comparable or lower systolic BP than unconditioned persons.

–Relative to $\dot{V}O_{2max}$, systolic BP is lower in conditioned persons than in unconditioned persons.

I.   MINUTE VENTILATION ($\dot{V}_E$)

–Also called **pulmonary ventilation,** $\dot{V}_E$ is calculated as:

tidal volume × breathing frequency

–**Normal resting** $\dot{V}_E$ is 6 L/min.

–**Normal maximal** $\dot{V}_E$ is a 15- to 25-fold increase over the resting value.

1. **Normal exercise response**

–During mild to moderate exercise, $\dot{V}_E$ is increased, primarily through increased tidal volume. During vigorous exercise, respiratory rate is also increased.

–The increase in $\dot{V}_E$ is directly proportional to $\dot{V}O_2$ and $\dot{V}CO_2$ increases during low-intensity exercise.

–At the anaerobic threshold (usually 47%–64% of $\dot{V}O_{2max}$ in most persons, 70%–90% of $\dot{V}O_{2max}$ in highly conditioned persons), $\dot{V}_E$ increases disproportionately, paralleling the abrupt rise in serum lactate concentrations.

2. **Adaptation to training**

–In response to cardiorespiratory training, **maximal** $\dot{V}_E$ **increases.**

–**Submaximal** $\dot{V}_E$ **commonly is not affected** but may be decreased in some clients due to decreased lactate production.

J.   TIDAL VOLUME

–is the volume of air entering the lungs with each breath.

–**Normal resting tidal volume** is 0.5 L/breath.

–**Maximal tidal volume** (or **vital capacity**) is 4 L/breath.

K.   RESPIRATORY RATE

–is the number of breaths per minute.

–**Normal resting respiratory rate** is 12 breaths/min.

–**Normal maximal respiratory rate** is 48 breaths/min.

–Breathing frequency is increased at maximal exercise with training.

L.   RESPIRATORY PATTERN

–Light exercise is generally associated with increased tidal volume and respiratory rate.

–Tidal volume and respiratory rate both increase until 70%–80% of peak exercise, after which increased respiratory rate is the primary response.

–Tidal volume frequently plateaus at 50%–60% of vital capacity.

–Respiratory rate increases 1- to 3-fold in most subjects, 6- to 7-fold in conditioned athletes.

M.   ANAEROBIC THRESHOLD

–is the point at which CO_2 production exceeds O_2 consumption ($\dot{V}CO_2/\dot{V}O_2 > 1.15$) and metabolic acidosis or anaerobic metabolism begins **(Figure 2-3)**

–can be determined through serial measurements of blood lactate or by assessment of expired gases, specifically pulmonary ventilation and CO_2 production.

1. **Healthy unconditioned persons** have an anaerobic threshold of approximately 55% of $\dot{V}O_{2max.}$

2. **Adaptation to training**

–The percentage of $\dot{V}O_{2max}$ at which the anaerobic threshold occurs increases with training. Conditioned persons can have an anaerobic threshold as high as 70%–90% of $\dot{V}O_{2max.}$

–Endurance training improves oxidative capacity of skeletal muscle by increasing the number and size of mitochondria, myoglobin content, oxidative enzyme levels, and capillary density.

–Conditioned persons have lower blood lactate levels than unconditioned persons at any fixed workload.

–At $\dot{V}O_{2max,}$ blood lactate levels are higher in conditioned persons than in unconditioned persons.

III. PHYSIOLOGICAL EFFECTS OF EXERCISE, POSTURE, AND DETRAINING

A. MODES OF EXERCISE TESTING

1. Treadmill exercise testing

–is weight-bearing.

–allows both running and walking.

–is more expensive, noisier, and less mobile than other modalities.

–$\dot{V}O_{2max}$ is 10%-20% higher and maximal heart rate is 5%-20% higher on a treadmill than on a cycle ergometer.

2. Cycle exercise testing

–is non–weight-bearing.

–permits accurate measurement of the work performed by assessing the resistance against the flywheel multiplied by the distance traveled.

–Decreased upper body motion allows easier BP assessment and ECG monitoring than with arm ergometry.

3. Arm exercise testing

–is non–weight-bearing.

–is useful for those participants unable to use their legs for treadmill or cycle ergometry.

–Typically, a lower functional capacity is achieved than with leg ergometry.

4. Stepping

–is weight-bearing.

–can be used as a field test to estimate cardiorespiratory fitness.

–is not practical for graded exercise testing.

B. DYNAMIC VERSUS STATIC EXERCISE

1. Dynamic (isotonic) exercise

–involves rhythmic, repetitive motion of large muscle groups.

–places a volume load on the myocardium, producing the training effect.

–Increased oxygen consumption, heart rate, and systolic BP parallel the intensity of the activity.

–Blood is shunted from viscera to working skeletal muscle, where oxygen extraction increases a-vO_2 difference.

2. Static (isometric) exercise

–involves sustained muscle contraction against a fixed load or resistance, with no change in the length of the involved muscle group or joint motion.

–places a significant pressure load on the heart, increasing $\dot{V}O_{2max}$ and elevating systolic BP.

–During muscle contractions greater than 20% of maximal voluntary contraction (MVC), heart rate and systolic BP increase. Stroke volume remains unchanged until > 50% MVC, where it may decrease.

–Usual signs of overexertion, such as tachycardia, sweating and dyspnea, are masked by low aerobic requirements.

–In clients with normal or near-normal aerobic fitness levels and left ventricular function, isometric exercise rarely produces angina, ST segment depression, or arrhythmias.

–Because it is difficult to avoid static effort in daily activities, a client's physiological responses (BP, heart rate, ECG) to static exercise should be evaluated to determine the safety of participation in various activities.

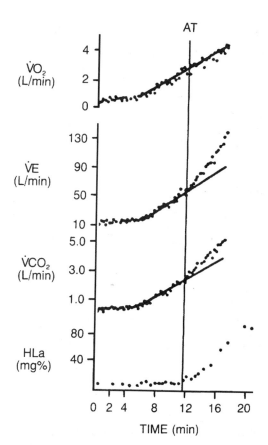

FIGURE 2-3 Relationship between intensity of exercise (oxygen consumption, $\dot{V}O_2$) and simultaneous abrupt nonlinear increases in serum lactate (HLa), CO_2 production ($\dot{V}CO_2$), and pulmonary ventilation ($\dot{V}_E$), occurring at the anaerobic threshold (AT). Exercise was instituted at minute 4. (Adapted from Davis JA, Vodak P, Wilmore JH et al: Anaerobic threshold and maximal aerobic power for three modes of exercise. *J Appl Physiol* 41:544–550, 1976.)

C. ARM EXERCISE VERSUS LEG EXERCISE

–At a given workload, arm exercise results in higher $\dot{V}_E$, $\dot{V}O_2$, respiratory exchange ratio, and blood lactate concentration and lower stroke volume and anaerobic threshold than leg exercise.

–At equivalent workloads, systolic BP is higher with arm exercise than with leg exercise, reflecting greater peripheral resistance.

–Because the arms have less mass than the legs, $\dot{V}O_{2max}$ during arm exercise is only 64%–80% of the $\dot{V}O_{2max}$ during leg exercise.

–A client's prescribed target heart rate for leg training should be reduced by approximately 10 beats/min for arm training.

–Arm and leg exercise can achieve similar cardiovascular adaptations to exercise.

D. SPECIFICITY

–The concept of **specificity** has implications for persons with orthopedic limitations.

–Little or no **crossover benefit** is achieved from arm to leg training or vice versa.

–Endurance training with one limb or set of limbs leads to increased $\dot{V}O_{2max}$ and anaerobic threshold and decreased heart rate, pulmonary ventilation, ventilatory equivalent, BP, and perceived exertion during submaximal training in conditioned limbs.

–Most physiological training effects can be attributed to extracardiac or peripheral factors, such as altered blood flow and cellular and enzymatic adaptations in the conditioned limb alone. There is, however, some evidence of increased $\dot{V}O_{2max}$ or reduced submaximal heart rate in the unconditioned limbs of both normal and cardiac clients, suggesting some central circulatory adaptations to endurance training.

–Initial fitness level, along with the intensity, frequency, and duration of activity, are important factors in predicting the effects of conditioning on untrained limbs.

E. ELECTROPHYSIOLOGY

–The myocardium responds to the electrical stimulus generated by the heart's **action potential.**

–Positive charges crossing myocardial cell membranes cause **depolarization** (Figure 2-4;

Table 2-4). Depolarization occurs during phase 0 of the action potential and generates the QRS complex on the ECG.

–The difference between the positive and negative charges, the **transmembrane potential,** normally ranges from –80 to –90 mV.

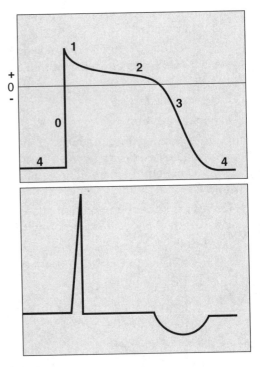

FIGURE 2-4 Changes in membrane potential over time. (From *ACSM's Resource Manual for Guidelines for Exercise Testing and Prescription,* 3rd ed. Baltimore, Williams & Wilkins, 1998, p 398.)

Table 2-4. Normal Sequence of Depolarization and the ECG Correlation

Sinoatrial node	Silent
Atrial depolarization	P wave
Atrioventricular node	PR interval
His bundle	PR interval
Purkinje fibers	PR interval
Ventricular muscle depolarization	QRS complex
Ventricular isoelectric period	ST segment
Ventricular muscle repolarization	T wave

(From *ACSM's Resource Manual for Guidelines for Exercise Testing and Prescription,* 3rd ed. Baltimore, Williams & Wilkins, 1998, p 404.)

–**Repolarization** (restoration of the transmembrane potential) occurs during phases 2 and 3 of the action potential. On the ECG, repolarization is represented by the ST segment and the T wave.

F. WARM-UP AND COOL-DOWN

1. **Warm-up exercises** redistribute blood flow from the trunk to peripheral areas, decrease resistance in tissues to enhance movement, and increase tissue temperature and energy production.

    –Between 5 and 10 minutes of warm-up at a heart rate moderately higher than resting level will prepare the body for increasing demands during the conditioning phase.

2. **Cool-down** allows the heart rate and blood pressure to return to resting levels, redistributes blood flow, and gradually allows for adequate venous return while heart rate decreases.

G. POSTURE during exercise affects venous return and preload, particularly during brief bouts of physical activity.

1. **EDV** (see II B) is highest with the body recumbent and decreases progressively as position shifts from sitting and then to standing.

    a. During **exercise in the supine position,** EDV remains largely unchanged.

    b. During **exercise while upright,** EDV increases at an exercise intensity $< 50\%$ $\dot{V}O_{2max}$; at higher intensities, EDV and stroke volume may decrease.

2. **Prolonged upright exercise** at a constant work rate places an increased load on the heart, resulting in a progressive decrease in venous return and increase in heart rate.

    –For this reason, exercising on a recumbent cycle ergometer may be most appropriate for certain persons with cardiovascular disease.

H. EFFECTS OF DECONDITIONING

1. **Long periods of inactivity are associated with reversal of many adaptations of conditioning** (Table 2-5; Figure 2-5).

    a. $\dot{V}O_{2max}$ **declines** rapidly during the first month of inactivity, with a slower rate of decline in subsequent months.

b. Deconditioning also results in **decreased heart mass, stroke volume, blood volume, and bone mass.**

c. **Maximal and submaximal heart rates increase** markedly.

Table 2-5. **Responses of Highly Trained Individuals After 3 Months of Detraining Compared to Sedentary Controls**

	Sedentary Control	% of Sedentary Controls	
		Trained	Detrained 3 Months
$\dot{V}O_2$max (ml/kg/min)	43.3	143%*	117%†
Stroke volume (ml)	128	120%*	101%†
a-vO_2 diff at max (ml/100 ml)	12.6	122%	116%†
Citrate synthase activity (mol/kg/hr)			
Whole muscle of both fiber types	4.1	243%*	149%*†
Type I fibers	4.8	140%*	108%†
Type II fibers	2.6	246%*	180%†
Capillary density (cap/mm²)	318	146%*	150%*

Trained responses are expressed as a percentage of sedentary control values. * Higher (p < 0.05) than sedentary control. † Detrained lower than trained: p < 0.05. (Data from Coyle EF, et al. Time course of loss adaptations after stopping prolonged intense endurance training. *J Appl Physiol* 57:1857-1864, 1984; Coyle EF, Martin WH, Bloomfield SA, et al. Effects of detraining on responses to submaximal exercise. *J Appl Physiol* 59:853-859, 1985; Costill DL, et al. Metabolic characteristics of skeletal muscle during detraining from competitive swimming. *Med Sci Sports Exerc* 17:339-343, 1985.)

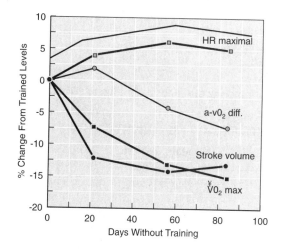

FIGURE 2-5 Effects of detraining on percent change in stroke volume during exercise, $\dot{V}O_{2max}$, maximal heart rate (HR), and maximal a-vO_2 difference. (Modified from Coyle EF et al: Time course of loss adaptations after stopping prolonged intense endurance training. *J Appl Physiol* 57:1857–1864, 1984.)

2. Deconditioning produces more marked effects than **reduced conditioning,** which may maintain cardiovascular and metabolic adaptations more effectively.

3. **Rapid reconditioning after deconditioning** appears to return muscle strength and size to the previously conditioned state.

4. **Guidelines** for working with severely deconditioned clients are presented in **Table 2-6.**

 Table 2-6. Guidelines for Exercise Professionals Working with Severely Detrained or Bed-Rested Individuals

Emphasize strength training of back and lower limb postural muscle groups
Back extensors
Quadriceps and associated hip extensors
Ankle extensors (soleus and gastrocnemius)
Use gradual, progressive, overload starting at appropriately low intensities
Incorporate training for postural stability and dynamic balance during walking, particularly if the client is elderly
Be aware of increased risk of bone fracture even after muscle strength is normalized, especially in osteopenic-prone individuals (estrogen-deficient women, elderly)

(From *ACSM's Resource Manual for Guidelines for Exercise Testing and Prescription,* 3rd ed. Baltimore, Williams & Wilkins, 1998, p 198.)

IV. CLINICAL APPLICATIONS OF EXERCISE

A. FACTORS TO CONSIDER WHEN DESIGNING AN EXERCISE PROGRAM

1. Activity restrictions
2. Primary and secondary medical diagnoses
3. Medications

   –Some medications (e.g., **beta antagonists** and **calcium antagonists**) reduce the heart rate response to exercise. Clients taking these medications often exhibit blunted exercise heart rates, achieving only 50%-60% of expected maximal levels.

   –In some clients, however, maximal functional capacity may be reduced from the decreased maximal heart rate caused by certain medications.

4. Physical conditioning
5. Orthopedic concerns
6. Exercise and activity preferences/personal goals

B. CLIENTS WITH HEART DISEASE

–Clients with heart disease typically have certain **limitations affecting their ability to exercise,** including reduced oxygen transport capacity and reduced contractile force of the left ventricle and resulting decreased ejection fraction.

–**Table 2-7** compares typical circulatory data in a person with heart disease and a healthy person.

–**Figure 2-6** shows the sequence of events that may lead to angina, ischemia, or arrhythmias as a result of intense exercise by a client with heart disease.

1. **Limits on exercise**

   –should be set based on the presence of any of the following key signs and symptoms:

   a. Onset of angina or other symptoms of cardiovascular insufficiency

   b. Plateau or decrease in systolic BP, systolic BP > 240 mm Hg, or diastolic BP > 110 mm Hg

   c. ST segment depression > 1 mm, horizontal or downsloping

   d. Radionuclide evidence of left ventricular dysfunction or onset of moderate to severe wall motion abnormalities during exertion

   e. Increased frequency of ventricular arrhythmias

   f. Other significant ECG disturbances (e.g., second- or third-degree heart block, atrial fibrillation, supraventricular tachycardia, complex ventricular ectopy)

   g. Other signs and symptoms of exercise intolerance, such as exertional hypotension, angina pectoris, myocardial ischemia, or electrical instability

2. **Clinical objectives of inpatient cardiac rehabilitation**

   a. To offset the deleterious psychological and physiological effects of bed rest

   b. To provide additional medical surveillance

   c. To identify any specific cardiovascular, physical, or cognitive impairments that may influence safety

   d. To enable the patient to return to activities of daily living within the limits imposed by the disease

Table 2-7. Hypothetical Circulatory Data at Rest and during Maximal Exercise for a Sedentary Man and a Patient with Heart Disease

Condition	Oxygen Consumption (l/min)	Oxygen Consumption (ml/kg/min)	Cardiac Output (l/min)	Heart Rate (beats/min)	Stroke Volume (ml/beat)	a-vO$_2$ Difference (ml/dl blood)
Sedentary man (70 kg)						
Rest	0.25	3.5[a]	6.1	70	87	4.0
Maximal exercise	2.50	35.0	17.7	190	93	14.0
Cardiac patient (70 kg)						
Rest	0.25	3.5[a]	6.1	82	74	4.0
Maximal exercise	1.50	21.5	10.4	165	66	13.6

[a] 3.5 ml/kg/min = 1 metabolic equivalent (MET); average resting metabolic rate expressed per unit body weight.
(From *ACSM's Resource Manual for Guidelines for Exercise Testing and Prescription,* 3rd ed. Baltimore, Williams & Wilkins, 1998, p 152.)

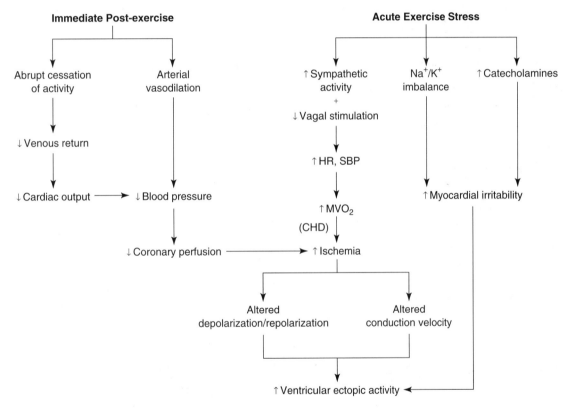

FIGURE 2-6 Physiologic alterations accompanying acute exercise and recovery, and their possible sequelae. (From *ACSM's Resource Manual for Guidelines for Exercise Testing and Prescription,* 3rd ed. Baltimore, Williams & Wilkins, 1998, p 152.)

e. To prepare the patient and the support system at home to optimize recovery following hospital discharge

3. **Clinical objectives of outpatient cardiac rehabilitation**

    a. To provide appropriate supervision to ensure detection of problems and potential complications, and to provide timely feedback to the referring physician to enhance effective medical management

b. Contingent on clinical status, to return the patient to premorbid vocational and/or recreational activities, to modify these activities as necessary, or to find alternative activities

c. To develop and help the patient implement a safe and effective home exercise program and recreational lifestyle

d. To provide patient and family education to maximize secondary prevention through increased anginal threshold, improved cardiorespiratory function, and risk factor modification

C.   CLIENTS WITH PULMONARY DISEASE

–Clients with a **ventilatory limitation on exercise** become fatigued when the limits of breathing reserve are reached.

1. **Limitations on exercise**
   a. Reduced maximal ventilatory volume (MVV) due to obstructed air flow
   b. Diminished lung volumes
   c. Increased physiologic dead space, necessitating a higher minute ventilation at peak exercise to maintain gas exchange
   d. Arterial oxygen desaturation

2. **Risks of exercise participation**
   a. Oxygen desaturation
   b. Hyperventilation

3. **Objectives of exercise training**
   a. Increased functional capacity
   b. Increased functional status
   c. Reduced severity of dyspnea
   d. Improved quality of life

D.   OBESE CLIENTS

1. **Limitations on exercise**
   a. Orthopedic problems
   b. Heat intolerance
   c. Dyspnea
   d. Movement restrictions
   e. Anxiety

2. **Risks of exercise participation**
   a. Elevated cardiac output, oxygen consumption, minute ventilation, BP, and heart rate
   b. Increased risk of heart disease and diabetes
   c. Increased risk of orthopedic injury

3. **Objectives of exercise training**
   a. Reduce body fat
   b. Increase lean body mass
   c. Increase metabolic rate

E.   CLIENTS WITH DIABETES MELLITUS

1. **Limitations on exercise**
   a. Autonomic and peripheral neuropathies
   b. Reduced functional capacity

   c. Increased progression of atherosclerosis
   d. Obesity

2. **Risks of exercise participation** include hypoglycemic reaction.

3. **Objectives of exercise training** include improved blood glucose control.

F.   CLIENTS WITH PERIPHERAL VASCULAR DISEASE

1. **Limitations on exercise**
   a. Claudication
   b. Fatigue

2. **Risks of exercise participation**
   a. Coronary artery disease
   b. Leg pain

3. **Objectives of exercise training** include reduced severity of intermittent claudication.

G.   CLIENTS WITH CONGESTIVE HEART FAILURE

1. **Limitations on exercise**

   –result from the inability to eject a sufficient stroke volume during ventricular systole. Clients are diagnosed with either systolic dysfunction or diastolic dysfunction.
   a. **Systolic dysfunction** is due to poor left ventricular contractile function (ejection fraction < 50%).
   b. **In diastolic dysfunction,** the ventricle does not fill at a normal diastolic pressure, resulting in inadequate left ventricular volume, slow filling, or elevated ventricular diastolic pressure.

2. **Risks of exercise participation**
   a. Reduced exercise capacity
   b. Fatigue and weakness
   c. Dyspnea, especially with exertion
   d. Orthopnea and/or paroxysmal nocturnal dyspnea

3. **Objectives of exercise training**
   a. Increased functional capacity due to increased a-vO_2 difference
   b. Improved quality of life
   c. Decreased resting heart rate
   d. Decreased leg vascular resistance and increased leg blood flow

H.   CLIENTS WITH HYPERTENSION

1. **Limitations on exercise** include an excessive rise in BP.

2. **Risks of exercise participation**
   a. ST segment abnormalities caused by use of diuretics and resulting hypokalemia
   b. Left ventricular hypertrophy
   c. Valsalva's maneuver, causing a spike in systolic BP

3. **Objectives of exercise training**
   a. Reduced resting systolic and diastolic BP
   b. Reduced systolic BP at submaximal workloads

I. **CLIENTS WITH HYPERLIPIDEMIA**

1. **Limitations on exercise**
   a. Underlying atherosclerosis
   b. Underlying obesity, diabetes, or insulin resistance

2. **Objectives of exercise training**
   a. Reduced triglyceride levels
   b. Reduced postprandial lipemia
   c. Decreased low-density lipoprotein (LDL) cholesterol level
   d. Increased high-density lipoprotein (HDL) cholesterol level

REVIEW TEST

DIRECTIONS: Carefully read all questions and select the BEST single answer.

1. Myocardial oxygen consumption is best estimated from
   (A) maximal oxygen consumption.
   (B) rate–pressure product.
   (C) cardiac output.
   (D) heart rate.

2. During mild to moderate exercise, pulmonary ventilation increases primarily as a result of increased
   (A) tidal volume.
   (B) breathing frequency.
   (C) vital capacity.
   (D) total lung volume.

3. The anaerobic threshold occurs at the onset of
   (A) oxidative phosphorylation.
   (B) maximal oxygen consumption.
   (C) metabolic acidosis.
   (D) aerobic metabolism.

4. Which of the following statements about static exercise is accurate?
   (A) It results in reduced pressure on the heart.
   (B) It is inappropriate for any client with heart disease.
   (C) It involves rhythmic, continuous activity.
   (D) It results in increased heart rate and systolic blood pressure.

5. Which of the following statements regarding arm versus leg exercise is correct?
   (A) Target heart rate should not be used as a guide for arm exercise.
   (B) Target heart rate for leg exercise should be decreased by 10 beats/min.
   (C) Target heart rate for leg exercise should be increased by 10 beats/min.
   (D) Higher maximal oxygen consumption should be expected in arm exercise.

6. End-diastolic volume is highest when measured with the client in which position?
   (A) Recumbent
   (B) Sitting
   (C) Standing
   (D) Supine

7. Repolarization is represented by the
   (A) QRS complex.
   (B) T wave.
   (C) P wave.
   (D) delta wave.

8. Which of the following are byproducts of aerobic metabolism?
   (A) Carbon dioxide and water
   (B) Oxygen and water
   (C) Adenosine triphosphate and oxygen
   (D) Hydrogen and oxygen

9. Cardiac output is a function of
   (A) heart rate, preload, afterload, and contractility.
   (B) heart rate and systolic blood pressure.
   (C) stroke volume and end-diastolic volume.
   (D) maximal oxygen consumption and arteriovenous oxygenation difference.

10. The prescribed exercise regimen for an obese client typically includes
    (A) high-intensity movements.
    (B) low-impact aerobic activity.
    (C) ballistic exercise.
    (D) high-intensity strength training.

11. Which of the following describes a normal postexercise blood pressure (BP) response?
    (A) Elevated systolic and diastolic values compared to pre-participation values
    (B) Progressive decline in systolic BP
    (C) Progressive increase in systolic BP
    (D) Exaggerated decrease in diastolic BP

12. Clinical objectives of outpatient cardiac rehabilitation include
    (A) modifying risk factors.
    (B) lowering the anginal threshold.
    (C) reducing high-density lipoprotein cholesterol.
    (D) minimizing secondary prevention.

13. Stroke volume is defined as
    (A) the product of cardiac output and total peripheral resistance.
    (B) the difference between end-diastolic volume and end-systolic volume.
    (C) the product of preload and heart rate.
    (D) the product of cardiac output and arterial-venous oxygen difference.

14. Which of the following precautions is indicated for individuals diagnosed with hypertension?
    (A) Never undergo a stress test.
    (B) Stop all antihypertensive medications while exercising.
    (C) Engage in heavy resistance training.
    (D) Engage in low-intensity exercise.

15. Which of the following instructions is appropriate for a client with diabetes?
    (A) Inject insulin into the active muscle.
    (B) Increase the insulin dose before exercising.
    (C) Eat carbohydrate snacks before a long exercise session.
    (D) Exercise during the peak of insulin activity.

16. Which of the following physical limitations is most common in clients with peripheral vascular disease?
    (A) Localized muscular fatigue
    (B) Low cardiac output
    (C) Chronotropic insufficiency
    (D) Exaggerated heart rate in response to exercise

17. Persons with hypertension are at risk for which of the following during exercise?
    (A) Chronotropic intolerance
    (B) Exaggerated systolic blood pressure (BP) elevation
    (C) Significant diastolic BP decrease
    (D) Peripheral neuropathy

18. For a client with chronic obstructive pulmonary disease (COPD), the main risk during exercise is
    (A) oxygen desaturation.
    (B) atrial fibrillation.
    (C) hypoglycemia.
    (D) angina pectoris.

19. As a result of exercise training, cardiac output becomes
    (A) higher at any given workload.
    (B) lower at any given workload.
    (C) essentially unchanged at any given workload.
    (D) diminished due to reduced stroke volume.

20. During exercise, stroke volume increases as a result of
    (A) the Frank-Starling mechanism.
    (B) increased heart rate.
    (C) increased ejection fraction.
    (D) increased pulmonary artery pressure.

ANSWERS AND EXPLANATIONS

1–B. Determinants of myocardial oxygen consumption ($M\dot{V}O_2$) include heart rate, myocardial contractility, and the tension or stress in the ventricular wall. Ventricular wall tension reflects a combination of systolic blood pressure (BP) and ventricular volume and is inversely related to myocardial wall thickness. During exercise, heart rate is the major contributor to myocardial oxygen demand, and oxygen supply is facilitated by increased coronary blood flow, which is enabled by decreased vascular resistance. Investigators have reported an excellent correlation between measured $M\dot{V}O_2$ and the rate–pressure product (heart rate x systolic BP). Heart rate alone has limited ability to assess $M\dot{V}O_2$, especially when systolic BP is elevated.

2–A. Pulmonary ventilation ($\dot{V}_E$), the volume of air exchanged per minute, generally approximates 6 L/min at rest in the average sedentary adult male. At maximal exercise, however, $\dot{V}_E$ often increases 15- to 25-fold over resting values. $\dot{V}_E$ is a function of tidal volume and respiratory rate. During mild to moderate exercise, $\dot{V}_E$ increases, due primarily to increasing tidal volume, whereas increases in respiratory rate are more important to augment $\dot{V}_E$ during vigorous exercise.

3–C. The anaerobic threshold represents the onset of metabolic acidosis. Anaerobic threshold can be determined by serial measurements of blood lactate or can be noninvasively assessed by expired gases during exercise testing, specifically pulmonary ventilation and carbon dioxide (CO_2). Anaerobic threshold indicates the peak work rate or oxygen consumption at which the body's energy demands can be met by aerobic metabolism. Metabolic acidosis can be attributed to the buffering of lactate by sodium bicarbonate so that CO_2 is released in excess of muscle metabolism, providing an additional stimulus for ventilation. Accordingly, values for V_E and CO_2 increase out of proportion to the exercise performed.

4–D. During static (or isometric) exercise, heart rate increases in relation to the tension exerted, and an abrupt and precipitous increase in systolic blood pressure (BP) occurs. The increased heart rate and systolic BP (rate–pressure product) results in increased myocardial oxygen demand. Static exercise involves sustained muscle contraction against a fixed load or resistance with no change in the length or the involved muscle group or joint motion. Because static exertion is present in normal activities, it is not contraindicated in all cardiac clients, but it must be performed in a safe and controlled setting.

5–B. Maximal oxygen consumption during arm exercise in men and women is 64%–80% of that during leg exercise. Similarly, maximal cardiac output is lower during arm exercise than during leg exercise, whereas maximal heart rate, systolic blood pressure, and rate–pressure product are comparable or slightly lower during arm exercise. The latter have relevance to arm exercise training recommendations, particularly training intensity. Accordingly, an arm exercise prescription that assumes a maximal heart rate equivalent to leg exercise testing may result in overestimation of the training heart rate. As a general guideline, the prescribed heart rate for leg training should be reduced by approximately 10 beats/min for arm training.

6–A. End-diastolic volume (EDV) depends on heart rate, filling pressure, and ventricular compliance. Posture affects venous return and preload, particularly during brief bouts of physical exertion. At rest, EDV is highest in the recumbent position, and decreases progressively with movement to sitting and then to standing.

7–B. The electrical activity recorded during atrial depolarization is termed the P wave. Depolarization of the myocardial cells of the ventricles generates the QRS complex. The T wave represents repolarization of the ventricles.

8–A. Aerobic production of adenosine triphosphate (ATP) combines two complex metabolic processes: the Krebs cycle and the electron transport chain. During the Krebs cycle, hydrogen is produced and carbon dioxide (CO_2) is removed. Oxidative phosphorylation uses oxygen as the final hydrogen acceptor to form CO_2 and water. The final products of cellular respiration, as measured by direct calorimetry, are heat, CO_2, and water.

9–A. The product of heart rate and stroke volume determines cardiac output. Stroke volume is equal to the difference between end-diastolic volume (EDV) and end-systolic volume (ESV). EDV is determined by heart rate, filling pressure, and ventricular compliance (preload). ESV is determined by contractility and afterload.

10–B. Low-impact aerobic exercise reduces the risk of orthopedic injury while expending calories. High-intensity movements, ballistic exercise, and high-intensity strength training all increase the risk of injury in an obese client.

11–B. During graded exercise, systolic blood pressure (BP) increases with increased workload, resulting from increased cardiac output. On completion of exercise, systolic BP declines gradually, due to decreasing demand by skeletal tissue for increased cardiac output and oxygen delivery.

12–A. A major objective of outpatient cardiac rehabilitation programs is to help clients reduce modifiable risk factors associated with future cardiovascular complications. Applicable

strategies may include stress management, smoking cessation, and dietary modification.

13–B. Stroke volume is the amount of blood ejected from the left ventricle during cardiac systole. This volume is a fraction of the end-diastolic volume (the amount of blood originally in the left ventricle just before ventricular systole). The remaining blood not ejected by the left ventricle is the end-systolic volume.

14–D. Hypertensive clients may undergo stress testing as long as blood pressure (BP) is well controlled. Antihypertensive medications should be taken as prescribed to avoid a hypertensive response to exercise. Also, because many antihypertensive medications affect the heart's response to exercise, not taking prescribed medication may result in an inappropriate target heart rate. Heavy resistance training may exacerbate hypertension. Low- to moderate-intensity exercise reduces the risk of a hypertensive response to exercise and appears to lower BP to the same or a greater extent than higher-intensity exercise.

15–C. Carbohydrate and caloric intake should be increased before a long exercise session, commonly by eating a high-carbohydrate snack. Insulin should never be injected directly into active exercising muscles. Insulin dosage may be decreased before exercise; it should never be increased. Exercising during the peak of insulin activity is not recommended.

16–A. Persons with peripheral vascular disease experience local muscle fatigue due to reduced blood flow to active muscle tissue. This is a direct consequence of the buildup of atherosclerotic plaque in peripheral arteries. Low cardiac output, chronotropic insufficiency, and exaggerated heart rate in response to exercise may occur in clients with peripheral vascular disease but are not as common as localized muscle fatigue.

17–B. Although elevated systolic blood pressure (BP) with exercise is expected, this elevation is typically exaggerated in persons with hypertension. Thus, it is important to routinely evaluate the exercise BP response in this client population to ensure that BP does not exceed safe limits. Chronotropic intolerance and decreased diastolic BP are more common in clients with hypotension. Peripheral neuropathy is a complication of diabetes mellitus.

18–A. Oxygen desaturation during exercise is a sign of exercise-induced hypoxia and is the primary risk of exercise in clients with chronic obstructive pulmonary disease (COPD), as it can lead to metabolic acidosis. Atrial fibrillation, hypoglycemia, and angina pectoris may occur in some clients during exercise but are unrelated to COPD.

19–C. The product of heart rate and stroke volume determines cardiac output. Cardiac output in healthy adults increases linearly with increased work rate, from a resting value of approximately 5 L to a maximum of 20 L during upright exercise. At exercise intensities of up to 50% of maximal oxygen consumption, the increase in cardiac output is facilitated by increases in heart rate and stroke volume. At higher intensities, the increase in cardiac output results almost solely

from a continued increase in heart rate. Cardiac output remains essentially unchanged at any given workload.

20-A. In healthy adults, stroke volume at rest in the upright position generally varies between 60 and 100 ml/beat, with a maximum stroke volume of 100 to 200 ml/beat. During exercise, stroke volume increases curvilinearly with the work rate until it reaches near maximum at a level equivalent to approximately 50% of aerobic capacity, increasing only slightly thereafter. Within physiological limits, enhanced venous return increases end-diastolic volume, stretching cardiac muscle fibers and increasing the force of contraction (Frank-Starling mechanism).

CHAPTER 3

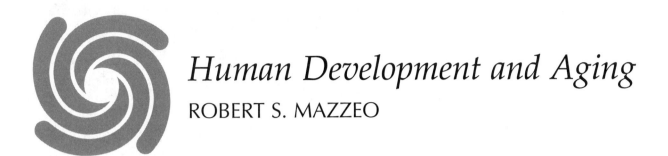

Human Development and Aging
ROBERT S. MAZZEO

I. OVERVIEW OF HUMAN GROWTH AND DEVELOPMENT

A. AGE GROUPS, as typically defined, are as follows:

  1. **Neonatal:** birth–3 weeks

  2. **Infancy:** 3 weeks–1 year

  3. **Early childhood:** 1–6 years

  4. **Middle childhood:** 7–10 years

  5. **Late childhood/prepuberty:** girls, 9–15 years; boys, 12–16 years

  6. **Adolescence:** the 6 years following puberty

  7. **Adulthood**

    –**Early adulthood:** 20–29 years

    –**Middle adulthood:** 30–44 years

    –**Later adulthood:** 45–64 years

  8. **Older adulthood**

    –**Old:** 65–74 years

    –**Older:** 75–84 years

    –**Very old/frail:** 85 years and older

B. SIGNIFICANT VARIABILITY exists in growth and development for a given chronological age group.

C. AGING IS A COMPLEX PROCESS involving the interaction of many factors, including genetics, lifestyle, and disease **(Figure 3-1).**

D. AN AGING POPULATION

  –The number or people in the United States over age 65 will reach 70 million by the year 2030, with those over age 85 the fastest-growing population segment **(Figure 3-2).**

E. AGE AND EXERCISE

  –A client's age must be taken into consideration when designing an exercise program. **Children, adolescents, and older adults have special physiological and behavioral characteristics** that must be considered in program design to ensure safety and effectiveness. A medical history and proper screening are recommended.

  –**Both aerobic and resistance training are recommended for older adults** to improve health, functional capacity, and overall quality of life.

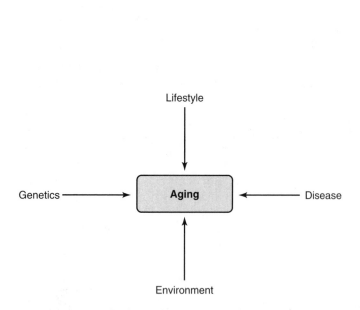

FIGURE 3-1 Factors that influence how we age. While genetics plays an important role, other factors, such as lifestyle (e.g., exercise patterns, diet, stress), environment, and disease states, also contribute to the aging process.

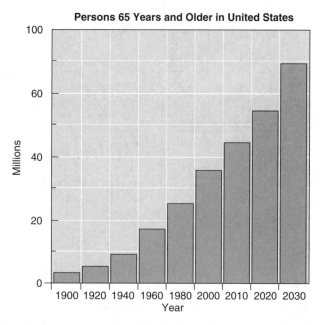

FIGURE 3-2 Estimation of the number of individuals who will be 65 years and older by the year 2000 and beyond. Note the exponential growth rate in this age group, making them the fastest-growing U.S. population segment.

II. AGE-RELATED PHYSIOLOGICAL CHANGES

A. CARDIOPULMONARY FUNCTION

1. **Changes in cardiac function**

   a. **Left ventricular hypertrophy** increases with aging, apparently related to increased afterload associated with increased peripheral resistance.

   b. **Decreased arterial compliance and increased arterial stiffness** with age can result in **elevated systolic and diastolic blood pressures** both at rest and during exercise.

   c. **Early left ventricular diastolic function** at rest and during exercise **decreases with age.**

2. **Changes in heart rate, stroke volume, and cardiac output**

   a. **Heart rate is higher in children** both at rest and during exercise, most likely as compensation for a lower stroke volume.

   b. Resting stroke volume and resting heart rate remain relatively unchanged with age.

   c. Decreases in both maximal heart rate (decline of 6–10 beats per decade) and maximal stroke volume cause a **significant decline in maximal cardiac output with age.**

3. **Changes in maximal oxygen uptake ($\dot{V}O_{2max}$)**

   $\dot{V}O_{2max}$ is a function of maximal cardiac output × maximal arterial-venous oxygen ($a–vO_2$) difference.

   $\dot{V}O_{2max}$ **remains relatively unchanged throughout childhood and adolescence.**

   $\dot{V}O_{2max}$ **typically declines by 5%–15% per decade after age 25,** related to decreases in both maximal cardiac output and maximal $a–vO_2$ difference. An individual's rate of decline can be slowed by regular physical activity (**Figure 3-3**).

4. **Changes in pulmonary function**

   a. **Residual volume increases** and **vital capacity decreases** with aging.

   b. **Lung compliance increases** with aging, as the lungs lose elastin fibers and elastic recoil.

   c. Aging brings a **20% increase in the work of respiratory muscles** but a **decrease in the strength** of these muscles.

5. **Application to exercise training in older adults**

   a. Reduced cardiopulmonary function with aging does not necessarily limit exercise performance in older adults, even though this population is prone to exercise-induced expiratory flow limitation.

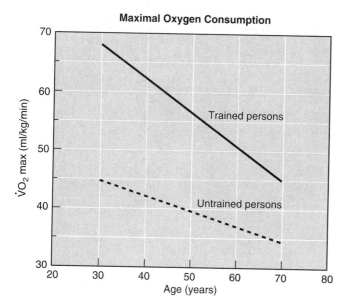

FIGURE 3-3 Changes in maximal oxygen consumption ($\dot{V}O_{2max}$) as a function of age in both conditioned and unconditioned individuals.

b. Regular aerobic training produces similar increases in $\dot{V}O_{2max}$ in younger adults and older adults (10%–30%).

  (1) In men, this increased $\dot{V}O_{2max}$ comes from improved central cardiovascular adaptations (e.g., increased cardiac output) and increased a–vO$_2$ difference.

  (2) In older women, the increased $\dot{V}O_{2max}$ appears to be solely the result of increased a–vO$_2$ difference.

B. MUSCULOSKELETAL FUNCTION

1. **Changes in muscle mass**

   a. An individual's **total number of muscle fibers** becomes fixed before adolescence.

   b. At **adolescence,** males exhibit more rapid muscle growth (**hypertrophy**) than females.

   c. A decline in muscle mass (**atrophy**) occurs with advancing age, due to a progressive decrease in the number and size of muscle fibers (**Figure 3-4**). This directly contributes to an **age-related decline in muscle strength.**

2. **Changes in muscle strength**

   a. **Muscle strength typically peaks in the mid-twenties** for both sexes and remains fairly stable through the mid-forties.

   b. **Muscle strength declines** approximately 15% per decade in the sixth and seventh decades and about 30% per decade thereafter.

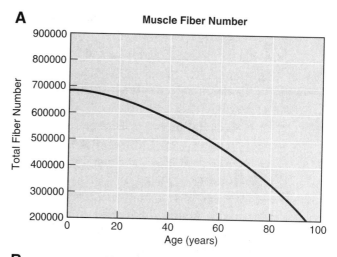

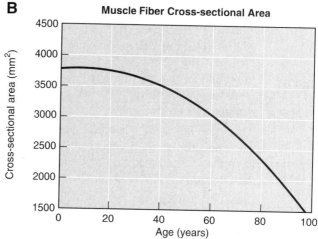

FIGURE 3-4 Alterations in muscle fiber number (A) and cross-sectional area (B) as a function of aging. A significant loss both in the number of fibers and fiber area begins around age 50–55.

3. **Bone changes**

   a. **In children,** problems with bone growth can develop as a result of strenuous exercise because the epiphysis is not yet united with the bone shaft.

   –**Epiphysitis** can occur with overuse.

   –**Fractures** can pass through the epiphyseal plate, disrupting normal bone growth.

   b. **Osteoporosis**

   –Advancing age brings a progressive decline in bone mineral density and calcium content in both men and women. In women, this loss is accelerated immediately after menopause.

   –As a result, **older individuals are more susceptible to bone fractures,** which are a significant cause of morbidity and mortality in the elderly.

   –**Hip fractures are the most common** and account for a large share of the disability, death, and medical costs associated with falls.

4. **Changes in joints, flexibility, and balance**

   a. **Connective tissue** (fascia, ligaments, tendons) **becomes less extensible** with age.

   b. **Degeneration of joints,** especially in the spine, occurs with advancing age.

   c. **Range of motion** (active and passive) **decreases** with age.

   d. A **progressive loss of flexibility** begins during young adulthood, related to disuse, deterioration of joints, and degeneration of collagen fibers.

   e. **Balance and postural stability are affected** by sensory and motor system changes. **Poor balance** is one **risk factor for falling.** (Other risk factors include medication use, diminished cognitive status, postural hypotension, and impaired vision.)

      –Age-related changes in the vestibular, visual, and somatosensory systems result in diminished feedback to the postural centers.

      –The muscle effectors may lack the capacity to respond appropriately to disturbances in postural stability.

5. **Application to exercise training in older adults**

   a. **Older adults exhibit strength gains from resistance training** that are similar to or even greater than those seen in younger adults. These strength gains are related to improved neurological function and, to a lesser extent, increased muscle mass.

   b. Regular **aerobic exercise enhances bone health,** particularly in postmenopausal women.

   c. **Resistance training** can offset the normal age-related declines in **bone health** by maintaining and sometimes improving bone mineral density.

   d. **Flexibility and balance can be improved,** and the risk of falling reduced, in older adults through an exercise program that incorporates resistance exercise, balance training, and stretching.

C. **BODY COMPOSITION**

1. **Body fat percentage** generally increases from childhood to early adulthood, to 15%–20% in males and 20%–25% in females. Thereafter, body fat percentage gradually increases with age (**Figure 3-5**), because of increasing fat mass and decreasing muscle mass.

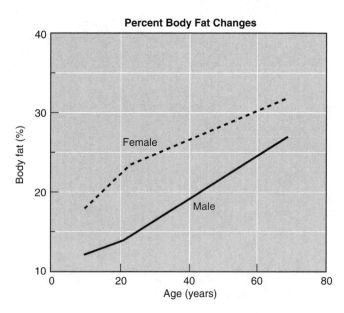

FIGURE 3-5 Changes in percent body fat as a function of age in males and females.

2. **Abdominal obesity** has reached epidemic proportions and plays a significant role in many diseases, including heart disease, cancer, and diabetes.

3. **Physiological changes associated with aging that contribute to unfavorable changes in body composition**

   a. **Inactivity is a primary factor in the increasing fat mass with age.** Energy expenditure from physical activity declines with age, and body fat mass increases when there is an imbalance between caloric intake and energy expenditure.

   b. **A progressive decline in skeletal muscle mass begins around age 50.**

      –During the developmental years, a positive nitrogen balance exists with deposition of protein into skeletal muscle and increasing muscle mass.

      –After age 50, however, individuals may enter into a state of negative nitrogen balance, contributing to a gradual loss of muscle mass.

   c. **A gradual decrease in basal metabolic rate is associated with aging.** Coupled with a more sedentary lifestyle, this typically results in a loss of lean muscle mass and a concurrent increase in the less metabolically active fat mass.

4. **Application to exercise training in older adults**

   a. Regular **aerobic exercise** has an obvious impact on energy balance by increasing energy expenditure.

b. Regular **resistance training** has positive anabolic effects in older individuals, leading to the preservation of skeletal muscle mass, which can help slow the age-related decline in basal metabolic rate.

D. THERMOREGULATION

1. Children

–Because of their immature thermoregulatory system, children consistently sweat less than adults, and thus may have difficulty making thermoregulatory adaptations in extreme temperature conditions.

2. Older adults

–Numerous factors can impair thermoregulation in older adults, including:

a. Reduced total body water

b. Decreased renal function with blunted sweat response

c. Decreased vascular peripheral response

d. Rapid dehydration

3. Application to exercise training in older adults

–Initial studies suggest that regular aerobic exercise may attenuate the decrease of peripheral sweat production known to occur with aging.

III. EXERCISE PRESCRIPTION IN OLDER ADULTS

A. GENERAL CONSIDERATIONS

–Most older adults are not sufficiently active and can greatly benefit from regular participation in a well-designed exercise program.

–Benefits of regular exercise include enhanced fitness, improved health status (due to reduction in risk factors associated with various diseases), increased independence, and an overall improvement in the quality of life.

B. MEDICAL SCREENING

1. A **complete medical history** and **screening for risk factors** should be done before an exercise program is prescribed for an older adult. Older clients with **preexisting medical problems** (e.g., heart disease, arthritis, diabetes) or who take medications that can affect response to exercise should be referred for **diagnostic exercise tolerance testing.**

2. **Consultation with and approval by a physician** is warranted before an older individual participates in a moderate or vigorous exercise program.

3. **Preprogram evaluation by an exercise specialist** is necessary to document initial measurements of muscle strength, aerobic fitness capacity, flexibility, and range of motion. Any impairment in cardiopulmonary, musculoskeletal, or sensory function should be identified.

C. EXERCISE ACTIVITY

1. Older individuals with age-related limitations in range of motion, orthopedic problems, restricted mobility, arthritis, or other diseases may need an exercise program focusing on **minimal or non-weight-bearing, low-impact activities** (e.g., swimming).

2. Because of the age-related alterations in cardiovascular capacity, muscle mass and strength, flexibility, and balance, a well-rounded program should incorporate **both aerobic and resistance training.**

D. EXERCISE FREQUENCY AND DURATION

1. It is generally recommended that older adults increase their frequency of exercise to 5–7 days per week to optimize cardiovascular health as well as balance and flexibility.

2. Exercise sessions of **20–60 minutes of continuous aerobic activity** are recommended for cardiovascular training. The specific **duration depends on the intensity of exercise;** high-intensity activity should be limited to shorter periods.

E. EXERCISE INTENSITY

1. Generally, **light- to moderate-intensity exercise** of extended duration is recommended for older adults engaging in aerobic training programs.

2. **For resistance training, higher relative intensity is recommended** to produce optimal training adaptations in muscle mass and strength.

REVIEW TEST

DIRECTIONS: Carefully read all questions and select the BEST single answer.

1. In terms of chronological age, early childhood is usually described as
   - (A) birth–3 weeks.
   - (B) 3 weeks–1 year.
   - (C) 1–6 years.
   - (D) 7–10 years.

2. Which age group is the fastest-growing segment of the U.S. population?
   - (A) Preadolescents
   - (B) Adolescents
   - (C) Adults age 65–85
   - (D) Adults over age 85

3. Increased afterload associated with increased peripheral resistance due to aging causes
   - (A) left ventricular hypertrophy.
   - (B) kidney failure.
   - (C) liver damage.
   - (D) liver failure.

4. An increase in both systolic and diastolic blood pressure at rest and during exercise often accompanies aging. Blood pressure usually increases because of
   - (A) increased arterial compliance and decreased arterial stiffness.
   - (B) decreased arterial compliance and increased arterial stiffness.
   - (C) decrease in both arterial compliance and arterial stiffness.
   - (D) increase in both arterial compliance and arterial stiffness.

5. Maximal oxygen uptake ($\dot{V}O_{2max}$) remains relatively unchanged throughout childhood. However, after age 25 years, it typically decreases by
   - (A) 0%–5% each decade.
   - (B) 5%–15% each decade.
   - (C) 15%–20% each decade.
   - (D) 15%–20% each year.

6. Cardiac output is a function of heart rate and stroke volume. In children, why is heart rate higher at rest and during exercise?
   - (A) Because in children, stroke volume is directly related to how much left ventricular stiffness reduces diastolic filling
   - (B) Because in children, cardiac output is regulated more by peripheral resistance than by any other variable
   - (C) Because children typically have a lower stroke volume than adults
   - (D) Because children typically have a more elevated peripheral resistance than adults

7. $\dot{V}O_{2max}$ is known to increase as a result of physical training in elderly persons. This occurs for all of the following reasons EXCEPT
   - (A) in men, the increase is a function of improved central and peripheral adaptations.
   - (B) in women, the increase is a function of improved peripheral adaptations.
   - (C) in both men and women, regular aerobic exercise slows the decline in $\dot{V}O_{2max}$ with aging.
   - (D) in both men and women, regular aerobic exercise speeds the decline in $\dot{V}O_{2max}$ with aging.

8. The total number of muscle fibers is fixed at an early age; however,
   - (A) at adolescence, males exhibit rapid hypertrophy of muscle.
   - (B) in comparison to males, females exhibit a more rapid hypertrophy of muscle.
   - (C) males lose muscle mass faster at an early age when they remain sedentary.
   - (D) males tend to exhibit muscle hypertrophy at a later age than females.

9. Strenuous exercise can predispose children to which of the following?
   - (A) Osteoporosis
   - (B) Osteoarthritis
   - (C) Malignant tumors
   - (D) Epiphysitis

10. Advancing age brings a progressive decline in bone mineral density and calcium content; this process is accelerated in women immediately following menopause. Which condition is commonly associated with this condition?
    (A) Osteoarthritis
    (B) Osteoporosis
    (C) Arthritis
    (D) Epiphysitis

11. All of the following musculoskeletal changes typically occur with advancing age EXCEPT
    (A) decreased flexibility.
    (B) impaired balance.
    (C) inhibited range of motion.
    (D) skeletal muscle hypertrophy.

12. Body fat generally increases with advancing age, particularly between childhood and early adulthood, because of
    (A) an exponential increase in caloric consumption.
    (B) a great increase in caloric consumption and a small decline in fat production.
    (C) body fat accumulation as a result of an imbalance between caloric intake and energy expenditure.
    (D) alterations in resting metabolic rate.

13. Which of the following factors does NOT impair an older individual's ability to thermoregulate?
    (A) Reduction in total body water
    (B) Decline in renal function
    (C) Decreased vascular peripheral responsiveness
    (D) Enhanced sweat response

14. A medical history as well as risk factor screening are important before prescribing an exercise program for older adults. Individuals who have been identified as having one or more risk factors for exercise participation should be referred
    (A) directly to the hospital and admitted for further evaluation.
    (B) in 1 month to the nearest exercise facility.
    (C) for diagnostic exercise tolerance testing.
    (D) immediately to a hospital emergency room.

15. Which of the following can an older person expect as a result of participation in an exercise program?
    (A) Overall improvement in the quality of life and increased independence
    (B) No changes in the quality of life but an increase in longevity
    (C) Increased longevity but a loss of bone mass
    (D) Loss of bone mass with a concomitant increase in bone density

16. Which of the following generally would be the preferred mode of exercise for an elderly person?
    (A) Jogging
    (B) Calisthenics
    (C) Swimming
    (D) Archery

17. An exercise program for elderly persons generally should emphasize increased
    (A) frequency.
    (B) intensity.
    (C) duration.
    (D) intensity and frequency.

18. For optimal cardiovascular as well as balance and flexibility adaptations, an elderly person generally should exercise how many days per week?
    (A) 1
    (B) 2
    (C) 3
    (D) 5–7

19. In response to regular resistance training,
    (A) older men and women demonstrate similar or even greater strength gains when compared to younger individuals.
    (B) younger men have greater gains in strength than older men.
    (C) younger women have greater gains in strength than older women.
    (D) younger men and women demonstrate similar or greater strength gains compared to older persons.

ANSWERS AND EXPLANATIONS

1–C. Typical age groupings/distinctions are neonatal, birth–3 weeks; infancy, 3 weeks–1 year; early childhood, 1–6 years; middle childhood, 7–10 years; late childhood/prepuberty, 9–15 years in females and 12–16 years in males; adolescence, the 6 years following puberty; adulthood, 20–64 years; older adulthood, 65 and older.

2–C. The number of individuals in the United States over age 65 will reach 70 million by the year 2030, with people over age 85 the fastest-growing segment of the population.

3–A. Left ventricular hypertrophy increases with age, apparently related to increased afterload associated with increased peripheral vascular resistance.

4–B. A decrease in arterial compliance and an increase in arterial stiffness with age can result in elevated systolic and diastolic blood pressure both at rest and during exercise.

5–B. A function of cardiac output and a–vO$_2$, $\dot{V}O_{2max}$ can remain relatively unchanged throughout adulthood. But without any exercise intervention, it decreases 5%–15% each decade after age 25. Both cardiac output and a–vO$_2$ decline with age; regular physical activity will help reduce these effects.

6–C. At rest and during exercise, heart rate is higher in children, from compensation for a lower stroke volume. Maximal heart rate and maximal stroke volume both decrease with age, causing a significant decline in maximal cardiac output.

7–D. Regular aerobic training produces similar increases in maximal oxygen consumption in younger and older adults. In men, this increase seems to be both central and peripheral, whereas in women, the changes seem to be peripheral. Men and women who participate in regular endurance exercise programs reduce the loss in maximal oxygen consumption with aging.

8–A. At adolescence, males exhibit rapid hypertrophy of muscle, disproportionately greater than that observed in females. The total number of muscle fibers seems to be fixed at an early age in both genders. Muscle mass declines (atrophy) with advancing age as a result of a progressive decrease in the number and size of fibers, with a greater selective loss of type II fibers.

9–D. Because in children the epiphysis is not yet united with the bone shaft, strenuous exercise can cause problems with bone growth. Epiphysitis can occur with overuse. Also, fractures can pass through the epiphyseal plate, leading to disruption in normal bone growth.

10–B. Advancing age brings a progressive decline in bone mineral density and calcium content. This loss is accelerated in women immediately after menopause. As a result, older adults are more susceptible to osteoporosis and bone fractures.

11–D. Connective tissue (fascia, ligaments, tendons) become less extensible with age. Degeneration of joints, especially the spine, occurs with advancing age, causing decreased range of motion along with a progressive loss of flexibility. Balance and postural stability are also affected due to age-related changes in both sensory and motor systems.

12–C. The energy expenditure related to physical activity declines with age making inactivity a primary factor responsible for the increase in fat mass with age. Body fat accumulates as a result of an imbalance between caloric intake and energy expenditure.

13–D. A number of factors can impair an older individual's ability to thermoregulate, including reduced total body water, declining renal function, decreased vascular peripheral responsiveness, rapid dehydration, and a blunted sweat response.

14–C. Awareness of preexisting medical problems and current medication use, gained through a medical history and risk factor screening, is necessary before an exercise program is prescribed. Persons with one or more risk factors should be referred for diagnostic exercise tolerance testing.

15–A. Most older adults are not sufficiently active. This population can benefit greatly from regular participation in a well-designed exercise program. Benefits include increased fitness, improved health status (reduction in risk factors associated with various diseases), increased independence, and an overall improvement in the quality of life.

16–C. For older adults, who often suffer from limited range of motion, orthopedic problems, restricted mobility, arthritis, and other disorders, an emphasis on minimal or non-weight-bearing, low-impact activities (such as swimming) is generally most appropriate.

17–A. Increased frequency of exercise is generally recommended for older adults to optimize cardiovascular as well as balance and flexibility adaptations. The recommended duration of exercise depends on the intensity of the activity; higher-intensity activity should be conducted over a shorter period.

18–D. An older person will benefit more from increased frequency of exercise than from increased intensity or duration of exercise. Recommended frequency is 5–7 days per week.

19–A. Muscle strength peaks in the mid-twenties for both genders and remains fairly stable through the mid-forties. Muscle strength declines approximately 15% per decade in the sixth and seventh decades and about 30% thereafter. However, older men and women demonstrate similar or even greater strength gains when compared with younger individuals in response to resistance training. The strength gains are related to improved neurological function and, to a lesser extent, by increased muscle mass.

CHAPTER 4

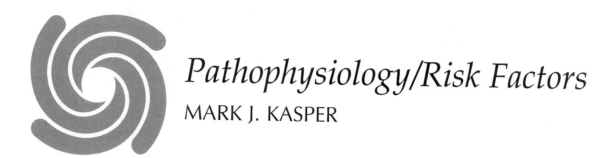

Pathophysiology/Risk Factors
MARK J. KASPER

I. CARDIOPULMONARY DISORDERS

A. PULMONARY DISEASE

1. **Chronic obstructive pulmonary disease (COPD)**

   –is a group of pulmonary disorders characterized by expiratory airflow obstruction, dyspnea (shortness of breath), and some degree of airway reversal or resolving of the condition. For example, an acute asthma attack can resolve spontaneously or as a result of medication (e.g., bronchodilator). COPD includes **bronchitis, emphysema, and asthma.**

   a. **Bronchitis**

      –In bronchitis, an **irritant** such as cigarette smoke or industrial pollution causes **inflammation and edema of the trachea and bronchial tubes.** The resultant mucosal hypertrophy with increased mucus secretion narrows and partially obstructs the airway. Impaired gas exchange leads to arterial hypoxemia (deficient blood oxygenation). **Arterial hypoxemia causes vasoconstriction** of smooth muscle in the pulmonary arterioles and venules, compounding the obstruction. Continued vasoconstriction **leads to pulmonary hypertension, right ventricular hypertrophy, and, ultimately, right heart failure** (cor pulmonale).

      –**Classic symptoms** of bronchitis include **chronic cough, sputum production, and dyspnea.**

   b. **Emphysema**

      –In emphysema, alveolar wall integrity is damaged by an irritant, such as cigarette smoke or pollution. **Alveolar destruction** results in loss of alveolar surface area, **impairing gas exchange and causing hypoventilation.** This process results in "wasted ventilation" (ventilation going to the lung units that have no capillaries) and these areas often referred to as "dead space" (places in the lungs where no perfusion occurs). Alveolar destruction is not uniform throughout the lung; some lung areas are better ventilated than others. Hypoventilation of the alveoli leads to **hypoxia and hypercapnia** (excess carbon dioxide in the blood), with extremely high minute ventilation. "Pink puffer" is the term commonly used to describe these individuals. To maintain adequate perfusion (as viewed by a "pink" rather than a blue or cyanotic skin color) an abnormally high minute ventilation ("puffer") is required. Destruction of alveoli also destroys small blood vessels of the pulmonary system, leading to **increased pulmonary resistance, elevated pulmonary arterial pressure, and, eventually, right heart failure.**

      –A **classic symptom** of emphysema is **dyspnea.**

   c. **Asthma**

      –is a reversible condition of increased responsiveness, or heightened sensitivity to an initiating factor or trigger, and obvious narrowing of the bronchial airways.

      –Narrowing of bronchial airways causes shortness of breath.

–An **initiating factor** (e.g., dust, pollen, hyperventilation) triggers an asthma attack by increasing calcium influx into mast cells, causing **release of chemical mediators** such as histamine. These mediators trigger **bronchoconstriction and an inflammatory response** (i.e., tissue swelling). Bronchoconstriction may also occur as a result of the chemical mediators directly stimulating the vagus nerve.

–Clinical manifestations of asthma include **dyspnea** and possibly **hypoxia** and **hypercapnia.**

–An **asthma attack can be self-limiting or may necessitate drug therapy** to prevent respiratory failure.

2. **Restrictive lung disease**

–includes **disorders that affect the alveolar tissue of the lung** (lung parenchyma), such as pulmonary fibrosis, sarcoidosis, alveolitis, and pneumothorax.

–can also be caused by **conditions that affect the spine** (e.g., scoliosis, ankylosing spondylitis) **or the muscles of respiration** (e.g., muscular dystrophy); obesity is another contributing factor.

–These disorders **compromise both resting and exercise lung volumes.**

–**Chronic restriction** can lead to dyspnea, hypoxia, hypercapnia, and respiratory failure.

3. **Pulmonary vascular disease**

   a. **Pulmonary embolism**

   –is a **moving blood clot** that typically lodges in a major branch of the pulmonary artery. Clots are **common in patients with congestive heart failure, atrial fibrillation, phlebitis** (inflammation of a vein), **and varicose veins.**

   –A **large pulmonary embolism can be instantly fatal;** a smaller clot may grow and increase pulmonary artery pressure, leading to right-sided heart failure.

   b. **Pulmonary edema**

   –is **excessive fluid retention in the lungs.**

   –can be caused by any factor that results in left heart failure, causing pooling of blood in the lungs.

   c. **Pulmonary hypertension**

   –is increased pressure within the pulmonary circulation (usually above 30 mm Hg systolic and 12 mm Hg diastolic).

   –**Possible causes** include:

   (1) Conditions of the left atrium, such as mitral valve stenosis or left ventricular failure

   (2) Ventricular or atrial septal defects (e.g., patent ductus arteriosus)

   (3) Any factor that increases pulmonary vascular resistance (right-sided heart failure), such as COPD or pulmonary embolism.

B. **CORONARY ARTERY DISEASE (CAD)**

   –The coronary arteries undergo anatomical changes due to genetic predisposition, the aging process, and multiple lifestyle risk factors.

   –**Figure 4-1** depicts the normal coronary artery wall.

   1. **Arteriosclerosis and atherosclerosis**

   –**Arteriosclerosis** is a normal loss of elasticity (or hardening) of the arteries that begins at birth and progresses throughout life.

   –**Atherosclerosis** is a form of arteriosclerosis characterized by accumulation of obstructive

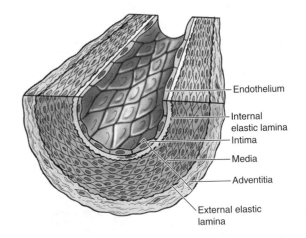

Endothelium
Internal elastic lamina
Intima
Media
Adventitia
External elastic lamina

FIGURE 4-1 The normal coronary artery wall. The **lumen** is the inside cavity or channel where blood flows. The **endothelium** is a single layer of cells that form a tight barrier between blood and the arterial wall. It resists thrombosis, promotes vasodilatation, and inhibits smooth muscle cells from migration and proliferation into the intima. Damage to the endothelium increases the susceptibility of the artery to atherosclerosis. The **intima** is a very thin, innermost layer of the artery wall. Comprised of predominantly connective tissue with some smooth muscle cells, it is where atherosclerotic lesions are formed. The thickest, middle layer of the artery wall, the **media** is comprised of predominantly smooth muscle cells. It is responsible for vasoconstriction or vasodilatation of the artery, and it can contribute to the atherosclerotic process through migration and proliferation of smooth muscle cells to the intima. The **adventitia** is the outermost layer of the artery wall. It provides the media and intima with oxygen and nutrients, and is not believed to have a significant role in the development of atherosclerosis. (With permission from Ross R, Glomset J: The pathogenesis of atherosclerosis. *N Engl J Med* 295:369, 1976.)

lesions in or beneath the artery wall. **Risk factors** include smoking, dyslipidemia, and hypertension.

  a. **Results of arterial injury** (Figure 4-2)

   (1) Endothelial cells lose their permeability, enabling cells and molecules to pass into the subendothelial space.

   (2) Endothelial cells lose their antithrombotic properties, resulting in **increased risk of clot formation and thrombus.**

   (3) Reduced secretion of vasodilating substances (e.g., endothelium-derived relaxing factor nitric oxide [EDRF-

NO]) leads to **increased vasoconstriction.**

   (4) Endothelial cells secrete platelet-derived growth factor, resulting in movement of smooth muscle cells into the intima.

   (5) Endothelial cells attract other key cells toward the intima that are involved in the development of atherosclerosis.

  b. **Response to arterial injury**

   (1) Platelets adhere at the site of injury and form a "cap" to protect and isolate the plaque within the injured arterial wall.

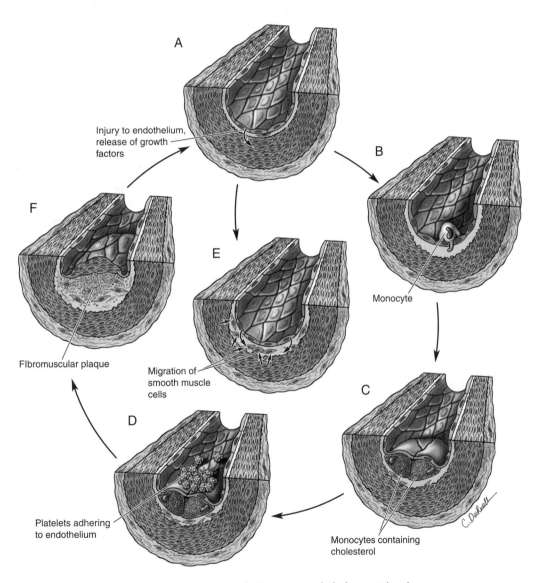

FIGURE 4-2 The atherosclerotic process-response to injury. **A,** Injury to endothelium with release of growth factors (small arrow). **B,** Monocytes attach to endothelium. **C,** Monocytes migrate to the intima, take up cholesterol, form fatty streaks. **D,** Platelets adhere to the endothelium and release growth factors. **F,** The result is a fibromuscular plaque. An alternative pathway is shown with arrows from **A** to **E** to **F,** with growth factor-mediated migration of smooth muscle cells from the media to the intima (**E**). (With permission from Ross R: The pathogenesis of atherosclerosis—an update. *N Engl J Med* 314:496, 1986.)

(2) Small thrombi develop.

(3) The release of additional growth factors and vasoactive substances continues.

(4) Monocytes adhere to the endothelium, move to the intima, and take up lipids, particularly low-density lipoproteins (LDL).

(5) Smooth muscle cells and connective tissue move from the media to the intima, producing fatty streaks or lesions.

(6) As the process continues, lesions increase in size to form a fibrous plaque.

(7) As the plaque enlarges, the vessel lumen becomes occluded, obstructing blood flow. Other complications include thrombus formation with occlusion, peripheral emboli, and weakening of the vessel wall.

(8) Atherosclerosis does not necessarily occur in a stable, linear manner. Some lesions develop slowly and are relatively stable. Other lesions progress very quickly due to frequent plaque rupture, thrombi formation, and intima changes.

(9) Regression is possible with aggressive multifactorial risk correction. Modest results have been observed.

2. **Myocardial ischemia**

   –is insufficient blood flow to the myocardium.

   –results when myocardial oxygen demand exceeds the oxygen supply.

   –is **an outcome of significant coronary atherosclerosis.**

   –is referred to as silent ischemia if not accompanied by angina pectoris.

3. **Angina pectoris**

   –is the **pain associated with myocardial ischemia.** The pain is located in the chest area, neck, cheeks, shoulder, or arms and is described as constricting, squeezing, burning, or a heavy feeling.

   a. **Classic (typical) angina** is initiated by provoking factors such as exercise or stress, excitement, cold or hot weather, or after meals, and is relieved by rest or nitroglycerin.

   b. **Vasospastic (variant or Prinzmetal's) angina** usually occurs at rest; it is due to coronary vasospasm and is initiated by vasoconstrictors produced by the injured endothelium.

4. **Acute myocardial infarction (MI)**

   –is the **irreversible necrosis of the myocardium resulting from prolonged ischemia.** Muscle fibers die in the center of the ischemic zone; fibrous tissue develops among the dead fibers. The area of necrosis may increase owing to residual ischemia, or it may decrease owing to collateral circulation.

   a. About 90% of MIs result from formation of an acute thrombus in an atherosclerotic coronary artery.

   b. Plaque rupture is a major cause of coronary thrombi.

   c. Endothelial dysfunction also contributes to vasoconstriction of the coronary artery through a reduction of vasodilator substances.

   d. **Thrombolytic therapy** with a specific clot-dissolving agent during acute MI may restore blood flow and limit myocardial necrosis. Administration within the first 1 to 2 hours after onset of MI yields the greatest benefit. Thrombolytic agents used include streptokinase and recombinant tissue plasminogen activator (t-PA).

   e. **Possible complications** of MI include:

      (1) Extension to another MI

      (2) Ventricular aneurysm

      –Necrotic muscle fibers of the heart degenerate, and the myocardial wall becomes very thin. During systole, these nonfunctional muscle fibers do not contract but rather bulge outward (aneurysm), increasing the risk of thrombus, ventricular arrhythmias, and heart failure.

      (3) Rupture

      –This involves the same mechanism as a ventricular aneurysm, but the ventricular wall breaks open.

      –Rupture causes pericarditis/cardiac tamponade if it occurs in the free wall of the ventricle.

      –Rupture causes congestive heart failure if it occurs in the ventricular septal wall.

      (4) Papillary necrosis

      –This necrosis of the papillary muscle(s) damages heart valve(s), resulting in heart failure or pulmonary edema.

(5) Expansion

–This is left ventricular dilation caused by weakening of the left ventricle due to necrotic muscle fibers. It can cause congestive heart failure.

C. SIGNS AND SYMPTOMS OF CARDIOPULMONARY DISEASE

–Major signs and symptoms suggestive of cardiovascular and pulmonary disease are listed in **Table 4-1.**

 Table 4-1. Major Symptoms or Signs Suggestive of Cardiopulmonary or Metabolic Disease

Symptom: Pain or discomfort in the chest or surrounding areas that appears to be ischemic in nature.
Clarification/Significance: One of the cardinal manifestations of cardiac disease, in particular coronary artery disease. Key features favoring an ischemic origin include:
  A. Character—constricting, squeezing, burning, "heaviness" or "heavy feeling"
  B. Location—substernal; across midthorax, anteriorly; in both arms, shoulders; in neck, cheeks, teeth; in forearms, fingers; in interscapular region
  C. Provoking factors—exercise, excitement, other forms of stress, cold weather, occurrence after meals.

Key features against an ischemic origin include:

  A. Character—dull ache; "knife-like," sharp, stabbing; "jabs" aggravated by respiration
  B. Location—in left submammary area; in left hemithorax
  C. Provoking factors—after completion of exercise, provoked by a specific body motion.

Symptom: Unaccustomed shortness of breath or shortness of breath with mild exertion.
Clarification/Significance: Dyspnea (defined as an abnormally uncomfortable awareness of breathing) is one of the principal symptoms of cardiac and pulmonary disease. It commonly occurs during strenuous exertion in healthy, well-trained persons and during moderate exertion in healthy, untrained persons. It should be regarded as abnormal, however, when it occurs at a level of exertion that is not expected to evoke this symptom in a given individual. Abnormal exertional dyspnea suggests the presence of cardiopulmonary disorders, in particular left ventricular dysfunction or chronic obstructive pulmonary disease.

Symptom: Dizziness or syncope.
Clarification/Significance: Syncope (defined as a loss of consciousness) is most commonly caused by a reduced perfusion of the brain. Dizziness and, in particular, syncope *during* exercise may result from cardiac disorders that prevent the normal rise (or an actual fall) in cardiac output. Such cardiac disorders are potentially life-threatening and include severe coronary artery disease, hypertrophic cardiomyopathy, aortic stenosis, and malignant ventricular arrhythmias. Although dizziness or syncope shortly *after* cessation of exercise should not be ignored, these symptoms may occur even in healthy persons as a result of a reduction in venous return to the heart.

Symptom: Orthopnea and paroxysmal nocturnal dyspnea.
Clarification/Significance: Orthopnea refers to dyspnea occurring at rest in the recumbent position that is relieved promptly by sitting upright or standing. Paroxysmal nocturnal dyspnea refers to dyspnea, beginning usually 2 to 5 hours after the onset of sleep, which may be relieved by sitting on the side of the bed or getting out of bed. Both are symptoms of left ventricular failure. Although nocturnal dyspnea may occur in persons with chronic obstructive pulmonary disease, it differs in that it is usually relieved after the person relieves himself or herself of secretions rather than specifically by sitting up.

Sign: Ankle edema.
Clarification/Significance: Bilateral ankle edema that is most evident at night is a characteristic sign of heart failure or bilateral chronic venous insufficiency. Unilateral edema of a limb often results from venous thrombosis or lymphatic blockage in the limb. Generalized edema (known as anasarca) occurs in persons with the nephrotic syndrome, severe heart failure, or hepatic cirrhosis. Edema around the eyes and of the face is characteristic of several conditions, including the nephrotic syndrome, acute glomerulonephritis, angioneurotic edema, hypoproteinemia, and myxedema.

Symptom/Sign: Palpitations or tachycardia.
Clarification/Significance: Palpitations (defined as an unpleasant awareness of the forceful or rapid beating of the heart) may be induced by various disorders of cardiac rhythm. These include tachycardia, bradycardia of sudden onset, ectopic beats, compensatory pauses, and accentuated stroke volume due to valvular regurgitation. Palpitations also often result from anxiety states and high cardiac output (or hyperkinetic) states, such as anemia, fever, thyrotoxicosis, arteriovenous fistula, and the so-called idiopathic hyperkinetic heart syndrome.

Symptom: Claudication.
Clarification/Significance: Intermittent claudication refers to the pain that occurs in a muscle with an inadequate blood supply (usually as a result of atherosclerosis) that is stressed by exercise. The pain does not occur with standing or sitting, is reproducible from day to day, is more severe when walking upstairs or up a hill, and is often described as a cramp, which disappears within 1 or 2 minutes after stopping exercise. Coronary artery disease is more prevalent in persons with intermittent claudication. Diabetics are at increased risk for this condition.

Sign: Known heart murmur.
Clarification/Significance: Although some may be innocent, heart murmurs may indicate valvular or other cardiovascular disease. From an exercise safety standpoint, it is especially important to exclude hypertrophic cardiomyopathy and aortic stenosis as underlying causes because these are among the more common causes of exertion-related sudden cardiac death.

These symptoms and signs must be interpreted in the clinical context in which they appear, because they are not all specific for cardiopulmonary or metabolic disease. (Data from American College of Sports Medicine: *Guidelines for Exercise Testing and Prescription,* 6th ed. Philadelphia, Lippincott Williams & Wilkins, 2000; Braunwald E, Isselbacher KJ, Petersdorf RG et al (eds): *Harrison's Principles of Internal Medicine.* New York, McGraw-Hill, 1988; and Braunwald E: The history. In *Heart Disease: A Textbook of Cardiovascular Medicine.* Edited by Braunwald E. Philadelphia, WB Saunders, 1988.)

II. RISK FACTORS FOR CORONARY ARTERY DISEASE

A. PRIMARY RISK FACTORS—NONMODIFIABLE

1. **Increasing age**

   –About 50% of MIs occur in persons over age 65, 45% in those age 45 to 65, and 5% in those under age 45.

2. **Male sex**

   –Up to age 50, men are roughly 3 times more prone to CAD than are women. The risk of CAD rises in women after menopause; men over age 50 are only about 1.5 times more prone to CAD than are postmenopausal women.

3. **Family history**

   –Children and siblings of a person with CAD are more likely to develop it themselves. The risk is greatest in those with the lowest overall CAD risk profile; for example, those with a family member who sustained an MI but did not have any of the traditional risk factors.

B. PRIMARY RISK FACTORS—MODIFIABLE

1. **Tobacco smoking**

   –Smokers are at roughly 2.5 times greater risk for CAD than nonsmokers, although individual risk varies with extent of exposure (lifetime dosage).

   –Smoking has both acute effects (e.g., increases myocardial oxygen demand) and chronic effects (e.g, endothelium damage) on the myocardium.

   –Smoking negatively influences other coronary artery disease risk factors (e.g., lowers high-density lipoproteins [HDLs]).

2. **Dyslipidemia**

   –There is a positive correlation between total cholesterol (TC) and low-density lipoprotein (LDL) levels, the amount of fat, saturated fat, and cholesterol in the diet, and CAD mortality and morbidity.

   –TC, LDLs, and triglycerides contribute to the atherosclerotic process, whereas high-density lipoproteins (HDLs) are cardioprotective. The Framingham Heart Study data suggest that the TC-to-HDL ratio may be the best predictor of CAD risk related to lipid values.

   –The National Cholesterol Education Program (NCEP) provides recommendations for the detection, evaluation, and treatment of high blood cholesterol in adults.

3. **Hypertension**

   –Blood pressure classifications of the 1997 Sixth Report of the Joint Committee on Prevention, Detection, Evaluation, and Treatment of High Blood Pressure are provided in Chapter 2, Table 2-3. Recommendations on treatment are also available from this document.

   –As the severity of hypertension increases, so does the risk of cardiovascular disease.

   –Hypertension has both acute effects (e.g., increased myocardial oxygen demand) and chronic effects (e.g, endothelium damage) on the myocardium.

4. **Physical inactivity**

   –Physical inactivity carries a risk for CAD similar to that of hypertension, dyslipidemia, and cigarette smoking.

   –Physical inactivity can influence other risk factors (e.g., increasing blood pressure, lowering HDL cholesterol, and decreasing the sensitivity to insulin resulting in elevated blood glucose levels).

   –Persons who are physically inactive post-MI have significantly higher mortality rates than more active individuals.

5. **Obesity**

   –In 1998, the American Heart Association classified obesity as a major, modifiable risk factor for CAD.

   –Obesity has a strong positive relationship with other risk factors for CAD, such as hypertension, dyslipidemia, and Type 2 diabetes mellitus.

   –The risk for CAD is greater in persons with central (android or upper body) obesity than in those with peripheral (gynoid or lower body) obesity. Waist-to-hip ratio (WHR) provides an index of central obesity. Health risk increases for WHR and standards for risk vary with age and gender.

   –A waist circumference alone of greater than 100 cm is an indicator of health risk.

   –A body mass index (BMI) of greater than 30 kg/m^2 has been defined as obesity.

   –Classification of disease risk can also be based on BMI and waist circumference.

6. **Diabetes mellitus**

   –Persons with diabetes mellitus are 2 to 4 times more likely to develop CAD than are those without diabetes; risk of MI is 50%

greater in diabetic men and 150% greater in diabetic women.

–Although aggressive blood glucose control can reduce microvascular complications (e.g., loss of eyesight), an associated reduction in CAD is questionable.

–Diabetes mellitus is commonly associated with central obesity, elevated triglyceride and LDL levels, and hypertension (known as "syndrome X" or the "metabolic syndrome").

–The 1997 Report of the Expert Committee on the Diagnosis and Classification of Diabetes Mellitus revised the diagnostic and classification criteria for diabetes mellitus.

C. **SECONDARY RISK FACTORS** include **psychosocial stress, postmenopausal status,** and **excessive alcohol consumption.**

III. DIAGNOSIS OF CORONARY ARTERY DISEASE

A. ELECTROCARDIOGRAPHY (ECG)

–is a valuable noninvasive diagnostic test that records cardiac electrical currents by means of placing electrodes placed on the body surface.

–can be administered with the patient resting or exercising.

–can detect rhythm and conduction disturbances, chamber enlargement, ischemia, and infarction.

1. Various changes and combinations of ST segment abnormalities, presence of significant Q waves, and absence of R waves point to acute, recent, or old MI.

   a. ST segment depression suggests subendocardial ischemia.

   b. ST segment elevation suggests transmural ischemia.

2. Certain cardiac conditions, illnesses, and medications may make interpretation of resting or exercise ECG difficult. More sensitive and specific tests (e.g., radionuclide imaging, echocardiography, coronary angiography) may be needed to confirm or rule out ischemia. (See Chapter 6, III F, for definitions of sensitivity and specificity in exercise testing.)

B. RADIONUCLIDE IMAGING

–is a more sensitive and specific test than exercise ECG.

–is useful when predictive value of positive ECG test is low or modest.

–is necessary in cases when resting ECG abnormalities (e.g., due to digoxin, left bundle branch block) mask the ST segment or the patient is unable to exercise (e.g., peripheral vascular disease, arthritis).

1. **Perfusion imaging**

   –This test evaluates the extent and location of myocardial perfusion defects, both transient (ischemic) and fixed (necrotic).

   a. A radioisotope such as thallium-201, technetium-99m, or sestamibi (Cardiolite) is injected intravenously while the patient exercises. In a **pharmacologic stress test,** the radioisotope is used in combination with dipyridamole, dobutamine, or adenosine to create stress for those unable to exercise.

   b. Images are taken immediately postexercise and 4 to 24 hours later using planar, single-photon emission computed tomography (SPECT), or positron emission tomography (PET) scans.

      –In a **normal heart,** full perfusion is revealed in both the initial and the delayed scans.

      –In an **ischemic heart,** unequal perfusion (a defect or cold spot) is seen in the initial scan, but reversal to full perfusion is seen in the delayed scan.

      –In a **necrotic heart,** both scans show unequal perfusion in areas where scarring has occurred.

   c. The sensitivity and specificity for each type of scan are as follows:

      –Planar: sensitivity 83%, specificity 88%

      –SPECT: sensitivity 89%, specificity 76%

      –PET: sensitivity 78%–100%, specificity 87%–97%.

2. **Radionuclide ventriculography (RVG)**

   –is commonly called a multiple gated acquisition scan (MUGA).

   –is used to assess heart wall motion abnormalities, ejection fraction, systolic and diastolic function, and cardiac output.

   a. In MUGA, a bolus (first-pass technique) of radioisotope is ejected in a central vein. In MUGA with pharmacologic testing (commonly done to assess complications of acute MI), dipyridamole, dobutamine, or adenosine is administered to create stress for those unable to exercise or in whom exercise might be overly demanding.

   b. The real-time exercise scans are recorded and compared to resting scans.

C. ECHOCARDIOGRAPHY

–is used to assess heart wall motion abnormalities, ejection fraction, systolic and diastolic function, and cardiac output by use of sound waves.

–is commonly used to detect valvular disease.

–Images are viewed while the patient exercises on a cycle ergometer or immediately after treadmill exercise. A radioactive isotope is not administered; however, pharmacologic stress echocardiography may be appropriate for those unable to exercise.

D. CORONARY ANGIOGRAPHY

–In coronary angiography, a catheter is inserted into the groin or arm and positioned in a heart chamber or at the origin of the coronary arteries. A dye with a vasodilator effect is injected and visualized radiographically.

–Coronary angiography is of most use in patients with a high pretest likelihood of CAD.

–It can be used to diagnose the presence and extent of atherosclerosis by imaging the arterial lumen.

–It can be used in combination with ventriculography to assess heart wall motion abnormalities, cardiac ejection fraction, systolic and diastolic function, and cardiac output.

IV. TREATMENT OF CORONARY ARTERY DISEASE

A. RISK FACTOR MODIFICATION

–Aggressive control of modifiable risk factors may reverse or reduce the progression of atherosclerosis.

B. PHARMACOLOGIC THERAPY

  1. Platelet inhibitors

–Platelet-inhibiting agents such as aspirin have been shown to significantly reduce mortality, cardiovascular events, acute thrombotic occlusion following angioplasty, and patency of saphenous graphs.

  2. Anti-ischemic agents

    a. Beta adrenergic blockers

–reduce ischemia by lowering myocardial oxygen demand for any given workload.

–lower blood pressure and control ventricular arrhythmias.

–reduce first-year mortality rate in post-MI patients by 20% to 35%.

    b. Calcium channel blockers

–reduce ischemia at any given workload by altering the major determinants of myocardial oxygen supply and demand. Some calcium channel blockers reduce resting and exercise heart rate. All calcium channel blockers reduce resting and exercise blood pressure.

–have not been shown to reduce post-MI mortality.

    c. Nitrates

–reduce ischemia by reducing myocardial oxygen demand with some increase in oxygen supply.

–are used to treat typical and variant angina.

–have not been shown to reduce post-MI mortality.

  3. Lipid-lowering therapy

–The goal is to reduce the availability of lipids to the injured endothelium.

–Lowering LDLs and TC has proven effective in influencing the progression and regression of atherosclerosis.

–There are various classifications of lipid-lowering drugs that work through different mechanisms:

    a. The **bile acid sequestrants** such as cholestyramine (Questran) and colestipol (Colestid) lower LDLs but tend to elevate triglycerides. They work by binding bile acids and reducing recirculation through the liver.

b. Niacin (Nicobid) lowers LDLs by inhibiting secretion of lipoproteins from the liver; it has no influence on triglycerides.

c. The **statin drugs** such as lovastatin (Mevacor), pravastatin (Pravachol) and simvastatin (Zocor) are also effective for lowering LDLs. They work by increasing the number of LDL receptors in the liver.

d. Drugs such as **gemfibrozil** (Lopid) and **clofibrate** (Atromid) are effective for lowering elevated triglyceride levels with a moderate reduction in LDLs. They work by promoting lipolysis of VLDL triglycerides.

C.   PERCUTANEOUS TRANSLUMINAL CORONARY ANGIOPLASTY (PTCA)

–In PTCA, a catheter with a deflated balloon is inserted into the narrowed portion of the coronary artery. The balloon is inflated, resulting in an enlarging of the inner diameter of the artery. The balloon is then deflated and the catheter removed. Over 70% of these procedures also involve the placement of a coronary artery stent.

–PTCA can be used in the acute MI stage for patients who are not candidates for thrombolytic therapy.

–PTCA is typically reserved for younger patients, those with single-vessel disease, and those with stenosis distal to the occluded artery.

–Restenosis occurs within 6 months in up to 50% of patients.

–PTCA carries a greater risk of revascularization than either a coronary artery stent or coronary artery bypass graph surgery.

D.   CORONARY ARTERY STENT

–A coronary artery stent is a slotted stainless steel tube that acts as a scaffold to hold the walls of the artery open, thereby improving blood flow and relieving the symptoms of CAD. The stent is mounted on a balloon catheter that is inserted into the artery, inflated/expanded at the blockage site, and permanently implanted in the artery.

–Candidates for stents are similar to those in need of PTCA, including those who experience restenosis after PTCA and those who underwent coronary artery bypass graft surgery who have stenosis of another artery.

–Restenosis occurs within 6 months in up to about 35% of patients.

–A coronary artery stent carries a lower rate of revascularization than does PTCA.

E.   CORONARY ARTERY BYPASS GRAFT SURGERY (CABGS)

–In CABGS, a saphenous vein is removed from the leg and attached to the base of the aorta and below the stenosis of a coronary artery. An internal mammary artery can also be used to attach below the stenosis.

–CABGS is reserved for patients with a poor prognosis for survival or those who are unresponsive to pharmacological treatment, stents, or PTCA (e.g., patients with angina, left main stenosis, multiple vessel disease, or left ventricular dysfunction).

–Arterial grafts are significantly superior to venous grafts in terms of patency (90% for arterial grafts vs. less than 50% for venous grafts at 10 years).

V. RISK STRATIFICATION FOR PATIENTS WITH CARDIOPULMONARY DISORDERS

A.   DEFINITION

–Risk stratification consists of placing an individual in a risk group based on the likelihood of untoward events.

B.   PURPOSE

–The purpose of risk stratification is to provide guidelines for monitoring and supervision during exercise training, and to make recommendations for occupational, recreational, or daily activity participation and any necessary restrictions.

C.   CRITERIA

–The criteria for risk stratification for cardiac patients are published by the American College of Physicians (ACP) and American Association of Cardiovascular and Pulmonary Rehabilitation (AACVPR) (**Table 4-2**), and the American Heart Association (AHA) (**Table 4-3**).

Table 4-2. American Association of Cardiovascular and Pulmonary Rehabilitation (AACVPR) Risk Stratification Criteria for Cardiac Patients

Low Risk	Moderate Risk	High Risk
• No significant left ventricular dysfunction (ejection fraction of > 50%) • No resting or exercise-induced complex arrhythmias • Uncomplicated MI; CABG; angioplasty, atherectomy, or stent: — Absence of CHF or signs/symptoms of postevent ischemia • Normal hemodynamics with exercise or recovery • Asymptomatic including absence of angina with exertion or recovery • Functional capacity of ≥ 7 METs[†] • Absence of clinical depression	• Moderately impaired left ventricular function (ejection fraction = 40%–49%) • Signs/symptoms including angina at moderate levels of exercise (5–6.9 METs) or in recovery **Moderate risk is assumed for patients who do not meet the classification of either high or low risk.**	• Decreased left ventricular function (ejection fraction of < 40%) • Survivor of cardiac arrest or sudden death • Complex ventricular arrhythmias at rest or with exercise • MI or cardiac surgery complicated by cardiogenic shock, CHF, and/or signs/symptoms of post-event/procedure ischemia • Abnormal hemodynamics with exercise (especially flat or decreasing systolic blood pressure or chronotropic incompetence with increasing workload) • Signs/symptoms including angina pectoris at low levels of exercise (< 5.0 METs) or in recovery • Functional capacity of < 5.0 METs* • Clinically significant depression
Low-risk classification is assumed when each of the descriptors in the category is present.		**High-risk classification is assumed with the presence of any one of the descriptors included in this category.**

*Note: If *measured* functional capacity is not available, this variable is not considered in the risk-stratification process.
Abbreviations: MI, myocardial infarction; CABG, coronary artery bypass graft surgery; CHF, congestive heart failure; METs, metabolic equivalents (1 MET = 3.5 mL·kg[-1]·min[-1]; resting oxygen consumption).
(Adapted from American Association of Cardiovascular and Pulmonary Rehabilitation: *Guidelines for Cardiac Rehabilitation and Secondary Prevention Programs,* 3rd ed. Champaign, IL, Human Kinetics, 1999.)

Table 4-3. American Heart Association (AHA) Risk Stratification Criteria*

Class A: Apparently Healthy

• (1) Individuals < age 40 who have no symptoms of or known presence of heart disease or major coronary risk factors and (2) individuals of any age without known heart disease or major risk factors and who have a normal exercise test
• Activity guidelines: No restrictions other than basic guidelines
• ECG and blood pressure monitoring: Not required
• Supervision required: None

Class B: Documented, stable cardiovascular disease with low risk for vigorous exercise but slightly greater risk than for apparently healthy individuals

• Moderate activity is not believed to be associated with increased risk in this group
• Includes individuals with (1) CAD (MI, CABGS, PTCA angina pectoris, abnormal exercise test, and abnormal coronary angiograms) whose condition is stable and who have the clinical characteristics outlined below; (2) valvular heart disease; (3) congenital heart disease; (4) cardiomyopathy; and (5) exercise test abnormalities that do not meet the criteria outlined in Class C below
• Clinical characteristics: (1) New York Heart Association (NYHA) class 1 or 2; (2) exercise capacity of > 6 METs; (3) no evidence of heart failure; (4) free of ischemia or angina at rest or on the exercise test at or below 6 METS; (5) appropriate rise in systolic blood pressure during exercise; (6) no sequential ectopic ventricular contractions; and (7) ability to satisfactorily self-monitor intensity of activity
• Activity guidelines: Activity should be individualized with exercise prescription by qualified personnel trained in basic CPR or with electronic monitoring at home
• ECG and blood pressure monitoring: Only during the early prescription phase of training, usually 6 to 12 sessions
• Supervision required: Medical supervision during prescription sessions and nonmedical supervision for other exercise sessions until the individual understands how to monitor his or her activity

Class C: Those at moderate to high risk for cardiac complications during exercise and/or unable to self-regulate activity or to understand recommended activity level

• Includes individuals with (1) CAD with the clinical characteristics outlined below; (2) cardiomyopathy; (3) valvular heart disease; (4) exercise test abnormalities not directly related to ischemia; (5) previous episode of ventricular fibrillation or cardiac arrest that did not occur in the presence of an acute ischemic event or cardiac procedure: (6) complex ventricular arrhythmias that are uncontrolled at mild to moderate work intensities with medication; (7) three-vessel disease or left main disease; and (8) low ejection fraction (< 30%)
• Clinical characteristics: (1) Two or more MIs; (2) NYHA class 3 or greater; (3) exercise capacity of <6 Mets; (4) ischemic horizontal or downsloping ST depression of 4 mm or more or angina during exercise; (5) fall in systolic blood pressure with exercise; (6) a medical problem that the physician believes may be life-threatening; (7) previous episode of primary cardiac arrest; and (8) ventricular tachycardia at a workload of <6 METs
• Activity guidelines: Activity should be individualized with exercise prescription by qualified personnel
• ECG and blood pressure monitoring: Continuous during exercise sessions until safety is established, usually in 6 to 12 sessions or more
• Supervision required: Medical supervision during all exercise sessions until safety is established

Class D: Unstable disease with activity restriction

• Includes individuals with (1) unstable ischemia; (2) heart failure that is not compensated; (3) uncontrolled arrhythmias; (4) severe and symptomatic aortic stenosis; and (5) other conditions that could be aggravated by exercise
• Activity guidelines: No activity is recommended for conditioning purposes. Attention should be directed to treating the subject and restoring him or her to class C or higher. Daily activities must be prescribed based on individual assessment by the subject's personal physician

(Modified from Fletcher GA, Balady G, Froelicher VF et al: Exercise standards: A statement for health care professionals from the American Heart Association. *Circulation* 91:580–615, 1995.)

VI. EFFECTS OF EXERCISE ON CARDIOPULMONARY AND OTHER DISORDERS

A. PULMONARY DISEASE

–Exercise can improve musculoskeletal and psychosocial factors that typically limit exercise in persons with pulmonary disease.

–Because pulmonary disease is commonly associated with CAD and CAD risk factors, exercise training can reduce the risk of CAD in persons with pulmonary disease.

B. CORONARY ARTERY DISEASE

–Exercise has been shown to help reduce mortality in persons with CAD. The **mechanisms responsible for a reduction in CAD deaths** are various, and include:

1. The effects of exercise on other risk factors

2. Reduction in myocardial oxygen demand at rest and at submaximal workloads (resulting in an increased ischemic and angina threshold)

3. Reduction in platelet aggregation

4. Improved endothelial-mediated vasomotor tone

C. OBESITY

–An increase in caloric expenditure through exercise, combined with a reduction in caloric intake, results in a caloric deficit. Over time, a caloric deficit results in reduction of overall body fat and a likely reduction in central fat deposits.

–**Decreased body fat,** especially reduced central obesity, **can reduce risk factors for CAD,** including dyslipidemia, type 2 diabetes mellitus, and hypertension.

–Exercising to induce a caloric deficit can preserve lean body mass. Dieting alone to produce a caloric deficit usually results in a loss of lean body mass. A **combination of exercise and diet is best** for initial and long-term weight loss and maintenance of target weight.

D. DYSLIPIDEMIA

1. **Exercise has the beneficial effect of lowering triglycerides and raising HDLs.**

   –Exercise increases the activity of lipoprotein lipase (LPL), which "breaks up" the very-low-density lipoprotein triglyceride. Triglyceride levels are then decreased when they are used by the skeletal muscles during exercise. In addition, any very-low-density lipoprotein remnants serve as precursors to HDLs, which are cardioprotective.

   –To induce these beneficial changes, the volume of aerobic activity is more important than the intensity of activity.

2. **Exercise can indirectly lower TC and LDLs.**

   –Lowering TC and LDLs is related more to caloric restriction and body fat reduction than to exercise training alone. However, because exercise training can result in body fat reduction, it can have an indirect effect on TC and LDL levels.

E. DIABETES MELLITUS

–Exercise can improve insulin sensitivity and glucose metabolism in people with type 1 diabetes mellitus.

–In people with type 2 diabetes mellitus, exercise can enhance fat loss, resulting in improved insulin sensitivity and glucose metabolism.

–Exercise can favorably alter other risk factors typically associated with diabetes mellitus, including dyslipidemia and hypertension, and thus decrease the overall risk of CAD.

F. HYPERTENSION

–By reducing circulating catecholamines, plasma renin, and heart rate, and by increasing vasodilator substances, exercise can reduce cardiac output (CO) and total peripheral resistance (TPR), and thus reduce blood pressure. An average reduction of about 10 mm Hg in both systolic and diastolic blood pressure has been observed in patients with mild to moderate hypertension as a result of aerobic exercise training.

–Exercise can reduce intra-abdominal visceral fat and hyperinsulinemia, resulting in a decrease of TPR.

G. PERIPHERAL ARTERY DISEASE

–Exercise training can improve oxygen extraction from the skeletal muscle. Elevation of oxygen extraction improves the relationship between oxygen supply and oxygen demand. When oxygen supply equals or exceeds oxygen demand, claudication is less likely to occur.

–Exercise may improve the mechanical efficiency of walking, which, together with changes in the oxygen supply-demand ratio, improves the ability to walk longer or at higher intensities.

–Maintenance of exercise training reduces the ill effects of deconditioning and risk factors associated with peripheral artery disease (e.g., hypertension, insulin resistance).

H. OSTEOPOROSIS

–Exercise reduces the deleterious effects of deconditioning and the risk factors for osteoporosis associated with physical inactivity.

–Exercise may help delay or halt the age-related decline in bone mass.

–Resistance training may be more beneficial than aerobic training.

–Adaptations in bone are site-specific to the limbs exercised.

VII. ENVIRONMENTAL RISK FACTORS AND EXERCISE

A. HEAT

1. High ambient temperature and high relative humidity increase the risk of **heat-related disorders** such as heat cramps, heat syncope, dehydration, heat exhaustion, and heat stroke. Persons with hypertension or diabetes, obese individuals, unfit persons, pregnant women, children, the elderly, and individuals taking certain medications or alcohol may have particular difficulty adapting to high ambient temperature and high humidity, and thus are at increased risk for heat-related disorders.

2. High ambient temperature and high humidity may produce **increased heart rate response** at submaximal workloads, and **decreased oxygen consumption** at maximal workloads.

3. The **wet bulb globe temperature** is an index of environmental heat stress that is derived from measures of ambient temperature, relative humidity, and radiant heat. It provides guidance for exercise prescription to minimize the risk of developing heat-related illnesses.

4. General **guidelines for safe exercising** in high ambient temperatures and humidity are listed in **Table 4-4**.

B. COLD

–Cold exposure results in vasoconstriction with resulting blood pressure elevation. The elevation in blood pressure increases the oxygen demand on the heart. This lowers the angina threshold in patients who are prone to angina, and **may provoke resting angina** (variant or Prinzmetal's).

–Breathing large volumes of cold, dry air may provoke **exercise-induced asthma,** general dehydration, and dryness or burning of the mouth and throat.

–**Use the wind chill equivalent,** not the actual temperature, when gauging the risk of hypothermia and frostbite.

C. ALTITUDE

1. The primary consideration in exercise prescription at high altitude is to **lower the exercise intensity** (absolute workload), for the following reasons:

   –Acute exposure to high altitudes causes an increase in pulmonary ventilation, heart rate, and cardiac output at submaximal workloads.

   –After acclimatization to high altitudes, persons generally experience a continued increase in pulmonary ventilation and heart rate response at submaximal workloads, but reduced cardiac output, stroke volume, and heart rate at maximal exercise.

   –Even after exposure and training, there is approximately a 10% reduction in maximal oxygen consumption per 1,000 meters of altitude above 1,500 meters. These changes may lower the angina threshold.

2. Individuals with pulmonary hypertension, congestive heart failure, unstable angina, recent myocardial infarction, or severe anemia may be at greater risk for traveling or exercising at high altitudes.

D. CARBON MONOXIDE

–Prolonged exposure to carbon monoxide can reduce maximal oxygen consumption.

–Individuals with CAD have a lower angina threshold and are prone to arrhythmias induced by carbon monoxide exposure.

 Table 4-4. General Guidelines for Safe Exercise in High Temperatures and Humidity

Decrease the intensity and possibly the duration of the exercise session; if necessary, schedule intermittent rest periods.

Exercise in cool areas (e.g., an air-conditioned room) or during a cooler time of day (e.g., early morning, evening).

Be familiar with and alert for signs and symptoms of heat-related disorders, and know the appropriate first aid procedures.

Wear minimal, loose-fitting, light-colored clothing.

Ensure adequate hydration before, during, and after exercise.

Reduce the risk of developing heat-related illness through a gradual acclimation to exercise in hot environments (approximately 2 weeks).

–Guidelines for exercise prescription include avoiding carbon monoxide exposure, or decreasing the intensity and duration of exercise during periods or in areas of high ambient carbon monoxide levels (e.g., heavy motor vehicle traffic).

VIII. INFLUENCE OF DRUGS ON EXERCISE

–Common classes of drugs and their effects on resting and exercise electrocardiogram, heart rate, blood pressure, symptomatology, and exercise capacity are listed in Chapter 8, Table 8-8.

REVIEW TEST

DIRECTIONS: Carefully read all questions and select the BEST single answer.

1. Angina that occurs at rest is termed
   (A) silent.
   (B) stable.
   (C) variant.
   (D) typical.

2. A group of pulmonary disorders characterized by expiratory air flow obstruction, dyspnea (shortness of breath), and some degree of airway reversal is known as
   (A) bronchitis.
   (B) asthma.
   (C) emphysema.
   (D) chronic obstructive pulmonary disease.

3. The primary effects of chronic exercise training on lipid values are
   (A) decreased triglycerides and increased high-density lipoproteins.
   (B) decreased total cholesterol and low-density lipoproteins.
   (C) decreased high-density lipoprotein and increased low-density lipoproteins.
   (D) decreased total cholesterol and increased high-density lipoproteins.

4. Which of the following would be the best recommendation for exercise training outdoors in a hot and humid environment?
   (A) Wait for approximately 2 weeks to become acclimated to the heat before exercising.
   (B) Use a mode of activity, such as bicycling or running, that would increase heat loss by convection.
   (C) Reduce the exercise intensity.
   (D) Increase evaporative cooling by wiping away sweat that forms on the body.

5. Which of the following best explains the pathophysiology of coronary artery disease?
   (A) Injury to the artery wall begins in the media.
   (B) Platelets and thrombi form in the adventitia.
   (C) The endothelium takes up lipids, especially low-density lipoproteins.
   (D) Atherosclerotic lesions are formed in the intima.

6. A cardiac patient is taking a beta blocker medication. During an exercise test, you would expect
   (A) Cardiolite to be administered, because beta blockers depress the ST segment on the resting ECG.
   (B) an increase in the angina threshold compared to a test without the medication.
   (C) no change in heart rate or blood pressure compared to a test without the medication.
   (D) a slight decrease or no effect on blood pressure compared to a test without the medication.

7. The aging-related loss of elasticity (or "hardening") of the arteries is known as
   (A) atherosclerosis.
   (B) arteriosclerosis.
   (C) atheroma.
   (D) adventitia.

8. A deficiency of blood flow to the myocardium, resulting when the oxygen demand exceeds oxygen supply, is known as
   (A) infarction.
   (B) angina.
   (C) ischemia.
   (D) thrombosis.

9. What procedure uses a clot-dissolving agent during acute myocardial infarction to restore blood flow and limit myocardial necrosis?
   (A) Percutaneous transluminal coronary angioplasty
   (B) Thrombolytic therapy
   (C) Radionuclide imaging
   (D) Coronary artery bypass graft surgery

10. All of the following are suggestive of cardiovascular and pulmonary disease *except*
    (A) palpations that occur at rest.
    (B) dyspnea during strenuous exertion.
    (C) syncope during moderate-intensity exercise training.
    (D) substernal burning during exertion that dissipates with rest.

11. Modifiable primary risk factors for coronary artery disease include
    (A) hypertension, dyslipidemia, increasing age, and cigarette smoking.
    (B) postmenopausal status, excessive alcohol consumption, psychosocial stress, and high low-density lipoprotein level.
    (C) obesity, diabetes mellitus, cigarette smoking, and physical inactivity.
    (D) cigarette smoking, dyslipidemia, hypertension, and psychosocial stress.

12. What is the current state of knowledge on progression or regression of atherosclerosis in human coronary arteries?
    (A) Regression of atherosclerosis has been observed in clinical studies.
    (B) Regression of atherosclerosis has yet to be observed in clinical studies.
    (C) Progression of atherosclerosis begins at puberty.
    (D) There is no difference in the rate of progression or regression between those who undergo usual medical care and those who aggressively control risk factors.

13. What is the correct term and definition to describe a potential complication that may occur after an acute MI?
    (A) Expansion—another MI
    (B) Aneurysm—bulging of the ventricular wall
    (C) Extension—left ventricular dilation
    (D) Rupture—coronary artery breaks open

14. The purpose of risk stratification for cardiac patients is to
    (A) determine prognosis.
    (B) assess disease severity.
    (C) make clinical judgments for behavioral, pharmacological, or surgical interventions.
    (D) provide guidelines for participant monitoring and supervision during exercise training.

15. A classic sign of subendocardial ischemia is
    (A) angina.
    (B) ST segment depression.
    (C) ST segment elevation.
    (D) a pathologic Q wave.

16. What is the one true statement when comparing coronary bypass graph surgery (CABGS) and percutaneous transluminal coronary angioplasty (PTCA)?
    (A) PTCA has a higher rate of repeat revascularization than CABGS.
    (B) PTCA is indicated for patients who are unresponsive to CABGS.
    (C) CABGS is indicated for stenosis that is distal to the artery, whereas PTCA is reserved for stenosis that is proximal to the artery.
    (D) PTCA is contraindicated during the acute myocardial infarcted stage.

17. A possible mechanism by which chronic exercise training may reduce resting blood pressure in hypertensive individuals is through
    (A) an increase in plasma renin.
    (B) a higher cardiac output.
    (C) a reduced heart rate.
    (D) a lower stroke volume.

18. An embolism
    (A) can increase pulmonary vascular resistance.
    (B) is excessive fluid retention.
    (C) can be triggered by a chemical mediator such as histamine.
    (D) is an outward bulging of the ventricular wall.

19. A sedentary lifestyle
    (A) has a risk similar to that of hypertension, high cholesterol, and cigarette smoking.
    (B) increases HDL cholesterol.
    (C) increases the sensitivity to insulin.
    (D) has little influence on post-MI mortality rates.

ANSWERS AND EXPLANATIONS

1–C. Variant, or Prinzmetal's, angina is a form of unstable angina that occurs at rest due to coronary vasospasm. Typical, or classic, angina is usually provoked by physical activity and is relieved by rest or nitroglycerin. Stable angina is a form of typical angina that is predictable in onset, severity, and means of relief. Silent angina is not a medical term used to describe chest pain.

2–D. Bronchitis, asthma, and emphysema are all forms of chronic obstructive pulmonary disease (COPD).

3–A. Chronic exercise training has its greatest benefit on lowering triglycerides and increasing high-density lipoproteins. Changes in total cholesterol or low-density lipoprotein cholesterol are influenced more by dietary habits and body weight than by exercise training.

4–C. Compared to a cool and dry environment, there is a higher metabolic cost at submaximal workloads when exercising in the heat and humidity. Thus, one should alter the exercise prescription by lowering the intensity of work. Evaporation of sweat cools the skin; therefore, wiping away sweat would decrease evaporative cooling and heat loss. Heat loss by convection, such as that which occurs when a breeze is created by running can be beneficial but not unless the workload of activity is reduced. One must exercise in the heat and humidity to become acclimated to the environment; it will not occur by being sedentary.

5–D. Atherosclerotic lesions are formed in the intima. Injury to the artery wall does not begin in the media but rather in the endothelial layer with subsequent platelet and clot formation. Monocytes adhere to the endothelium, move to the intima, and take up cholesterol. The adventitia is the outermost layer of the artery wall and is not involved in the development of atherosclerosis.

6–B. Beta blockers increase the angina threshold by reducing myocardial oxygen demand at rest and during exercise. This occurs through a reduction in chronotropic (heart rate) and inotropic (strength of contraction) responses. Blood pressure is also reduced at rest and during exercise by a reduction in cardiac output (reduced chronotropic and inotropic response) and a reduction in total peripheral resistance. Beta blockers do not produce ST segment changes on the resting ECG.

7–B. Arteriosclerosis is often associated with the aging process with its characteristic "hardening" of the arteries, which is actually a loss of arterial elasticity. Atherosclerosis is a form of arteriosclerosis characterized by an accumulation of obstructive lesions within the arterial wall. The adventitia, the outermost layer of the artery wall, provides the media and intima with oxygen and other nutrients.

8–C. An outcome of significant coronary atherosclerosis, ischemia occurs when the oxygen supply does not meet oxygen demand, resulting from decreased blood flow to the myocardium. This process often leads to angina (symptoms) or infarction caused by a thrombosis.

9–B. Administration of streptokinase or t-PA (recombinant tissue plasminogen activator) within the first 1–2 hours after myocardial infarction may dissolve the clot causing the injury. This type of therapy, called thrombolytic therapy, is designed to restore blood flow and limit myocardial necrosis.

10–B. Dyspnea (shortness of breath) commonly occurs during strenuous exertion in healthy, well-trained persons and during moderate exertion in healthy, untrained persons. It should be regarded as abnormal, however, when it occurs at a level of exertion that is not expected to evoke this symptom in a given individual. Underlying cardiac arrhythmias may cause palpitations, even at rest. Syncope is loss of consciousness and is abnormal at rest or during any level of exertion. The location (substernal), character (burning), and provoking factor (exertion that dissipates with rest) of substernal burning are features of classic ischemia.

11–C. The primary modifiable risk factors for CAD are tobacco smoking, dyslipidemia, hypertension, physical inactivity, obesity, and diabetes mellitus. The primary nonmodifiable risk factors for CAD are increasing age, male gender, and family history. Secondary risk factors for CAD include psychosocial stress, postmenopausal status, and excessive alcohol consumption.

12–A. Clinical studies of cardiac patients have shown that long-term aggressive control of CAD risk factors can reduce or halt the rate of progression and may actually result in regression of atherosclerotic plaque. Individuals who aggressively attack, reduce, and control risk factors are more likely to see favorable results than individuals who undergo usual medical care. The process of atherosclerosis begins at birth.

13–B. A ventricular aneurysm is a bulging of the ventricular wall. Expansion is dilation of the left ventricle while extension is another myocardial infarction. Rupture is an aneurysm that breaks open in the ventricular wall not the coronary artery.

14–D. The purpose of risk stratification for cardiac patients is to make appropriate recommendations regarding supervision during exercise training. Guidelines are available from the American Heart Association, American Association of Cardiovascular and Pulmonary Rehabilitation, and American College of Physicians. Although risk stratification is based on the likelihood of experiencing an untoward cardiac event, it does not attempt to predict prognosis, severity of disease, or treatment options. Different nomograms and tables are available for such information.

15–B. A classic sign of MI ischemia is ST segment alteration. ST segment depression suggests subendocardial ischemia, whereas ST segment elevation indicates transmural ischemia. Pathologic Q waves point to transmural MI. Angina is a classic symptom, not a sign, of ischemia.

16–A. Within 6 months, up to 50% of PTCA patients will be restenosed, whereas bypass grafts are dysfunctional somewhere in the range of 10% to 60% at 10 years. CABGS is indicated for patients who are unresponsive to other treatments, including PTCA, and for patients with proximal disease, especially left main stenosis, whereas PTCA is typically done for distal occlusions. PTCA can be used during the early stages of acute MI, especially in individuals who are not candidates for thrombolytic therapy. In-hospital mortality rates for CABGS and PTCA are similar.

17–C. Blood pressure is the product of cardiac output and total peripheral resistance. A benefit of exercise training is a reduction in cardiac output and total peripheral resistance at any given workload including rest. A lower cardiac output is probably due to a reduction in heart rate as a result of an increased stroke volume and arteriovenous oxygen difference. Plasma renin is a catalyst for vasoconstriction. It is reduced, not increased, with exercise training.

18–B. Pulmonary patients and apparently healthy individuals have a linear increase in heart rate to oxygen consumption. The pulmonary patient will be limited by some mechanism that ultimately results in inefficient pulmonary gas exchange. An attempt to correct for this factor will be shown by a high ventilation per unit of oxygen consumed (VE/VO_2), a high percentage of pulmonary ventilation to maximal voluntary ventilation (VE/MVV), and a high respiratory rate.

19–A. The risk ratios of hypertension (2.1), high cholesterol (2.4), cigarette smoking (2.5) and physical inactivity (1.9) are similar. Physical inactivity results in a lowering of HDL cholesterol and a decrease in the sensitivity of insulin (higher plasma glucose values). Studies have shown that in post MI patients a regular exercise training program can significantly reduce mortality rates as compared to less active post MI individuals.

CHAPTER 5

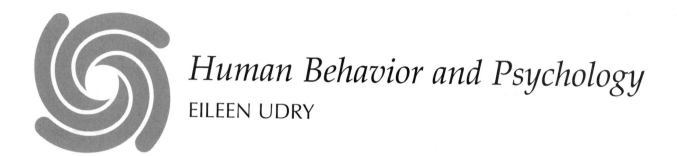

Human Behavior and Psychology
EILEEN UDRY

I. FOUNDATIONAL INTERPERSONAL SKILLS FOR THE EXERCISE SPECIALIST

–Effective interpersonal skills are not limited to what the exercise specialist says, but also include **how well the exercise specialist can listen to and assess the verbal and nonverbal communication** of program participants.

–Developing effective interpersonal skills serves **four purposes** for the exercise specialist: (1) developing rapport and conveying a sense of empathy; (2) assessing health-related functions; (3) facilitating change; and (4) assisting in the management of transient life crises.

A. DEVELOPING RAPPORT AND CONVEYING A SENSE OF EMPATHY

–Each patient should feel as if the exercise specialist understands the challenges he or she faces relative to rehabilitation and making health behavior changes. To this end, the exercise specialist should:

1. **Express acceptance.**

   –A tone of openness and acceptance toward participants should be fostered. Participants who feel they are being judged by the exercise specialist may not disclose important medical and/or lifestyle information.

2. **Use active listening; paraphrase the participant's response.**

   –Active listening allows the listener to make sure that he or she has accurately interpreted what the participant has said. It also conveys that the listener is sincerely attempting to understand what was said.

3. **Attend to nonverbal communication.**

   a. Nonverbal communication modes include:

      –**Kinesics** (body movements such as eye contact)

      –**Paralinguistics** (characteristics of speech, such as voice inflection and volume)

      –**Proxemics** (characteristics of interpersonal body placement, such as how much personal space individuals prefer)

   b. Nonverbal communication will sometimes provide information that is different from what the speaker expresses verbally. For instance, a patient states that "I followed my exercise plan *fairly* well while I was away," but, based on voice inflection, the exercise specialist might conclude that the patient actually was not able to follow the exercise plan "fairly well."

B. ASSESSING HEALTH-RELATED FUNCTIONS

–An exercise specialist who can communicate effectively is more likely to be able to obtain a complete health history from patients.

C. FACILITATING CHANGE

–The exercise specialist should serve as a facilitator rather than simply a prescriber of change. In this type of partnership, the **ultimate goal is for** patients to accept and maintain responsibility for their health behaviors.

–Patients may express **ambivalence** about making changes in health behaviors (e.g., adopting a low-fat diet, beginning an exercise program). To deal with a patient's ambivalence, the exercise specialist may find **gentle confrontation** useful; for example, "Jim, you need to help me understand you better. You say you want to exercise, yet your lack of attendance at sessions indicates otherwise."

D. ASSISTING IN THE MANAGEMENT OF TRANSIENT LIFE CRISES

–A patient may be experiencing emotional turbulence due to a transient life crisis, such as marital difficulty, financial problems, or a change in job status. Having good foundational interpersonal skills better enables the exercise specialist to make referrals to appropriate mental health professionals as needed.

II. PATIENT COPING AND CRISIS MANAGEMENT

–The exercise specialist should be able to recognize the various ways that patients typically respond to acute health stressors (e.g., a recent health setback) and to make necessary referrals when a patient demonstrates maladaptive forms of coping.

A. COMMON COPING REACTIONS

1. **Denial**

   –A patient experiencing **denial** is attempting to ignore, avoid, or minimize a problem.

   a. **Denial can be unhealthy** if it results in a delay or avoidance in seeking treatment for a problem (e.g., delay in diagnosis and treatment for a cardiac disorder).

   b. On the other hand, **in the short term denial may be a positive way to eliminate stress** in those circumstances in which an immediate solution to a problem is not possible (e.g., to alleviate worry about a possible job layoff, a situation out of one's control).

2. **Problem-focused coping**

   –The individual is attempting to define the problem, generate possible solutions, weigh the alternatives, and make a choice.

   –This form of coping is considered most appropriate when there is a solution to the stressor and the individual has a good deal of control over the situation. For example, a person may have received a medical diagnosis that he or she doesn't completely understand, and this lack of understanding may be unsettling. A problem-focusing coping reaction would be to consult one or more additional sources of medical information.

3. **Emotion-focused coping**

   –The individual attempts to regulate his or her emotional response to a stressful situation.

   –This type of coping reaction is more passive and nonphysical than problem-focused coping.

   –Emotion-focused coping is considered appropriate when a solution to a problem is not under the individual's control. For example, a cardiac patient may be detained in a waiting room before surgery, exposed to sights and sounds of the medical facility that are perceived as anxiety provoking. Under these conditions, using relaxation exercises to control his response to this uncontrollable situation would be an example of an emotion-focused reaction.

4. **Social-focused coping**

   –The individual attempts to include other people in the coping process.

   –For example, a person who has just received a medical diagnosis may seek out others with a similar diagnosis and solicit information and support from these individuals.

   –This coping reaction requires that the patient be able to adequately express his or her needs to others and behave in such a way as to elicit support and cooperation from others.

B. TYPES OF MALADJUSTMENT/ IMPAIRMENTS

–For various reasons, a participant in a rehabilitation program may feel unable to cope with the demands made on him or her. This perception may stem from the participant's recent change in health, or it may be the result of a long-term maladjustment problem that has just now come to light.

–The exercise specialist should be prepared to recognize the common types and symptoms of maladjustment or impairment and respond accordingly.

1. **Depression**

   a. **Symptoms** include feelings of being overwhelmed or helpless, tearfulness, withdrawal from usual social activities, loss of appetite or rapid weight gain, lack of sleep or change in sleep patterns (e.g., early morning awakening), fatigue, and excessive guilt feelings.

b. Incidence and course of action

–Depression affects approximately 5%–10% of all adults at some point in life.

–Patients hospitalized for myocardial infarction (MI) often report feeling depressed.

–Depression from acute health stressors typically subsides after several weeks or when usual activities are resumed.

–If depression either worsens or persists beyond 2–3 weeks, then referral to a primary care physician or a mental health professional is appropriate.

2. Anxiety

a. Symptoms include feeling "on edge" or "uptight" most of the time, rapid or shallow breathing, elevated heart rate, and panic attacks for no apparent reason (e.g., increased fear and physiological arousal when entering public or open spaces).

b. Courses of action include allowing the patient extra time and practice when learning a new skill, task, or procedure (e.g., a new exercise); having the patient exercise in a quiet, private setting whenever possible; and instructing the patient to focus on breathing and relaxation exercises.

3. Anger

a. Symptoms

–Illness or injury commonly produces stress. For many patients, this stress causes anxiety and depression; however, some (in particular, men), may react with feelings of anger.

b. Courses of action

–An angry or hostile patient often is more receptive to changing his or her behavior when given specific information linking anger to chronic health problems (e.g., cardiac dysfunction).

–The patient may benefit from relaxation exercises and stress management training, including interpersonal skill-building exercises that point out how he or she may be creating taxing social environments.

4. Cognitive impairments

–Stroke, organic brain disorders, and other neurologic problems may cause cognitive impairments such as memory loss, confusion,

unexpected changes in behavior, and/or difficulty in planning and organizing.

–Although not responsible for treating cognitive impairments, the exercise specialist should be alert for their sudden development, particularly in older adults and other patients at high risk, and make referrals as necessary.

5. Substance abuse and eating disorders

–Patients with substance abuse or eating disorders should be referred to mental health specialists.

C. GENERAL SIGNS OF MALADJUSTMENT

–Maladjustment may be identified and evaluated by exploring the following areas:

1. Have the patient's normal lifestyle patterns been disrupted as a result of the crisis?

2. Is the patient able to hold a job (as appropriate)?

3. Can the patient handle the responsibilities of daily living, such as keeping appointments, paying bills, and maintaining adequate nutrition?

4. Has the crisis disrupted the lives of others?

5. Is the patient's usual social support system intact, depleted, or absent?

6. Has the crisis significantly disrupted the patient's perception of reality?

D. RISK FACTORS FOR SUICIDE

–See **Table 5-1**.

Table 5-1. Risk Factors for Suicide

Although prediction of suicide is difficult, a patient's risk for suicide should be taken seriously if any of the following factors are noted:

Previous suicide attempt

Overt or indirect talk or threat of suicide

A current plan for how to commit suicide

The means to carry out the suicide plan

Depressed mood

Significant loss (e.g., spouse, job)

Sudden, unexpected change in attitude or behavior

Elderly male, isolated with chronic illness

Sense of loneliness, hopelessness, exhaustion, or "unbearable" psychological pain

Alcohol or drug use or intoxication

Failing health, particularly if previously independent

E. MAXIMIZING THE EFFECTIVENESS OF REFERRALS

–If the exercise specialist determines that a patient needs to be referred to a mental health professional, such a referral will tend to be most effective when:

1. The patient believes that the exercise specialist has a basic understanding of the problem.

2. The patient accepts the need for the referral and believes that his or her situation is likely to improve from the referral.

3. The exercise specialist is familiar with the mental health professional to whom the patient is being referred.

4. Follow-up and contact are made with the patient after the referral.

III. SOCIAL SUPPORT AND GROUP DYNAMICS

–Research shows that social influences can have a powerful effect in ensuring lasting changes in health behavior and on overall well-being.

–Patients may be positively or negatively influenced by "important others" (e.g., family members, close friends, other program participants).

–When the influence of important others is positive, it is termed **social support;** when negative, it is termed **negative social influence.**

A. SOCIAL SUPPORT

–is defined as the comfort, assistance, or information one receives through formal and informal contacts with individuals and groups.

1. **Types of social support**

   –**Tangible support** includes providing assistance with transportation and activities of daily living, such as meal preparation.

   –**Affectionate support** includes making one feel wanted and providing affection and love.

   –**Positive social interaction** involves engaging in enjoyable activities with others.

   –**Emotional/informational support** involves listening, giving advice, and sharing personal worries or concerns.

2. **Maximizing social support**

   –**Optimal matching** involves determining and, if possible, providing the specific type(s) and amount of social support that the patient needs. For example, emotional/informational support may be preferred before hospitalization for a health condition, and more tangible support may be needed following surgery and during rehabilitation.

   –If one support provider attempts to provide all forms of social support, he or she may experience feelings of being overextended, or **social resource bankruptcy.** The exercise specialist and other members of the patient's social network should guard against this form of depletion.

3. **Social support across the lifespan**

   a. **Middle-aged adults**

      –The **primary sources of social support** are spouses, friends, and coworkers.

      –Commonly provided **forms of support** include encouragement, participation in exercise and health activities, and provision of tangible assistance, such as child care and transportation.

      –Individuals generally are more likely to participate in physical activity when they have a companion (e.g., "buddy system").

   b. **Older adults**

      –**Primary sources of social support** are spouses, friends, and community social systems (e.g., senior centers).

      –Older adults benefit greatly from physical activity (perhaps more so than any other age group); however, they may face numerous social barriers to adopting and maintaining an active lifestyle, including insufficient encouragement from physicians, lack of peer involvement, or disapproval or absence of spouse. Thus, the development and maintenance of a social network that supports physical activity for an older adult may be challenging.

B. NEGATIVE SOCIAL INFLUENCE

–The negative influence of certain participants can undermine efforts to create a socially supportive atmosphere.

1. **Chronic complainers**

   –Patients who continually complain should be carefully interviewed. Some have legitimate medical conditions (e.g., joint or back problems) that cause pain during exercise, and their exercise program can be modified accordingly. Others will have complaints that stem from their dissatisfaction with the program; these concerns should be dealt with directly.

–A disruptive complainer may be asked to modify his or her behavior or leave the program.

   2. **Disrupters/comedians**

   –A patient with an extreme need for attention may be channeled into a productive leadership role within the group (e.g., taking attendance).

   –Any disrupter/comedian who poses a threat to others or detracts from the program's goals should be dealt with directly by the exercise specialist or group leader.

   3. **Overexerters**

   –Some patients work too hard during rehabilitation or physical activity, increasing the risk of injury and the chance of burn-out and consequent noncompliance with the program.

–An overexerter may benefit from instruction on how to pace the exercise program to avoid counterproductive excessive effort.

–Pairing an overexerter with a former overexerter who has modified his or her rehabilitation approach may be beneficial.

   4. **Underexerters**

   –Some patients do not work hard enough to benefit from prescribed rehabilitation.

   –Sedentary individuals typically go through a period of adjustment during which they must learn to tolerate increased levels of discomfort from exercise. Underexertion typically occurs during this period.

   –An underexerter can benefit from gentle but steady encouragement and/or pairing with a peer who is at a more advanced stage in a similar rehabilitation program.

IV. HEALTH BEHAVIOR CHANGE MODEL

–To explain why individuals succeed in or fail to make needed changes, a **health behavior change model** (Figure 5-1) has been synthesized from several existing theoretical frameworks (e.g., stages of change model, health belief model, social learning theory).

–In this model, health behavior change occurs in **three phases: antecedents, adoption, and maintenance.**

A. ANTECEDENTS

–Various factors can support, initiate, or hinder changes in health behaviors.

   1. **Information and instructions**

   –The exercise specialist must not assume that a patient has received appropriate health information. Although patients tend to follow physicians' instructions regarding physical

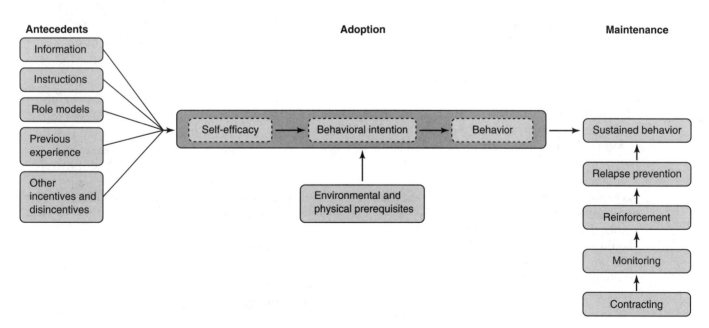

FIGURE 5-1 Integrated model of health behavior change. Health behavior change can be divided into antecedent, adoption, and maintenance phases. (With permission from *ACSM's Resource Manual for Guidelines for Exercise Testing and Prescription,* 3rd ed. Baltimore, Williams & Wilkins, 1998, p. 543.)

activity, relatively few physicians actually discuss physical activity programs with their patients.

–Patients' understanding of critical information needs to be carefully evaluated. Most people read only a small fraction of written instructional material. Moreover, 30%–40% of people read at the 7th-grade level or lower.

–The effectiveness of instructions is enhanced when accompanied by reminders and feedback, and when the instructional material is clear, simple, and concise.

2. **Role models**

–Family, friends, and others who have experienced similar circumstances can play a powerful role in facilitating change.

–Taped testimonials from successful past program participants can be useful when access to live role models is limited.

–Role models who demonstrate the actual strategies they used to make needed changes (e.g., dietary changes for weight loss) are particularly effective.

3. **Previous experience**

–Past behavior is a good predictor of future behavior. Thus, a person who has had a bad experience related to health behavior is likely to have reservations about adopting the same or a similar behavior in the future.

–Discussion of past health behaviors may provide an opportunity to examine and refute unreasonable beliefs or misconceptions about the behavior (e.g., "Older adults must always conserve their energy.").

4. **Incentives**

–Providing incentives for change influences a patient's **decisional balance** when weighing whether to participate in a program. A patient tends to engage in a behavior only when the perceived benefits (e.g., improved health and function) outweigh the costs (e.g., money, time, pain).

–Whenever possible, **the immediate benefits of a health behavior change** should be emphasized. For example, post-MI patients should focus on the immediate social benefits that they derive from being in a group rehabilitation setting, rather than the long-range medical benefits.

B. **ADOPTION**

–is the early phase of making a change or intending to make a change in a health behavior.

–This is often the most difficult phase of change. For example, persons trying to quit smoking often report feeling like they've lost a good friend.

1. **Environmental and physical prerequisites**

–Certain environmental and physical prerequisites typically must be met for health behavior change to occur (e.g., proper clothing and/or equipment, medical release).

2. **Self-efficacy and outcome efficacy**

–A person desiring to change a health behavior must have a **minimum level of self-efficacy**—confidence in one's ability to successfully engage in the activity (e.g., learn and perform a new exercise routine).

–Before an individual can change a behavior, he or she must have a certain **level of outcome efficacy**—belief that the change will lead to the desired outcome (e.g., "engaging in regular exercise will enhance quality of life.").

3. **Cues to action**

–are environmental and physical reminders that can stimulate change. Examples include reminder cards or calls, preparation of workout gear, and the presence of adverse symptoms (e.g., shortness of breath).

–Making a successful behavior change often involves substituting one behavior for another, rather than simply giving up a behavior. Cues to action should support this. For example, a cue to action for one smoker at the end of a meal was to prepare coffee to drink while having a cigarette. The substitute behavior chosen was walking the dog; thus, the new cue to action was placing the dog's leash in plain view.

4. **Goal setting and behavioral intention**

–Goals should be flexible, individualized, and realistic.

–A combination of short-term (specific) and long-term goals is generally most effective.

–It can be helpful to have the patient rate his or her confidence in the ability to reach a specific goal (from 0%–100%). A confidence level of 70% or higher indicates an appropriate goal; a lower level suggests the need for a revised, more realistic goal.

C. **MAINTENANCE**

–Once a behavioral change is made, various strategies will increase the likelihood of maintaining the change.

1. **Relapse prevention**

–The patient should identify and prepare for periods when disruption of the changed behavior is more likely; for example, an exercise routine tends to get disrupted during holiday seasons, but reminder phone calls from a friend may encourage continued participation.

–Once a lapse has occurred, additional effort will be needed to resume the behavioral change.

2. **Reinforcement**

–Positive reinforcement is a powerful way to sustain behavioral change. A wide range of reinforcers can be useful (e.g., attention, awards, food).

–Reinforcers tend to be idiosyncratic. The exercise specialist should strive to understand a patient's specific preferences/motivators.

–Generally, the farther an individual is from achieving his or her target goal, the more useful are external rewards and incentives (because the activity itself is not yet intrinsically reinforcing).

3. **Monitoring and self-monitoring**

–Sustained behavioral change is often correlated with the extent to which the individual uses self-monitoring strategies, which indicates a willingness to take personal responsibility for his or her health.

–**Self-reporting measures,** such as log sheets and diaries, can help the exercise specialist and patient monitor progress and solve problems.

–Monitoring/self-monitoring can also be tied to goal setting and reinforcement (e.g., accomplishments can be reviewed and a reward provided).

4. **Contracting**

–**Contracts** are extensions of goal setting and self-monitoring that take written form.

–Contracts should not be unrealistic or rigid but should outline possible solutions to a problem, a planned course of action, and consequences of achieving and not achieving a goal.

REVIEW TEST

DIRECTIONS: Carefully read all questions and select the BEST single answer.

1. As a form of nonverbal communication, kinesics involves attending to
   (A) characteristics of interpersonal body placement, such as how much interpersonal space individuals prefer.
   (B) body movements, such as eye contact.
   (C) characteristics of speech, such as voice inflection and volume.
   (D) management of transient life crises.

2. Which of the following statements about the role of the exercise specialist as a facilitator of change is true?
   (A) The goal is for patients to accept and maintain responsibility for their health behavior.
   (B) The goal is for the exercise specialist to use an aggressive and confrontational approach to stimulate change in patients.
   (C) The exercise specialist does not have to attend to patients' nonverbal communication.
   (D) The exercise specialist probably will not be able to help patients make significant lifestyle changes.

3. The use of active listening
   (A) tends to make patients feel as if they are being judged.
   (B) focuses on the use of denial as a coping mechanism.
   (C) allows the listener to make sure that he or she has accurately interpreted what the patient (or speaker) has said.
   (D) is a way to exercise when counseling patients about exercising.

4. Which of the following best describes problem-focused coping?
   (A) The individual is attempting to include other people in the coping process.
   (B) The individual is attempting to ignore, avoid, or minimize a problem.
   (C) The individual is attempting to regulate his or her emotional response to a stressful situation.
   (D) The individual is attempting to define the problem, generate possible solutions, and weigh alternatives.

5. Which of the following is *not* considered a symptom of depression?
   (A) Change in sleep pattern
   (B) Crying
   (C) Feelings of hopelessness
   (D) Hearing voices

6. Which of the following statements about depression in exercise program participants is *not* true?
   (A) It is often reported by patients hospitalized for MI.
   (B) It is not considered appropriate for the exercise specialist to suggest a referral to a primary care physician or mental health professionals if the depression persists for more than 2–3 weeks.
   (C) When depression stems from acute health stressors, it typically subsides after several weeks and/or resumption of normal activities.
   (D) It affects approximately 5%–10% of adults during their lifetime.

7. Which of the following is *not* considered a symptom of generalized anxiety disorder?
   (A) Autonomic hyperactivity (e.g., sweating, dry mouth)
   (B) Scanning (e.g., constantly feeling keyed up or on edge)
   (C) Motor tension (e.g., restlessness, trembling)
   (D) A feeling of being in control

8. Although predicting suicide is difficult, which of the following patients generally would be considered to be at the greatest risk for suicide?
   (A) An elderly man isolated with an acute illness
   (B) An elderly man isolated with a chronic illness
   (C) An elderly woman isolated with a chronic illness
   (D) An elderly woman isolated with an acute illness

9. When referring a program participant to a mental health professional, the exercise specialist can maximize the effectiveness of the referral by
   (A) conveying limited understanding of the problem to the patient.
   (B) being familiar with the professional to whom the patient is being referred.
   (C) not maintaining contact with the participant after the referral.
   (D) avoiding discussing the patient's case with the professional to whom the patient is referred.

10. The concept that patients may need different amounts and types of social support depending on the timing and the nature of the stressor refers to
    (A) social resource bankruptcy.
    (B) negative social influence.
    (C) emotional/informational support.
    (D) optimal matching.

11. Providing a patient with assistance in meal preparation following surgery is an example of which type of social support?
    (A) Affectionate support
    (B) Positive social interaction
    (C) Tangible support
    (D) Emotional/informational support

12. A difference between middle-aged adults and older adults relative to their most salient sources of social support is that
    (A) older adults tend to rely more on community social systems.
    (B) middle-aged adults tend to rely more on community social systems.
    (C) older adults tend to receive a great deal of encouragement from physicians to exercise.
    (D) older adults tend to rely more on peers for support.

13. When dealing with a program participant who appears to be a "chronic complainer," all of the following actions are recommended *except:*
    (A) carefully interviewing the individual about any legitimate concerns, such as a limiting medical condition.
    (B) if program concerns are the basis of the complaint, dealing with such concerns through direct discussions with the participant.
    (C) if discussions with the chronic complainer do not result in a satisfactory solution, possibly requesting that the individual make other program arrangements.
    (D) discussing the importance of pacing and being careful not to exercise beyond the recommended upper limit.

14. Which of the following has been identified as a useful strategy for dealing with a program participant identified as a disrupter/comedian?
    (A) Discuss the concept of pacing during exercise.
    (B) Channel the individual's need for attention into a productive leadership role within the group, such as taking attendance.
    (C) Ignore the situation, as it will probably resolve itself.
    (D) Deal with any concerns about the program through direct discussions with the individual.

15. Important phases of making a health behavior change are
    (A) intrinsic and extrinsic motivation.
    (B) adoption and maintenance.
    (C) antecedents, adoption, and maintenance.
    (D) direct and buffering.

16. The term "decisional balance" refers to
    (A) the processes that patients engage in when deciding whether to adopt or continue to engage in a health behavior.
    (B) the outcome expectancies of individuals relative to health behavior changes.
    (C) the self-efficacy levels of program participants.
    (D) whether or not the program participant feels that he or she is receiving social support for a behavior change.

17. Which of the following statements about providing information or educational material to help people make behavior changes is true?
    (A) The information should be stated in simple language, because more than 30% of the general population reads at or below the 7th-grade level.
    (B) Most people receive information about physical activity from their physicians.
    (C) Most people will read more than 90% of the information provided to them and demonstrate an adequate understanding of this information.
    (D) People who seem to benefit the most from the information will not ignore it.

18. Which of the following statements about relapse and relapse prevention is true?
    (A) A single behavior (e.g., smoking one cigarette) never precedes a total relapse.
    (B) Having the participant write down what he or she will do in the face of exercise barriers (e.g., illness, vacation) is an effective way to reduce the chance of relapse.
    (C) A participant who has relapsed will not need additional effort to overcome the lapse.
    (D) There is only one way to prevent relapse, through goal setting.

19. Which of the following statements about the principles of reinforcement is *not* correct?
    (A) Reinforcers tend to be universal (i.e., most participants will agree on what is reinforcing).
    (B) The farther a participant is from achieving his or her goals, the more likely that external rewards will be effective.
    (C) A narrow range of positive reinforcers should be used.
    (D) Continued adherence to a program usually results from behavioral success, rather than from education and instruction.

20. Which of the following is NOT considered to be an example of "generalization training" as it pertains to facilitating sustained exercise adherence?
    (A) Including family or significant others in exercise sessions
    (B) Requiring unsupervised home sessions from the early stage of the program
    (C) Adding additional exercises before graduation that are easily maintained in the home environment
    (D) Informing people of the general benefits of exercise

ANSWERS AND EXPLANATIONS

1–B. Kinesics refers to body movements, such as eye contact. Proxemics refers to characteristics of interpersonal body placement, such as how much interpersonal space individuals prefer. Paralinguistics refers to characteristics of speech, such as voice inflection and volume.

2–A. When the exercise specialist serves as facilitator rather than prescriber of change, the goal is for participants to accept and maintain responsibility for their health behavior. This approach does not rely on an aggressive approach, although gentle confrontations may be necessary to deal with patient ambivalence. The facilitator, rather than prescriber, of change approach is thought to be very useful in terms of helping participants make significant long-term lifestyle changes.

3–C. Active listening, or paraphrasing the participant's response, allows the listener to make sure that he or she has accurately interpreted what the participant has said. When used correctly, active listening lets the participant feel as if the listener is sincerely attempting to understand what was said rather than being judged. Active listening does not focus on denial as a coping mechanism, but involves genuine engagement in the communication process.

4–D. A person using problem-focused coping is attempting to define the problem, generate possible solutions, and weigh alternatives. In social-focused coping, the individual attempts to include others in the coping process. Denial is characterized by attempting to ignore, avoid, or minimize a problem. Emotion-focused coping is evident when the individual is attempting to regulate his or her emotional response to a stressful situation.

5–D. Depression may be marked by various symptoms including a change in sleep patterns, crying, feelings of hopelessness, fatigue, excessive guilt, loss of appetite, and rapid weight gain. Hearing voices is generally a sign of some form of mental disruption other than depression.

6–B. When program participants appear to be struggling with depression lasting longer than 2–3 weeks, it is considered appropriate for the exercise specialist to suggest a referral to a primary care physician or mental health professional. Depression is relatively common in patients hospitalized from MI and will affect some 5%–10% of all adults at some point. If the depression stems from acute health stressors, it typically will subside after several weeks and/or as more activities of daily living can be resumed.

7–D. Generalized anxiety disorder is characterized by increases in autonomic hyperactivity, scanning, and increased muscle tension. Individuals with this disorder often report a loss of feelings of control.

8–B. Prediction of suicide is not an exact science, although the possibility of suicide should always be taken seriously. Elderly men who are isolated and have a chronic illness are considered a greater risk for suicide than either women or men with an acute illness.

9–B. The effectiveness of a referral to a mental health professional tends to be enhanced when (1) the exercise specialist is familiar with the individual to whom the patient is being referred, (2) the patient believes that the exercise specialist has a basic understanding of the problem, (3) follow-up and contact are made with the patient after the referral, and (4) the patient accepts the need for the referral and believes that his or her situation is likely to improve based on the referral.

10–D. The optimal matching approach to social support suggests that individuals may need different amounts and types of social support, depending on the timing and the nature of the stressor. Social resource bankruptcy can occur when a social support provider attempts to provide all forms of social support, which can lead to feelings of being overextended. Negative social influence refers to the negative influence associated with some interpersonal interactions. Emotional/informational support is a specific type of positive social support that involves listening, giving advice, and/or sharing personal worries or concerns.

11–C. Tangible support involves providing assistance with activities of daily living (e.g., meal preparation, transportation). Affectionate support includes making an individual feel wanted and cared for by providing affection and love. Positive social interaction involves sharing enjoyable activities with others. Emotional/informational support includes listening, giving advice, and sharing personal worries or concerns.

12–A. It is important to take into account lifespan issues when considering social support among program participants. To this end, older adults tend to rely more on community social resources than middle-aged adults. A barrier that older adults experience relative to adopting and maintaining an active lifestyle is that they often receive insufficient encouragement from their physicians (and/or receive disapproval or have an absent spouse).

13–D. Answers A, B, and C are strategies that are suggested for dealing with a chronic complainer. The discussion of pacing and overexertion are suggested strategies for dealing with program participants who do not comply with the program guidelines (i.e., noncompliers) by virtue of overexerting.

14–B. When dealing with a program participant who is a disrupter/comedian, it can be helpful to channel the individual's need for attention into a productive leadership role within the group. If the disrupter/comedian's behavior poses a threat to others or is inconsistent with the goals of the program, direct discussions with the individual should occur. Discussions of pacing are more appropriate for individuals who are overexerters rather than disrupters/comedians.

15–C. The three important phases of making health behavior change include antecedents, adoption, and maintenance. Intrinsic and extrinsic motivation refer to two forms of motivations that may influence the intensity and direction of individual behavior, but these forms of motivation are distinct from the phases of health behavior change. The direct and buffering explanations have been forwarded as explanations for why social support is thought to be helpful in reducing stress.

16–A. An individual considering whether to adopt or continue to engage in a health behavior engages in "decisional balance," weighing the perceived costs and benefits of the behavior. Outcome expectancies refer to the belief that engaging in a health behavior will lead to the desired outcome. Self-efficacy refers to the extent to which an individual feels confident that he or she can engage in an activity.

17–A. The information that is provided to participants should be provided in simple language, because more than 30% of the population reads at or below the 7th-grade reading level. Additionally, most people only read 10%–15% of the information provided unless they are extremely interested in the topic. In terms of people sources of information on health-related matters, whereas medical sources are viewed as highly credible, relatively few physicians provide patients with information related to behaviors such as physical activity. Finally, it seems to be true that people who would seem to benefit most from information often will ignore it.

18–B. Having participants write down what they would do when facing a barrier to exercise (e.g., illness, vacation) is an effective way to reduce relapse. It has been observed that even a single cigarette may lead to a total relapse in smoking cessation. When relapse occurs, a patient may require additional effort to overcome the lapse.

19–A. When considering the use of reinforcers, it should be recognized that a wide range of reinforcers may be effective (e.g., attention, food, awards). However, the exercise specialist needs to be aware that reinforcers tend to be idiosyncratic rather than universal—that is, what is reinforcing to one person may not be so for another. A program participant in the early stages of making a behavior change likely will need to rely more on the use of external rewards, because the behavior is not yet intrinsically rewarding. Finally, continued adherence to a program usually results from behavioral success rather than education and instruction. This helps explain why many people, despite being knowledgeable about exercise, do not exercise.

20–D. Generalization training involves expanding behavior in a setting or a set of circumstances to a different setting to link the behavior with cues or "stimuli" in the second setting that may facilitate adherence. The other responses are all examples of using generalization training. Simply informing people of the general benefits of exercise is not a strategy that expands people's behavioral repertoire.

CHAPTER 6

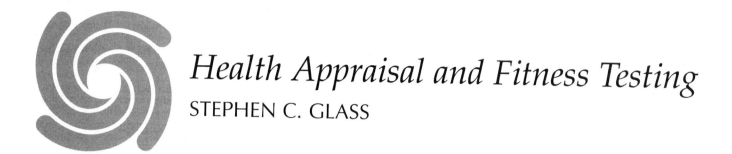

Health Appraisal and Fitness Testing
STEPHEN C. GLASS

I. PRETEST CONSIDERATIONS

A. HEALTH APPRAISAL

–Essential information is required before exercise testing to identify any necessary modifications of test protocols, risk factors for/contraindications to testing, or the need for referral to a physician.

1. **Health history**

   a. **Present history**

      –Known disease and/or symptoms of disease

      –Activity level

      –Dietary behaviors (including caffeine and alcohol intake)

      –Smoking/tobacco use

      –Medication use (including recreational drugs), drug allergies

   b. **Past history**

      –Cardiorespiratory problems

      –Orthopedic problems

      –Recent illnesses/hospitalizations

      –Exercise history

      –Work history

   c. **Family history**

      –Onset of heart disease in first-degree relative before age 55 (men) or 65 (women)

      –Other significant disorders, including diabetes, hyperlipidemia, stroke, and sudden death

   d. **Health screening questionnaire**

      –A pre-participation health screening tool, such as the **Physical Activity Readiness Questionnaire (PAR-Q)**, should be completed before exercise testing (**Figure 6-1**).

2. **Physical assessment and laboratory tests**

   a. **Resting heart rate**

      –After the client has been sitting quietly for 5 minutes, the pulse is palpated at the radial or carotid artery for 30 seconds; normal resting heart rate is 60–100 beats per minute (bpm).

   b. **Resting blood pressure**

      –Because blood pressure can fluctuate, accurate blood pressure assessment should be based on two or more measurements; findings are compared to published standards (see Chapter 4, Table 4-2).

      –Blood pressure should be measured with the client in both the supine and standing positions to screen for postural hypotension.

   c. **Lung capacity**

      –Tests of lung capacity assess airway patency and airflow volume and rate during one breath.

      (1) Forced vital capacity (FVC)

      –is the volume of air expired following a maximal inspiration.

      –assesses the degree of restrictive pulmonary disease.

      (2) Forced expiratory capacity at 1 second (FEV_1)

      –is the proportion of the FVC expired in 1 second.

      –assesses the degree of airway obstruction.

Physical Activity Readiness
Questionnaire - PAR-Q
(revised 1994)

PAR - Q & YOU

(A Questionnaire for People Aged 15 to 69)

Regular physical activity is fun and healthy, and increasingly more people are starting to become more active every day. Being more active is very safe for most people. However, some people should check with their doctor before they start becoming much more physically active.

If you are planning to become much more physically active than you are now, start by answering the seven questions in the box below. If you are between the ages of 15 and 69, the PAR-Q will tell you if you should check with your doctor before you start. If you are over 69 years of age, and you are not used to being very active, check with your doctor.

Common sense is your best guide when you answer these questions. Please read the questions carefully and answer each one honestly: check YES or NO.

YES	NO		
☐	☐	1.	Has you doctor ever said that you have a heart condition <u>and</u> that you should only do physical activity recommended by a doctor?
☐	☐	2.	Do you feel pain in your chest when you do physical activity?
☐	☐	3.	In the past month, have you had chest pain when you were not doing physical activity?
☐	☐	4.	Do you lose your balance because of dizziness or do you ever lose consciousness?
☐	☐	5.	Do you have a bone or joint problem that could be made worse by a change in your physical activity?
☐	☐	6.	Is your doctor currently prescribing drugs (for example, water pills) for your blood pressure or heart condition?
☐	☐	7.	Do you know of <u>any other reason</u> why you should not do physical activity?

If
you
answered

YES to one or more questions

Talk with your doctor by phone or in person BEFORE you start becoming much more physically active or BEFORE you have a fitness appraisal. Tell your doctor about the PAR-Q and which questions you answered YES.

- You may be able to do any activity you want—as long as you start slowly and build up gradually. Or, you may need to restrict your activities to those which are safe for you. Talk with your doctor about the kinds of activities you wish to participate in and follow his/her advice.
- Find out which community programs are safe and helpful for you.

NO to all questions

If you answered NO honestly to <u>all</u> PAR-Q questions, you can be reasonably sure that you can:

- start becoming much more physically active—begin slowly and build up gradually. This is the safest and easiest way to go.
- take part in a fitness appraisal—this is an excellent way to determine your basic fitness so that you can plan the best way for you to live actively.

DELAY BECOMING MUCH MORE ACTIVE:
- if you are not feeling well because of a temporary illness such as a cold or a fever—wait until you feel better; or
- if you are or may be pregnant—talk to your doctor before you start becoming more active.

Please note: If your health changes so that you then answer YES to any of the above questions, tell your fitness or health professional. Ask whether you should change your physical activity plan.

Informed Use of the PAR-Q: The Canadian Society for Exercise Physiology, Health Canada, and their agents assume no liability for persons who undertake physical activity, and if in doubt after completing this questionnaire, consult your doctor prior to physical activity.

You are encouraged to copy the PAR-Q but only if you use the entire form

NOTE: If the PAR-Q is being given to a person before he or she participates in a physical activity program or a fitness appraisal, this section may be used for legal or administrative purposes.

I have read, understood and completed this questionnaire. Any questions I had were answered to my full satisfaction.

NAME _____

SIGNATURE _____ DATE _____

SIGNATURE OF PARENT _____ WITNESS _____
or GUARDIAN (for participants under the age of majority)

© Canadian Society for Exercise Physiology
Société canadienne de physiologie de l'exercice

Supported by: [flag] Health Santé
Canada Canada

FIGURE 6-1 PAR-Q form. (Reprinted from the 1994 revised version of the Physical Activity Readiness Questionnaire (PAR-Q and YOU). The PAR-Q and YOU is a copyrighted, pre-exercise screen owned by the Canadian Society for Exercise Physiology.)

(3) Maximal voluntary ventilation (MVV)

–is the maximal volume of airflow per minute possible.

–represents the mechanical limit of pulmonary function.

d. **Blood tests**

–Various blood tests may shed light on the client's current health status and may help guide exercise programming. Typically, blood samples are drawn following an overnight fast; values are expressed in either mg/dl or mmol/L.

(1) Total cholesterol

–is the total amount of cholesterol in the blood; it includes all cholesterol fractions.

(2) Low-density lipoprotein (LDL)

–is a cholesterol-carrying protein that tends to deposit cholesterol on arterial walls, greatly accelerating atherosclerosis.

–LDLs are also thought to act as free radicals and cause damage to cell walls; **high levels mean increased risk.**

(3) High-density lipoprotein (HDL)

–is a cholesterol-carrying protein that tends to remove cholesterol from the blood.

–HDLs are also thought to remove cholesterol from cell walls, possibly reversing the progression of atherosclerosis; **high levels are desirable.**

(4) Fasting glucose

–is a measure of blood glucose level without the influence of a meal.

–High levels are indicative of impaired glucose tolerance.

B. CONTRAINDICATIONS AND RISK STRATIFICATION

1. Contraindications to exercise testing

–Some clients have risk factors that outweigh the potential benefits derived from exercise testing (**Table 6-1**).

a. Absolute contraindications apply to clients for whom exercise testing should not be performed until the situation or condition has stabilized.

b. Relative contraindications apply to clients who might be tested if the potential benefit from exercise testing outweighs the relative risk of testing.

2. Risk stratification

–Clients can be initially classified into three risk strata for exercise testing: low risk, moderate risk, and high risk.

a. Low risk

(1) This category includes apparently healthy individuals who are asymptomatic and have no more than one coronary risk factor for coronary artery disease (CAD); see **Table 6-2**.

(2) Other low-risk criteria are as follows:

–Uncomplicated myocardial infarction

–Functional capacity > 6–8 metabolic equivalents (METs) 3 or more weeks following a clinical event

–No ischemia or complex arrhythmias

–No significant left ventricular dysfunction (ejection fraction > 50%)

b. Moderate risk

(1) These clients have signs or symptoms suggesting possible cardiopulmonary or metabolic disease and/or two or more risk factors for CAD.

(2) Other moderate-risk criteria are as follows:

–Functional capacity < 6–8 METs 3 weeks after a clinical event

–Shock or congestive heart failure during a recent MI

–Moderate left ventricular dysfunction (ejection fraction 31%–49%)

 Table 6-1. Contraindications to Exercise Testing

Absolute

A recent significant change in the resting ECG suggesting significant ischemia, recent myocardial infarction (within 2 days) or other acute cardiac event

Unstable angina

Uncontrolled cardiac arrhythmias causing symptoms or hemodynamic compromise

Severe symptomatic aortic stenosis

Uncontrolled symptomatic heart failure

Acute pulmonary embolus or pulmonary infarction

Acute myocarditis or pericarditis

Suspected or known dissecting aneurysm

Acute infections

Relative*

Left main coronary stenosis

Moderate stenotic valvular heart disease

Electrolyte abnormalities (e.g., hypokalemia, hypomagnesemia)

Severe arterial hypertension (i.e., systolic BP of > 200 mm Hg and/or a diastolic BP of > 110 mm Hg) at rest

Tachyarrhythmias or bradyarrhythmias

Hypertrophic cardiomyopathy and other forms of outflow tract obstruction

Neuromuscular, musculoskeletal, or rheumatoid disorders that are exacerbated by exercise

High-degree atrioventricular block

Ventricular aneurysm

Uncontrolled metabolic disease (e.g., diabetes, thyrotoxicosis, or myxedema)

Chronic infectious disease (e.g., mononucleosis, hepatitis, AIDS)

* Relative contraindications can be superseded if benefits outweigh risks of exercise. In some instances, these individuals can be exercised with caution and/or using low-level end points, especially if they are asymptomatic at rest. (Modified from Gibbons RA, Balady GJ, Beasely JW et al: ACC/AHA guidelines for exercise testing. *J Am Coll Cardiol* 30:260–315, 1997.)

–Exercise-induced ST segment depression of 1–2 mm

–Reversible ischemic defects

c. High risk

(1) These clients have known cardiac, pulmonary, or metabolic disease.

(2) Other indicators of high risk are as follows:

–Severely depressed left ventricular function (ejection fraction < 30%)

Table 6-2. Coronary Artery Disease Risk Factor Thresholds for Use With ACSM Risk Stratification

Risk Factors	Defining Criteria
Positive	
Family history	Myocardial infarction, coronary revascularization, or sudden death before 55 years of age in father or other male first-degree relative (i.e., brother or son), or before 65 years of age in mother or other female first-degree relative (i.e., sister or daughter)
Cigarette smoking	Current cigarette smoker or those who quit within the previous 6 months
Hypertension	Systolic blood pressure of ≥ 140 mm Hg or diastolic ≥ 90 mm Hg, confirmed by measurements on at least 2 separate occasions, or on antihypertensive medication
Hypercholesterolemia	Total serum cholesterol of > 200 mg/dl (5.2 mmol/L) or high-density lipoprotein cholesterol of < 35 mg/dl (0.9 mmol/L), or on lipid-lowering medication. If low-density lipoprotein cholesterol is available, use > 130 mg/dl (3.4 mmol/L) rather than total cholesterol of > 200 mg/dl
Impaired fasting glucose	Fasting blood glucose of ≥ 110 mg/dl (6.1 mmol/L) confirmed by measurements on at least 2 separate occasions (7)
Obesity*	Body Mass Index of ≥ 30 kg/m² (8), or waist girth of > 100 cm (9)
Sedentary lifestyle	Persons not participating in a regular exercise program or meeting the minimal physical activity recommendations † from the U.S. Surgeon General's report (10)
Negative	
High serum HDL cholesterol ‡	> 60 mg/dl (1.6 mmol/L)

*Professional opinions vary regarding the most appropriate markers and thresholds for obesity; therefore, exercise professionals should use clinical judgment when evaluating this risk factor.
†Accumulating 30 minutes or more of moderate physical activity on most days of the week.
‡It is common to sum risk factors in making clinical judgments. If high-density lipoprotein (HDL) cholesterol is high, subtract one risk factor from the sum of positive risk factors because high HDL decreases CAD risk.
(Adapted from Expert Panel on Detection, Evaluation, and Treatment of High Blood Cholesterol in Adults. Summary of the second report of the National Cholesterol Education Program (NCEP) expert panel on detection, evaluation, and treatment of high blood cholesterol in adults (Adult Treatment Panel II). *JAMA* 269:3015–3023, 1993.)

–Resting complex ventricular arrhythmias exertional hypotension

–Survival of cardiac arrest

–Exercise-induced ST segment depression > 2 mm

C. INFORMED CONSENT

–Any supervised exercise testing and training program has an ethical and legal obligation to inform the client of the purposes, procedures, risks, and benefits of the tests or activities.

–The **informed consent form** must state that the client has had an opportunity to ask questions about the procedures and has been given adequate information with which to provide informed consent.

–**If the client is a minor,** written consent must also be obtained from a parent or legal guardian.

–**Release of any testing information** that may be seen by others and/or is used for research purposes must also be granted through informed consent.

–Informed consent does not prevent legal action arising out of cases of **negligence.**

D. CLIENT PREPARATION

1. **Client teaching** includes a description of the test and specific and general instructions, such as

   –Avoid eating, smoking, and consuming alcohol or caffeine within 3 hours before testing

   –Avoid exercise or other strenuous physical activity on the day of the test

   –Get adequate sleep the night before the test

   –Wear comfortable, loose-fitting clothing

2. **Preparing for ECG monitoring** involves abrading the client's skin with a rough pad or sandpaper to remove dead skin cells, followed by cleansing with alcohol and scrubbing with gauze, and then applying the ECG electrodes using the anatomical landmarks described in Chapter 1.

II. FITNESS TESTING

A. BODY COMPOSITION

−Assessment of body composition provides information on the amount of visceral body fat (a major CAD risk), overall body fat, and fat-free body mass.

1. Hydrostatic (underwater) weighing

a. Principle

−This method is based on **Archimedes's principle,** that a body immersed in water is buoyed by a counterforce equal to the weight of the water displaced. Because bone and muscle are more dense than water, and fat is less dense than water, a person with more fat-free body mass weighs more in water than a person of the same weight with a greater percentage of body fat.

b. Procedure

(1) The client is suspended from a scale in water and breathes out all of his/her air (residual volume can be indirectly measured or estimated and subtracted). The client holds his/her breath for 5 seconds while weight is recorded.

(2) Body density is then determined through the following formula:

$$Body\ Density = \cfrac{Weight\ in\ air}{\left[\cfrac{(Weight\ in\ air - Weight\ in\ water)}{Density\ of\ water} - \substack{Residual \\ Volume}\right]}$$

(3) Equations are then used to **convert body density into body fat percentage;** the two most common equations are:

$\%\ fat = (457/Body\ Density) - 414.2$[1]

$\%\ fat = (495/Body\ Density) - 450$[2]

c. Sources of error

−Inaccurate measurement or estimation of lung residual volume

−The great variability in bone density among individuals

[1]Equation from Brozek J, Grande F, Anderson J, Keys A: Densitometric analysis of body composition: Revision of some quantitative assumptions. *Ann NY Acad Sci* 110:113–140, 1963.
[2]Equation from Siri WE: Body composition from fluid spaces and density. *Univ Calif Donner Lab Med Phys Rep,* March 1956. Published with permission from University of California-Berkeley.

2. Skinfold measurements

a. Principle

−This technique assumes a relationship between subcutaneous fat and overall body fat, a predictable pattern of body fat distribution for men and for women, and a given fat-free density.

−**Age** is accounted for because of changes in body fat distribution with age. With aging, more fat is stored internally, thus altering the meaning of a given skinfold measure.

−**Body fat equations** are specific to age, gender, and ethnicity (**Table 6-3**).

b. Procedure

−The **measurement technique** involves using the thumb and index finger to grasp a fold of skin 1 cm above the site being measured (**Table 6-4**), placing the caliper jaws perpendicular to the fold, and recording the measurement on the caliper.

−Two measurements are taken at each site; if these vary by more than 1 cm, then a third measurement is taken and the two closest measurements are averaged.

c. Sources of error

−Improper site identification

−Inaccurate calipers

−Poor technique

−A client who doesn't fit norms for standard equations (e.g., odd body fat distribution)

3. Body mass index (BMI)

−This basic weight-for-height ratio can be quickly determined using a standard nomogram. The results are compared to a standard table to classify obesity according to BMI value (**Table 6-5**).

−BMI is commonly used in large population studies. It has been found to correlate with incidence of certain chronic diseases, such as hyperlipidemia.

−**BMI should not be used to assess an individual's body fat** during a fitness assessment, because it does not take into account fat-free density and skeletal mass.

4. Waist-to-hip ratio (WHR)

−A simple index of upper versus lower body fat distribution, WHR provides a predictor of

Table 6-3. Skinfold Prediction Equations

	Ethnicity	Gender	Age	Equation
1	Black	Males	18–61	Db (g/cc) = 1.1120 – 0.00043499 (Σ 7SKF chest, abdomen, thigh, triceps, subscapular, suprailiac, midaxillary) + 0.00000055 (Σ 7SKF)^2 – 0.00028826 (age).
2	Black	Females	18–55	Db (g/cc) = 1.0970 – 0.00046971 (Σ 7SKF chest, abdomen, thigh, triceps, subscapular, suprailiac, midaxillary) + 0.00000056 (Σ 7SKF)^2 – 0.00012828 (age).
3	White	Males	18–61	Db (g/cc) = 1.109380 – 0.0008267 (Σ 3SKF chest, abdomen, thigh) + 0.0000016 (Σ 3SKF)^2 – 0.0002574 (age).
4	White	Females	18–55	Db (g/cc) = 1.0994921 – 0.0009929 (Σ 3SKF triceps, suprailiac, thigh) + 0.0000023 (Σ 3SKF)^2 – 0.0001392 (age).
5	Hispanic	Females	20–40	Db (g/cc) = 1.0970 – 0.00046971 (Σ 3SKF chest, abdomen, thigh, triceps, subscapular, suprailiac, midaxiliary) + 0.00000056 (Σ 7SKF)^2 – 0.00012828 (age).
6	Black & white	Males	≤ 18	%BF = 0.735 (Σ 2SKF triceps, calf) + 1.0.
7	Black & white	Males (SKF > 35 mm)	≤ 18	%BF = 0.735 (Σ 2SKF triceps, subscapular) + 1.6.
8	Black & white	Males (SKF > 35 mm)	≤ 18	%BF = 0.783 (Σ 2SKF triceps, subscapular) – 0,008 (Σ 2SKF)^2 + 1*.
9	Black & white	Females	≤ 18	%BF = 0.610 (2SKF triceps, calf) + 5.1.
10	Black & white	Females (SKF > 35 mm)	≤ 18	%BF = 0.546 (Σ 2SKF triceps, subscapular) + 9.7.
11	Black & white	Females (SKF > 35 mm)	≤ 18	%BF = 1.33 (Σ 2SKF triceps, subscapular) – 0.013 (Σ 2SKF)^2 – 2.5.

(Adapted from Heyward VH, Stolarcyzk LM: Applied Body Composition Assessment. Champaign, IL, Human Kinetics, 1996, pp 173–185.) * = intercept substitutions based on maturation and ethnicity for boys:

Age	Black	White
Prepubescent	–3.2	–1.7
Pubescent	–5.2	–3.4
Postpubescent	–6.8	–5.5

Table 6-4. Standardized Description of Skinfold Sites and Procedures

Skinfold Site

Abdominal	Vertical fold; 2 cm to the right side of the umbilicus
Triceps	Vertical fold; on the posterior midline of the upper arm, halfway between the acromion and olecranon processes, with the arm held freely to the side of the body
Biceps	Vertical fold; on the anterior aspect of the arm over the belly of the biceps muscle, 1 cm above the level used to mark the triceps site
Chest/Pectoral	Diagonal fold; one-half the distance between the anterior axillary line and the nipple (men) or one-third of the distance between the anterior axillary line and the nipple (women)
Medial Calf	Vertical fold; at the maximum circumference of the calf on the midline of its medial border
Midaxillary	Vertical fold; on the midaxillary line at the level of the xiphoid process of the sternum. (An alternate method is a horizontal fold taken at the level of the xiphoid/sternal border in the midaxillary line.)
Subscapular	Diagonal fold (at a 45° angle); 1 to 2 cm below the inferior angle of the scapula
Suprailiac	Diagonal fold; in line with the natural angle of the iliac crest taken in the anterior axillary line immediately superior to the iliac crest
Thigh	Vertical fold; on the anterior midline of the thigh, midway between the proximal border of the patella and the inguinal crease (hip)

Procedures:

- All measurements should be made on the right side of the body
- Caliper should be placed 1 cm away from the thumb and finger, perpendicular to the skinfold, and halfway between the crest and the base of the fold
- Pinch should be maintained while reading the caliper
- Wait 1 to 2 s (and not longer) before reading caliper
- Take duplicate measures at each site and retest if duplicate measurements are not within 1 to 2 mm
- Rotate through measurement sites or allow time for skin to regain normal texture and thickness

(From *ACSM's Guidelines for Exercise Testing and Prescription*, 6th ed. Philadelphia, Lippincott Williams & Wilkins, 2000, p. 65.)

Table 6-5. Panel on Energy, Obesity, and Body Weight Standards Classification of Obesity According to BMI Values

20–24.9 kg/m²	Desirable range for adult men and women
25–29.9 kg/m²	Grade 1 obesity
30–40 kg/m²	Grade 2 obesity
> 40 kg/m²	Grade 3 obesity (morbid obesity)

(From *ACSM's Guidelines for Exercise Testing and Prescription*, 5th ed. Baltimore, Williams & Wilkins, 1995, p 59.)

Table 6-6. Waist-To-Hip Circumference Ratio (WHR) Standards for Men and Women

		Disease Risk Related to Obesity			
	Age	Low	Moderate	High	Very High
Men	20–29	< 0.83	0.83–0.88	0.89–0.94	> 0.94
	30–39	< 0.84	0.84–0.91	0.92–0.96	> 0.96
	40–49	< 0.88	0.88–0.95	0.96–1.00	> 1.00
	50–59	< 0.90	0.90–0.96	0.97–1.02	> 1.02
	60–69	< 0.91	0.91–0.98	0.99–1.03	> 1.03
Women	20–29	< 0.71	0.71–0.77	0.78–0.82	> 0.82
	30–39	< 0.72	0.72–0.78	0.79–0.84	> 0.84
	40–49	< 0.73	0.73–0.79	0.80–0.87	> 0.87
	50–59	< 0.74	0.74–0.81	0.82–0.88	> 0.88
	60–69	< 0.76	0.76–0.83	0.84–0.90	> 0.90

(With permission from Heyward VH, Stolarcyzk LM: Appied Body Composition Assessment. Champaign, IL, Human Kinetics, 1996, p 82.)

disease risk related to fat distribution. Waist circumference and hip circumference are measured; then WHR is calculated using a standard nomogram and compared to available standards **(Table 6-6)**.

5. **Bioelectrical impedance analysis (BIA)**

–This quick, noninvasive method of measuring fat and fat-free body mass is relatively inexpensive and does not require a highly skilled technician. In the most common form of BIA, four electrodes are placed on the client's skin (typically two on the right hand and two on the right foot), and a high-frequency, low-level excitation current is sent through the body. Because electrical conductivity varies based on the fat content of tissue (fat-free tissue is a good conductor, whereas fat is not), the measured resistance to current flow reflects body composition.

6. **Near-infrared interactance**

–This technique, based on principles of light absorption and reflection, uses near-infrared spectroscopy to measure body composition. A fiberoptic probe is placed on a body site (e.g., biceps), and the infrared beam penetrates the skin; the measurement of reflected light is related to subcutaneous fat.

7. **Dual-energy X-ray absorptiometry**

–In this technique, an emitter passes photons at two different energies (one deep, one shallow) through body tissue, and a scanner analyzes the energy that passes through the tissue. A computer calculates fat, bone, and muscle tissue based on pixel strength.

B. CARDIORESPIRATORY FITNESS

1. **Purpose of assessment**

–To measure variables such as heart rate, blood pressure, and oxygen uptake (VO_2) during exercise, in order to evaluate the body's ability to absorb, distribute, and utilize oxygen, and to help screen for CAD.

–To collect baseline and follow-up information for charting a client's fitness program progress

to help motivate a client by establishing and meeting reasonable fitness goals.

2. **Protocol selection**

–Test selection is influenced by the purpose and goals of the exercise test and also by characteristics of the client being tested.

a. **Maximal testing**

–A maximal exercise test can be most effective in detecting CAD and accurately measuring $\dot{V}O_{2max}$ (using on-line measurements of expired gases or estimated using prediction equations).

–The choice of maximal testing should be based on the reason for the exercise test (e.g., CAD screening or functional capacity measurement).

–Maximal testing is expensive, and guidelines for testing various populations and age groups should be followed **(Table 6-7)**.

b. **Submaximal testing**

–Submaximal exercise tests are used extensively to assess fitness, evaluate changes in fitness following a training program, and provide an estimate of $\dot{V}O_{2max}$ used to establish an initial training program.

–Submaximal testing estimates $\dot{V}O_{2max}$ based on the assumed linear relationship between heart rate and $\dot{V}O_2$. Heart rate is measured at multiple

Table 6-7. ACSM Recommendations for (A) Current Medical Examination* and Exercise Testing Prior to Participation and (B) Physician Supervision of Exercise Tests

	Low Risk	Moderate Risk	High Risk
A.			
Moderate exercise[†]	Not necessary‡	Not necessary	Recommended
Vigorous exercise[§]	Not necessary	Recommended	Recommended
B.			
Submaximal test	Not necessary	Not necessary	Recommended
Maximal test	Not necessary	Recommended‖	Recommended

*Within the past year (see reference 2).
†Absolute moderate exercise is defined as activities that are approximately 3–6 METs or the equivalent of brisk walking at 3 to 4 mph for most healthy adults (13). Nevertheless, a pace of 3 to 4 mph might be considered to be "hard" to "very hard" by some sedentary, older persons. Moderate exercise may alternatively be defined as an intensity well within the individual's capacity, one which can be comfortably sustained for a prolonged period of time (~45 min), which has a gradual initiation and progression, and is generally noncompetitive. If an individual's exercise capacity is known, relative moderate exercise may be defined by the range 40%–60% maximal oxygen uptake.
‡The designation of "Not necessary" reflects the notion that a medical examination, exercise test, and physician supervision of exercise testing would not be essential in the preparticipation screening; however, they should not be viewed as inappropriate.
§Vigorous exercise is defined as activities of > 6 METs. Vigorous exercise may alternatively be defined as exercise intense enough to represent a substantial cardiorespiratory challenge. If an individual's exercise capacity is known, vigorous exercise may be defined as an intensity of > 60% maximal oxygen uptake.
‖When physician supervision of exercise testing is "Recommended," the physician should be in close proximity and readily available should there be an emergent need.
(From *ACSM's Guidelines for Exercise Testing and Prescription*, 6th ed. Philadelphia, Lippincott Williams & Wilkins, 2000, p 27.)

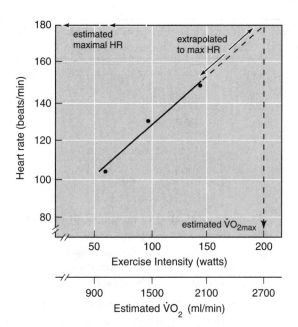

FIGURE 6-2 Heart rate obtained from at least two (more are preferable) submaximal exercise intensities may be extrapolated to the age-predicted maximal heart rate. A vertical line to the intensity scale estimates maximal exercise intensity from which an estimated $\dot{V}O_{2max}$ can be calculated. (Redrawn with permission from *ACSM's Guidelines for Exercise Testing and Prescription*, 5th ed, p 65.)

workloads during the test, and $\dot{V}O_{2max}$ at an estimated maximum heart rate is calculated **(Figure 6-2)**.

–**Submaximal testing is based on several assumptions:**

(1) Measurements are made while the client is at steady state.

(2) There is a linear relationship between heart rate and $\dot{V}O_{2max}$.

(3) Maximal heart rate is similar for all individuals in a given age group.

(4) Mechanical efficiency is the same for all clients.

c. **Discontinuous and continuous protocols**

(1) In a **discontinuous test protocol,** the test is momentarily stopped, measurements are obtained, and the test is then resumed. Discontinuous protocols are usually used only in special circumstances, because of the lengthy time required for such a test. Examples include:

–individuals being tested using arm ergometry, stopping for blood pressure measurement.

–clients with claudication who develop leg pain and need rest periods.

(2) A **continuous test protocol,** the most common form, involves multiple stages of increasing work intensity with no stoppages.

d. **Protocol selection for overweight clients**

–During weight-bearing exercise, a client's absolute oxygen costs are directly proportional to his or her body mass.

–In some cases, weight-supported exercise, such as cycle ergometry, is preferred for an overweight client to minimize orthopedic stress and reduce the risk of injury.

e. **Protocol selection for children**

–**Physical fitness testing** is common in school-based physical education programs to evaluate skill-related fitness and, most importantly, health-related fitness **(Tables 6-8 and 6-9)**.

–**Clinical exercise testing** is also performed to screen for preexisting cardiorespiratory disease in children.

–**Challenges** involved in testing children include the difficulty in assessing

Table 6-8. Field Fitness Testing for Children*

Fitness/Health Component	Field Test
Aerobic capacity	1-mile walk/run
Muscular strength and endurance	Curl-ups
	Pull-ups/push-ups
Flexibility	Sit-reach/V-sit reach
Agility	Shuttle run
Body composition	Body mass index/skinfolds

*For detailed descriptions of specific test items, the reader is referred to the following publications: *Fitnessgram: The Test Administration Manual.* Dallas, Institute for Aerobics Research, 1994; and President's Council on Physical Fitness and Sports: *The Presidential Physical Fitness Award Program.* Washington, DC, 1997.
(From *ACSM's Guidelines for Exercise Testing and Prescription,* 6th ed. Philadelphia, Lippincott Williams & Wilkins, 2000, p 218.)

 Table 6-9. Protocols Suitable for Graded Exercise Testing of Children

Modified Balke Treadmill Protocol

Subject	Speed (mph)	Initial Grade (%)	Increment (%)	Stage Duration (min)
Poorly fit	3.00	6	2	2
Sedentary	3.25	6	2	2
Active	5.00	0	2.5	2
Athlete	5.25	0	2.5	2

The McMaster Cycle Test

Height (cm)	Initial Load (watts)	Increments (watts)	Step Duration (min)
< 120	12.5	12.5	2
120–139.9	12.5	25	2
140–159.9	25	25	2
≥ 160	25	50 (boys)	2
		25 (girls)	

(Adapted from Skinner J: *Exercise Testing and Exercise Prescription for Special Cases,* 2nd ed. Philadelphia, Lea & Febiger, 1993.)

changes in physical fitness as a result of training or maturation.

–Exercise testing is **contraindicated** in children with acute inflammatory disease, myocardial infarction, pulmonary disease, renal disease, hepatitis, uncontrolled congestive heart failure, or severe systemic hypertension, and in those using any medication that affects the cardiovascular response to exercise.

f. **Protocol selection for the elderly**

–Exercise testing in the elderly must take into account **age-related changes** in cardiovascular and other physiological variables, including maximal heart rate, maximal cardiac output, maximal oxygen uptake, resting and exercise blood pressure, residual volume, vital capacity, reaction time, muscular strength, bone mass, flexibility, glucose tolerance, and body fat percentage.

–Other factors to consider include the great **variations in physiological status** in elderly clients due to differing levels of activity and the presence of underlying disease.

–Modifications to standard test protocols may be needed for severely deconditioned clients or those with physical limitations.

–Given the longer adaptation time to a workload in the elderly compared to younger adults, a **prolonged warm-up phase is recommended.**

g. **Protocol selection for clients with cardiorespiratory disorders**

–Exercise testing may help differentiate exercise-induced breathlessness from dyspnea due to cardiorespiratory disease.

–Oxygen uptake, ventilation, and oxygen saturation should be measured during exercise testing, because desaturation is possible during exercise.

–Test protocol selection should be individualized, because each client will respond differently; protocols should be adjusted to achieve a test duration of 8–12 minutes.

3. **Modes of exercise testing**

a. **Field tests**

–These tests can be administered with minimal equipment and in clients with varying conditions.

(1) **Cooper 12-minute test**

–The subject must cover the greatest distance possible during the 12-minute test period. $\dot{V}O_{2max}$ is estimated based on the distance covered.

(2) **1.5-mile test**

–The subject must cover 1.5 miles as rapidly as possible. $\dot{V}O_{2max}$ is estimated based on this time.

(3) **Rockport walking test**

–This submaximal test requires the client to walk 1 mile as fast as possible, with heart rate measured for 15 seconds immediately posttest. $\dot{V}O_{2max}$ is predicted based on gender, time, and heart rate.

(4) Limitations

–Although these tests are easy to administer, they have certain limitations:

(a) An individual's motivation may influence test performance and thus the accuracy of the test.

(b) Clients unaccustomed to the test may pace themselves inappropriately, which may affect results

(c) Because the client is not monitored (i.e., heart rate, blood pressure, symptoms), clients at risk or older clients should not be tested using this method.

b. **Nuclear/radionuclide imaging**

–In these exercise tests, radioactive substances are injected into the bloodstream to visualize aspects of the circulatory system more closely; this technique helps increase test sensitivity and specificity.

(1) Perfusion imaging

–During the last minute of a standard stress test, thallium-201 is injected into the bloodstream. Thallium-201 enters myocardial cells in proportion to the amount of blood flow to those cells, and emits energy detectable with a scintillation counter.

–Images of the myocardium can be constructed immediately following a stress test and 4–24 hours later. Areas with little or no perfusion immediately following a test indicate areas of ischemia; any "cold spots" remaining 4–24 hours later indicate necrotic tissue.

–Areas of reversible ischemia will reperfuse and cold spots will disappear in later testing.

–**Single-photon emission computed tomography (SPECT)** enhances sensitivity and also allows for multidimensional viewing.

(2) Ventriculography

–To visualize the resting and exercise cardiac function related to cardiac output, ejection fraction,

and wall motion, a test such as a **multiple gated acquisition study (MUGA)** is performed. Technetium 99n (TC 99) is injected into the bloodstream, where it attaches to red blood cells. Areas where the blood pools, such as the ventricles, are visualized by the technetium emissions. Changes in ejection fraction or wall motion abnormalities may be indicative of a failing heart or compromised blood flow through the coronaries.

c. **Exercise echocardiography**

–This technique uses ECG monitoring to identify the cardiac cycle, along with high-frequency sound waves to evaluate cardiac wall motion and pump function. Measurements can be made during or immediately after stationary cycle ergometry.

d. **Pharmacologic testing**

–In some instances, a client is not able to complete an exercise stress test owing to muscular limitations, neurological disability, peripheral vascular disease, or other conditions that prevent the client from achieving a sufficient work intensity to provide an accurate cardiovascular assessment.

–**Two common tests** are used that do not involve exercise, but rather use drug-induced changes in cardiovascular work.

(1) Dipyridamole (Persantine) perfusion imaging

–Infusion of dipyridamole causes vasodilation of normal coronary arteries, with little effect on narrowed arteries.

–Dipyridamole is often used in conjunction with a nuclear imaging agent (e.g., thallium) and a nuclear imaging technique (e.g., thallium scanning, SPECT).

–Arteries are visualized before and after drug administration and the findings compared.

(2) Dobutamine testing

–Dobutamine infusion elevates heart rate and increases myocardial oxygen demand.

–When used in concert with echocardiography, dobutamine testing can elicit heart wall motion abnormalities.

e. Holter ECG monitoring

–This test is used to track ECG abnormalities during the course of a day.

–Generally, a single-lead ECG is connected to a battery pack and a recorder.

–ECG monitoring is done continuously for up to 24 hours and recorded. The client records his or her activities during the day, as well as any symptoms experienced during these activities.

–ECG tracings are reviewed and compared with the client's activity log to identify precipitating events for ECG abnormalities.

C. MUSCULAR FITNESS

1. **Muscular strength assessment**

   a. **Purposes**

   –To determine maximum strength in order to create a prudent strength training program.

   –To monitor progress and revise the strength training program.

   –To determine physical strength for performing standardized work tasks (i.e., pre-employment screenings).

   b. **Resistance training methods**

   –In **isotonic (free-weight) training,** the weight is held constant through the range of motion (ROM); speed can vary with client movement.

   –In **isokinetic training,** the speed of movement is kept constant through the ROM; force can vary with client movement.

   –In **variable-resistance training,** the weight is altered using mechanical assistance to compensate for changes in the muscle's ability to generate force due to changes in the lever system.

   –In **isometric (static) training,** the joint angle remains constant while force is exerted.

   c. **Strength-testing devices**

      (1) Cable tensiometer

      –This device measures static strength by measuring force exerted while pulling on a steel cable. Various limbs can be tested, and varying the length of the cables can assess different joint angles.

      (a) Advantages: It can assess strength for almost all major muscle groups, and results are reliable.

      (b) Disadvantage: Strength is assessed statically, so results may not apply to dynamic movements in demonstrating strength.

      (2) Dynamometer

      –This is a more portable static strength-testing device that generally tests leg, back, and forearm strength.

      (a) Advantages: Portable, less cumbersome than cable tensiometers, and numerous clients can be tested quickly.

      (b) Disadvantages: Only a limited number of muscle groups can be tested; reliability is questionable.

      (3) Strain gauge

      –Thin electroconductive material is placed over machined metal parts and connected to an electrical source. As force is exerted, the gauge is bent or deformed, altering its electrical conductivity; measurement of the change in conductivity reflects the amount of force generated.

      –For example, a strain gauge is installed on the crank arm of a cycle ergometer pedal; as the cyclist pushes on the crank (pedals), the arm bends, changing the strain gauge's conductivity and allowing measurement of force.

   d. **One-repetition maximum (1-RM) testing**

   –assesses the maximum amount of weight that can be lifted one time for a given exercise.

   –begins with a weight that the client can lift easily. Following a successful lift, the client rests for 2–3 minutes, 5–10 pounds of weight are added, and the client lifts again.

   –Generally, 4–6 trials are needed to determine the 1-RM.

      (1) Advantages

      –It is easy to administer, and multiple muscle groups can be tested.

      –The same equipment used for testing can often be used for training.

      –It also provides a measure of dynamic strength, which is most applicable to real-world settings.

      (2) Disadvantages

      –In unconditioned clients, posttest muscle soreness is likely.

–Strength is limited by the weakest point in the ROM.

–The tester needs to take into account the skill involved with each lift, and ensure that the client can safely and effectively perform the lifts.

e. Special considerations

–Muscle force varies over joint ROM because of changes in joint angle; therefore, dynamic muscle strength testing (1-RM) is not useful for establishing strength throughout the ROM.

–Acceleration and inertia can both influence the performance of a dynamic strength test; thus dynamic strength testing should be standardized with regard to velocity.

–Body position must be stabilized to isolate the muscle group being tested.

2. Muscular endurance assessment

–These techniques assess the client's ability to exert a submaximal force repeatedly.

a. Static endurance

–A submaximal force is held for as long as possible; time is measured as an index of endurance performance.

–The same devices used to assess static strength can be used. In addition, measuring the drop in force with time will give an index of fatigue/muscular endurance.

b. Dynamic endurance

–Maximum repetitions completed at a set percentage of 1-RM and/or body weight, taking into account the size of the muscle mass being assessed (e.g., chest endurance, 50% 1-RM or 60% of body weight; biceps endurance, 50% 1-RM or 15% of body weight).

–**Isokinetic endurance** measures the number of repetitions completed above 50% of maximal torque.

–**Calisthenic tests** include sit-ups, push-ups, and pull-ups. The number of repetitions is assessed with the client lifting his or her own body weight.

–Clients who are not physically fit may be able to complete only a few repetitions; thus, these tests may be more useful for assessing strength than for assessing endurance.

3. Flexibility assessment

–Flexibility assessment provides information on joint ROM. Poor flexibility can contribute to skeletal muscle injury, low back pain, and impaired ability to perform activities of daily living (ADL) and other activities, such as sports.

a. Procedure

–Depending on the joint, **flexion, extension, rotation, abduction, adduction, supination, pronation, or deviation can be assessed** (Table 6-10 and Figure 6-3).

–The client should **warm up** before flexibility testing by lightly exercising the joint to be tested; this promotes a more accurate measure of flexibility and reduces the risk of injury.

–Measurements are taken with the limb starting in an anatomically neutral position to improve reliability.

–**Repeated measurements** of flexibility are essential to ensure accurate assessment of ROM.

b. Measurement devices

–Portable and cost-effective, **goniometers** consist of two arms that intersect at a disc that can measure 360° of movement. One arm is held on the stationary portion of the limb, while the other moves with the portion of the joint that moves.

–**Inclinometers/fleximeters** are either handheld or attached to a limb, head, or trunk to measure ROM. These devices, which have a high measurement reliability, are excellent to use when a goniometer is not feasible.

–**Tape measures** can accurately measure lateral trunk flexion and lumbar flexion as well as changes in ROM in the carpometacarpal and interphalangeal joints.

Table 6-10. Range of Motion of the Major Joints

Joint	Motion	Average Ranges (degrees)	Joint	Motion	Average Ranges (degrees)
Spinal			Thumb	Abduction	0–60
Cervical	Flexion	0–60		Flexion	
	Extension	0–75		Carpal-metacarpal	0–15
	Lateral flexion	0–45		Metacarpal-phalangeal	0–50
	Rotation	0–80		Inter-phalangeal	0–80
Thoracic	Flexion	0–50		Extension	
	Rotation	0–30		Carpal-metacarpal	0–20
Lumbar	Flexion	0–60		Metacarpal-phalangeal	0–5
	Extension	0–25		Interphalangeal	0–20
	Lateral flexion	0–25	Fingers	Flexion	
Upper Extremity				Metacarpal-phalangeal	0–90
Shoulder	Flexion	0–180		Proximal Interphalangeal	0–100
	Extension	0–50		Distal Interphalangeal	0–80
	Abduction	0–180		Extension	
	Adduction	0–50		Metacarpal-phalangeal	0–45
	Internal rotation	0–90	**Lower Extremity**		
	External rotation	0–90	Hip	Flexion	0–100
Elbow	Flexion	0–140		Extension	0–30
Forearm	Supination	0–80		Abduction	0–40
	Pronation	0–80		Adduction	0–20
Wrist	Flexion	0–60		Internal rotation	0–40
	Extension	0–60		External rotation	0–50
	Ulnar deviation	0–30	Knee	Flexion	0–150
	Radial deviation	0–20	Ankle	Dorsiflexion	0–20
				Plantar flexion	0–40
			Subtalar	Inversion	0–30
				Eversion	0–20

(From *ACSM's Resource Manual for Guidelines for Exercise Testing and Prescription*, 3rd ed. Baltimore, Williams & Wilkins, 1998, p 369.)

Hip Flexibility Screening

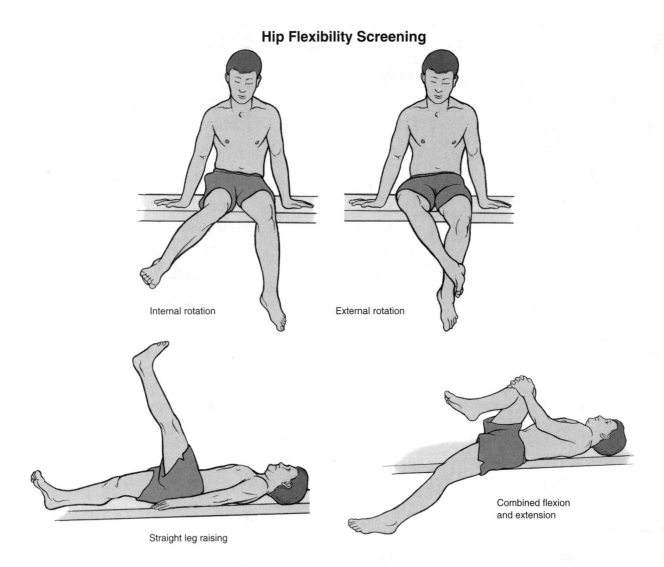

Internal rotation

External rotation

Straight leg raising

Combined flexion and extension

Neck and Trunk Flexibility Screening

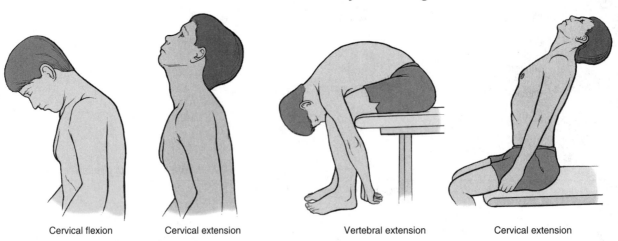

Cervical flexion

Cervical extension

Vertebral extension

Cervical extension

FIGURE 6-3 *Top:* **Hip flexibility screening.** *Internal rotation* involves flexing the hip and knee and moving the leg as far to the side as possible by rolling the thigh. *External rotation* involves moving the leg as far as possible past the midline by rolling the thigh outward. *Straight leg raising* consists of keeping the contralateral lower extremity in full extension while lifting the other extremity without bending the knee. Note limited hamstring flexibility. In the *combined test of hip flexion and extension,* one bent hip and knee are brought as close to the chest as possible, while allowing the other limb to drop over the edge of the table into extension (Thomas Test for hip extension). *Bottom:* **Neck and trunk flexibility screening.** In *cervical flexion,* the chin should touch the chest. *Cervical extension* involves bending the head as far as possible posteriorly. In *vertebral flexion,* with the hips and knees bent, the trunk should touch the anterior thighs. *Vertebral extension* involves backward movement of the trunk as far posterior as possible without hip extension. (Modified from *ACSM's Resource Manual for Guidelines for Exercise Testing and Prescription,* 3rd ed. Baltimore, Williams & Wilkins, 1998, pp 372–373.)

III. CLINICAL EXERCISE TESTING

A. INDICATIONS

1. **Predischarge exercise testing following myocardial infarction**

   –This is done to determine minimal standards of functional capacity, to **evaluate the client's ability to perform ADL.**

   –Testing is also conducted to evaluate the effectiveness of medications and the client's hemodynamic response to exercise.

   –This testing can reassure the client (and family members) of the client's capacity for physical work.

2. **Postdischarge exercise testing following myocardial infarction or cardiac surgery**

   –Testing can demonstrate the **degree of improvement since discharge;** maximal testing is usually conducted 3–6 weeks after the event.

   –Results are used to design an exercise program, identify signs or symptoms, and to aid decisions on medication adjustments.

3. **Diagnostic testing and determination of disease severity and prognosis**

   –Maximal testing with measures of heart rate, blood pressure, and ECG is the most cost-effective screening tool for detecting signs and symptoms of heart disease.

   –Individuals diagnosed with heart disease are also tested to determine the presence and extent of myocardial ischemia, and to provide information on prognosis.

   –Disease severity can be inferred from the shape or slope of the ST depression (up-sloping, flat, or down-sloping), as well as the magnitude of depression.

   –In addition, left ventricular function can be evaluated through measurements of maximal MET capacity as well as maximal systolic blood pressure achieved.

4. **Functional capacity testing**

   –Testing is useful in determining appropriate levels of activity, determining aerobic fitness, and providing feedback related to fitness improvements as part of a training program.

B. EXERCISE TEST MODALITIES AND PROTOCOLS

1. **Treadmill**

   –In this common test modality, the client walks or runs at a predetermined pace on a treadmill whose grade can be adjusted.

   –By raising the grade of the treadmill, the tester increases stress on the client. ECG and blood pressure readings evaluate the effects of this stress.

   a. In the **Bruce protocol,** work rate is increased in 3-MET increments in 3-minute stages by gradually increasing both the grade and speed of the treadmill. Although this protocol is widely used, it may not be appropriate for less-fit individuals.

   b. For clients who can complete only a submaximal protocol, the **modified Bruce protocol** may be used. This involves gradually increasing the grade while maintaining a constant low speed (1.7 mph).

   c. A variation of the Bruce protocol is the **ramp protocol,** which uses both grade and speed increases, but at a slower pace than in the Bruce protocol, to increase work rate.

   d. Other treadmill protocols include the **Balke-Ware, Naughton** (both most appropriate for less-fit clients), and **Ellestad** (appropriate for fit clients).

2. **Cycle ergometer**

   –Cycle ergometry has several advantages over the treadmill: it keeps the upper body stable, ensuring more accurate ECG and blood pressure measurements; supports the client's body weight, making it more appropriate for clients with poor balance; and allows work rate to be set more precisely.

   –Protocols can be easily individualized; most use stage durations of 2–5 minutes and work rate increments of 15–50 watts.

C. MEASUREMENTS

1. **Heart rate and blood pressure** are measured repeatedly before, during, and after the exercise test (Table 6-11).

2. Ideally, three **ECG leads** are monitored, one each from the lateral, inferior, and anterior views. One of those leads should be V_5 to pick up most ST segment changes.

3. Monitoring for any **clinical signs** (e.g., changes in gait, skin color, or responsiveness) that may develop during the test helps identify test termination criteria and enhances client safety.

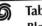

Table 6-11. Sequence of Measures for Heart Rate, Blood Pressure, Rating of Perceived Exertion (RPE), and Electrocardiogram (ECG) During Exercise Testing

Pretest

1. 12-lead ECG in supine and exercise postures

2. Blood pressure measurements in the supine position and exercise posture

Exercise*

1. 12-lead ECG recorded during last 15 seconds of every stage and at peak exercise (3-lead ECG observed/recorded every minute on monitor)

2. Blood pressure measurements should be obtained during the last minute of each stage†

3. Rating scales: RPE at the end of each stage, other scales if appicable

Posttest

1. 12-lead ECG immediately after exercise, then every 1 to 2 minutes for at least 5 minutes to allow any exercise-induced changes to return to baseline

2. Blood pressure measurements should be obtained immediately after exercise, then every 1 to 2 minutes until stabilized near baseline level

3. Symptomatic ratings should be obtained using appropriate scales as as long as symptoms persist after exercise

* In addition, these referenced variables should be assessed and recorded whenever adverse symptoms or abnormal ECG changes occur.
† Note: An unchanged or decreasing systolic blood pressure with increasing workloads should be retaken (i.e., verified immediately).
(From *ACSM's Guidelines for Exercise Testing and Prescription,* 6th ed. Philadelphia, Lippincott Williams & Wilkins, 2000, p 102.)

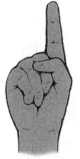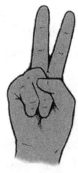

1 ONSET OF DISCOMFORT
You notice chest sensation.

2 MODERATE DISCOMFORT
You feel the pain increasing.

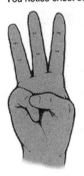

3 MODERATELY SEVERE
The discomfort would cause
you to rest or take nitroglycerin.

4 SEVERE DISCOMFORT

FIGURE 6-4 Nonverbal rating scale for exertional chest discomfort. The scale is particularly useful with gas exchange techniques. A rating of 3 is the appropriate endpoint. (Reprinted with permission from *ACSM's Resource Manual for Guidelines for Exercise Testing and Prescription,* 3rd ed. Baltimore, Williams & Wilkins, 1998, p 359.)

4. The client's subjective report of **rating of perceived exertion (RPE)** reflects his or her perception of work effort during testing.

   –RPE can help determine the test endpoint, as well as information to be used in a future exercise prescription.

   –The client is instructed to report his or her perception of effort during the last minute of each work stage, generally using a scale of 1–10 or 6–20.

5. **Perceptual scales** (e.g., 1–4, with 1 representing minimal discomfort and 4 severe discomfort), allow the client to express his or her degree of perceived angina or dyspnea during testing; this can be done nonverbally with hand signals (**Figure 6-4**).

D. INDICATIONS FOR TERMINATING AN EXERCISE TEST are classified as **absolute or relative** (Table 6-12).

E. POSTEXERCISE PERIOD

–**Active recovery,** involving walking or riding the cycle ergometer with a light load for 3–6 minutes, helps maintain venous return and prevents blood pooling, hypotensive response, and compromised cardiac output.

–Heart rate, ECG, and blood pressure are monitored, and the client is instructed to lie supine until ST changes have returned to baseline and heart rate falls below 100 bpm.

F. INTERPRETATION OF RESULTS

–The value of a stress test depends on proper test performance, careful client monitoring, and understanding the sensitivity and specificity of the test to make informed decisions regarding further testing or exercise prescription.

–**Prognostic implications** are based on sensitivity and specificity.

1. **Sensitivity** refers to the percentage of cases in which exercise testing accurately identifies the presence of CAD.

   a. **Current sensitivity** for detecting CAD using the exercise stress test **is about 70%.**

Table 6-12. Indications for Terminating Exercise Testing

Absolute Indications

Drop in systolic blood pressure of ≥ 10 mm Hg from baseline blood pressure despite an increase in workload, when accompanied by other evidence of ischemia

Moderate to severe angina

Increasing nervous system symptoms (e.g., ataxia, dizziness, or near syncope)

Signs of poor perfusion (cyanosis or pallor)

Technical difficulties monitoring the ECG or systolic blood pressure

Subject's desire to stop

Sustained ventricular tachycardia

ST elevation (≥ 10 mm) in leads without diagnostic Q-waves (other than V_1 or aVR)

Relative Indications

Drop in systolic blood pressure of ≥ 10 mm Hg from baseline blood pressure despite an increase in workload, in the absence of other evidence of ischemia

St or QRS changes such as excessive ST depression (> 2 mm horizontal or downsloping ST-segment depression) or marked axis shift

Arrhythmias other than sustained ventricular tachycardia, including multifocal PVCs, triplets of PVCs, supraventricular tachycardia, heart block, or bradyarrhythmias

Fatigue, shortness of breath, wheezing, leg cramps, or claudication

Development of bundle-branch block or intraventricular conduction delay that cannot be distinguished from ventricular tachycardia

Increasing chest pain

Hypertensive response*

---

*Systolic blood pressure of more than 250 mm Hg and/or a diastolic blood pressure of more than 115 mm Hg.
(Reprinted with permission from Gibbons RA, Balady GJ, Beasely JW et al: ACC/AHA guidelines for exercise testing. *J AM Coll Cardiol* 30:260–315, 1997.)

Table 6-13. Factors That Lower Sensitivity (False-Negatives)

Failure to reach 85% age-predicted maximal heart rate

Medicines that decrease MVO_2 (e.g., beta & calcium channel blockers)

Medicines that increase myocardial oxygen supply (e.g., nitrates)

Equivocal tests called normal

Failure to use other test data in test interpretation (e.g., chronotropic and inotropic responses, symptoms, and dysrhythmias)

Single vessel disease

Good collateral circulation

Insufficient number of monitoring leads to detect ST changes

Increased criteria for abnormal ST depression (e.g., 0.2 mV rather than 0.1 mV)

Technical or observer error

MVO_2 = myocardial oxygen uptake
(From *ACSM's Resource Manual for Guidelines for Exercise Testing and Prescription*, 3rd ed. Baltimore, Williams & Wilkins, 1998, p 242.)

Table 6-14. Factors That Lower Specificity (False-Positives)

Categorization of upsloping ST depression as abnormal

An abnormal resting ECG (e.g., LBBB, nonspecific ST-T abnormality)

Medications that produce ST-T changes (e.g., digitalis)

Cardiac hypertrophy or cardiomyopathy

Hypertension

Female gender

Mitral valve prolapse

Low prevalence of CAD in test population

Wolff-Parkinson-White syndrome

Pectus excavatum

Pre-exercise hyperventilation

Patients with vasospasm

Hypokalemia and anemia

Technical or observer error

LBBB = left bundle branch block
From *ACSM's Resource Manual for Guidelines for Exercise Testing and Prescription*, 3rd ed. Baltimore, Williams & Wilkins, 1998, p 242.

b. **Sensitivity is enhanced by the following factors:**

–The client exercises to near-maximal levels of exertion.

–Multiple-lead ECG is used.

–Other criteria besides ECG are assessed (e.g., blood pressure response, symptoms)

c. A **false-negative** stress test indicates a normal, or negative stress test (i.e., no signs of CAD) in individuals who actually have CAD (**Table 6-13**).

2. **Specificity** refers to the percentage of cases in which the exercise test accurately rules out CAD.

–Using standard criteria for detecting CAD, the exercise stress test has about an 84% specificity (84% of healthy people tested show no signs or symptoms of CAD)

–A **false-positive** stress test indicates CAD in individuals who actually do not have CAD (**Table 6-14**).

REVIEW TEST

DIRECTIONS: Carefully read all questions and select the BEST single answer.

1. A good measure of lung obstruction in clients with asthma is
   (A) residual volume.
   (B) forced expiratory volume at 1 second.
   (C) forced vital capacity.
   (D) maximal voluntary ventilation.

2. A client with a functional capacity of 7 METS, an ejection fraction of 37%, and 1 mm ST depression on exertion
   (A) should not exercise until his or her ejection fraction is > 50%.
   (B) is considered a low risk.
   (C) is considered a moderate risk.
   (D) is considered a high risk.

3. The most accurate screening method for signs and symptoms of coronary artery disease is a
   (A) maximal exercise test with a 12-lead ECG.
   (B) submaximal exercise test with a 12-lead ECG.
   (C) discontinuous protocol, stopping at 85% of maximal heart rate.
   (D) continuous protocol, stopping at 85% of maximal heart rate.

4. What is the best test to help determine ejection fraction at rest and during exercise?
   (A) Angiogram
   (B) Thallium stress test
   (C) Single proton emission computer tomography test
   (D) Multiple gated acquisition (blood pool imagery) study

5. A "cold spot" that is detected in the inferior portion of the left ventricle during a stress test and resolves 3 hours later most likely indicates
   (A) an old inferior myocardial infarction.
   (B) a myocardial infarction that is healing.
   (C) reversible myocardial ischemia.
   (D) the need for multiple bypass surgery.

6. What is the best test of cardiovascular function for a client who is obese, has claudication in his legs, and has limited mobility owing to neurological damage from uncontrolled diabetes?
   (A) Dipyridamole or dobutamine testing and assessment of cardiovascular variables
   (B) Discontinuous treadmill exercise test
   (C) Resting echocardiogram
   (D) Continuous submaximal cycle ergometer test

7. Although 12-lead testing is the optimal ECG configuration, if only one lead can be used, which one should it be?
   (A) Lead II
   (B) Lead AV_L
   (C) Lead V_5
   (D) Lead V_1

8. Which of the following is an indication for terminating an exercise test?
   (A) The client requests test termination.
   (B) The respiratory exchange rate exceeds 0.95.
   (C) The maximal heart rate exceeds 200 bpm.
   (D) The rating of perceived exertion exceeds 17 on the standard scale.

9. Given the sensitivity of the exercise ECG, stress testing conducted on 100 cardiac rehabilitation clients with documented coronary artery disease (CAD) would be expected to produce what results?
   (A) All 100 clients would show ECG indicators of CAD.
   (B) About 50 clients would show ECG indicators of CAD.
   (C) About 30 clients would show ECG indicators of CAD.
   (D) About 70 clients would show ECG indicators of CAD.

10. What action should you take for a 55-year-old client who has three risk factors for heart disease and complains of fatigue on exertion?
   (A) Conduct a submaximal stress test without the presence of a physician.
   (B) Conduct a maximal diagnostic stress test in the presence of a physician.
   (C) Use a questionnaire to evaluate activity and not conduct a test.
   (D) Start the client exercising slowly and test after 6 weeks.

11. For a client taking a beta blocker who has lowered resting blood pressure and heart rate, which of the following statements is true?
   (A) A submaximal test will provide the best estimate of the client's fitness.
   (B) A submaximal test may underestimate the client's fitness.
   (C) A submaximal test may overestimate the client's fitness.
   (D) The client should be tested only when not taking the medication.

12. Altering the weight lifted using mechanical assistance to compensate for strength differences at different joint angles is an example of
    (A) variable resistance training.
    (B) isotonic resistance training.
    (C) isokinetic resistance training.
    (D) isometric resistance training.

13. A client completes only two pushups before becoming fatigued. Which of the following statements regarding this client's muscular endurance is true?
    (A) The client has very limited muscular endurance.
    (B) A pushup test was a good assessment tool for this client.
    (C) The client needs to lose weight to improve his muscular endurance.
    (D) An alternative test of muscular endurance should be used for this client.

14. Which of the following statements about underwater weighing is true?
    (A) It can divide the body into bone, muscle, and fat components.
    (B) It is a test that assumes standard densities for bone, muscle, and fat.
    (C) It will divide the body into visceral and subcutaneous fat components.
    (D) It is a direct method of body composition assessment.

15. Two individuals have the same body weight, gender, ethnic background, and skinfold measurement results. One is 25 years old; the other, 45. Given this scenario, which of the following statements is accurate?
    (A) They both have the same percentage of body fat.
    (B) The 25-year-old is fatter.
    (C) The 45-year-old is fatter.
    (D) Who is fatter cannot be determined from the information given.

16. Lead V_1 is located at the
    (A) fifth intercostal space, left sternal border.
    (B) midclavicular line, fourth intercostal space.
    (C) fourth intercostal space, right sternal border.
    (D) midclavicular line, lateral to the xiphoid process.

17. Following termination of a stress test, a 12-lead ECG is
    (A) monitored immediately, then every 1–2 minutes until exercise-induced changes are at baseline.
    (B) monitored immediately, then at 2 and 5 minutes after the test.
    (C) monitored immediately only.
    (D) monitored and recorded only if any signs or symptoms arise during recovery.

18. The vertical fold on the posterior midline of the upper arm, halfway between the acromion and olecranon processes with the arm held freely to the side of the body, is the
    (A) biceps.
    (B) chest.
    (C) triceps.
    (D) midaxillary.

19. An inactive 38-year-old man with 26% body fat
    (A) requires a physician's evaluation before initiating an exercise program.
    (B) does not require a physician's supervision to complete an exercise test.
    (C) requires a physician's supervision to complete an exercise test.
    (D) is considered at increased risk for coronary artery disease.

20. For a client who has a contraindication for exercise testing but could benefit greatly from the information gained through testing, which of the following statements is true?
    (A) The contraindication is considered a relative contraindication.
    (B) The contraindication is considered an absolute contraindication.
    (C) The client should not be tested until the contraindication is resolved.
    (D) A submaximal test is the only test that the client should complete.

21. A client who has a measured forced vital capacity of 3.5 L and was able to expel 3.1 L within 1 second has
    (A) an obstructive defect.
    (B) a restrictive defect.
    (C) an FEV_1 of 3.1.
    (D) an FEV_1 of 89%.

ANSWERS AND EXPLANATIONS

1–B. Forced expiratory capacity at 1 second (FEV_1) is the proportion of the forced vital capacity that is expired in one second. This is a measure of the level of obstruction present in the airway. Residual volume is the volume of air that remains in the lungs following a maximal expiration. Forced vital capacity (FVC) is the volume of air that is expired following a maximal inspiration; this volume identifies the level of restrictive disease present in an individual. Maximal voluntary ventilation (MVV) is the maximal volume of airflow per minute possible; it represents the mechanical limit of pulmonary function.

2–C. Moderate risk individuals have signs or symptoms that suggest possible cardiopulmonary or metabolic disease and/or two or more risk factors. Other moderate risk criteria include: functional capacity < 6–8 METs 3 weeks after a clinical event; shock or congestive heart failure during a recent MI; moderate left ventricular dysfunction (ejection fraction 31%–49%); exercise-induced ST-segment depression of 1–2 mm; and reversible ischemic defects.

3–A. A maximal stress test requires the heart to work at its peak capacity. If heart disease is present, then signs and/or symptoms should be detected. A submaximal test may not stress the heart sufficiently to allow detection of ischemia.

4–D. A multiple gated acquisition study (MUGA) may be performed to assess resting and exercise cardiac function related to cardiac output, ejection fraction, and wall motion. In this test, technetium 99n is injected into the blood stream, where it attaches to red blood cells. Areas where the blood pools, such as the ventricles, are visualized by the technetium emissions.

5–C. During a standard stress test, a client is connected to an intravenous line. During the last minute of exercise, thallium-201 is injected into the blood stream. Thallium enters myocardial cells in proportion to the amount of blood flow to those cells, and emits energy detectable with a scintillation counter. Images of the myocardium can be constructed immediately following a stress test and 4–24 hours later. Areas with little or no perfusion immediately following a test indicate areas of ischemia. Persistence of these "cold spots" for 4–24 hours later indicates necrotic tissue. Areas of reversible ischemia will reperfuse, and cold spots will disappear in later testing.

6–A. In some instances clients are not able to complete a stress test because of muscular limitations, neurological disability, peripheral vascular disease, or other conditions that prevent the client from achieving a sufficient work intensity to provide an accurate cardiovascular assessment.

7–C. During the test, three leads should be monitored, one each from the lateral, inferior, and anterior views. Research has shown that one of these leads should be V_5, as it will pick up most ST segment changes.

8–A. Criteria are classified as absolute or relative indications. These criteria are based both on measured physiological responses and on symptoms displayed by the client. However, under any test condition, if the client requests that the test be stopped, then it must be stopped.

9–D. Sensitivity refers to the percentage of cases in which exercise testing accurately identifies the presence of CAD. While the exercise ECG is not completely sensitive to detecting CAD, it is the most cost-effective first-line screening tool. Current sensitivity for detecting CAD using the exercise stress test is about 70%.

10–B. A maximal exercise test can be most effective in detecting CAD as well as allowing the technician to measure maximal oxygen uptake ($\dot{V}O_{2max}$). Therefore, when screening for CAD, a maximal diagnostic stress test (ECG, physician supervision) is recommended.

11–C. Submaximal testing estimates $\dot{V}O_{2max}$ based on the assumed linear relationship between heart rate and $\dot{V}O_2$. Heart rate is measured at multiple workloads during the test, and $\dot{V}O_{2max}$ at an estimated maximal heart rate is calculated. Submaximal testing is based on several assumptions:
–Measurements are done while the client is at steady state.
–The relationship between heart rate and $\dot{V}O_2$ is linear.
–Maximal heart rate is similar for any given age.
–A beta blocker will change the reliability of the assumption, showing a lower heart rate for a given workload, thus predicting a higher achievable workload (and thus $\dot{V}O_{2max}$).

12–A. In variable resistance training, the weight is altered using mechanical assistance to compensate for changes in the muscle's ability to generate force due to changes in the lever system. In isotonic (free-weight) training, the weight is held constant through the range of motion (ROM). Speed can vary based on client movement. In isokinetic training, the speed of movement is held constant through the ROM. Force can vary based on client movement. In isometric (static) training, the joint angle remains the same while force is exerted.

13–D. Calisthenic tests include sit-ups, push-ups, and pull-ups. The number of repetitions is assessed with the client lifting his or her own body weight. However, poorly conditioned clients may be able to perform very few repetitions, and thus these tests may be a demonstration more of strength than of endurance.

14–B. Underwater weighing is based on the concept that the human body can be divided into a fat component and fat-free component. Fat is expressed relative to body weight (this includes all fat). This is an indirect method of measurement, because fat is not actually separated by dissection.

15–C. Age is accounted for in skinfold equations because of the changes in body fat distribution with age. With aging, more fat is stored internally, altering the meaning of a given skinfold measure. Thus the same skinfold for an older man indicates a higher relative body fat than a younger man of equivalent size and sum of skinfold.

16–C. The position for lead V_1 is located by palpating along the intercostal spaces to the fourth space; the electrode is placed along the right sternal border.

17–A. The 12-lead ECG should be recorded immediately after exercise, then every 1–2 minutes for 5 minutes or until exercise-induced ECG changes are at baseline.

18–C. The question stem describes the triceps site used in skinfold measurements to determine body composition. The biceps, chest/pectoral area, and midaxillary area are also skinfold sites used in assessing body composition. See Table 6-4 for descriptions of skinfold sites.

19–B. Because the client is under age 40 and has only one risk factor (inactivity), ACSM guidelines indicate that a physician's supervision during a stress test is not required.

20–A. *Relative contraindications* include clients who might be tested if the potential benefit from exercise testing outweighs the relative risk. *Absolute contraindications* refer to individuals for whom exercise testing should not be performed until the situation or condition has stabilized.

21–D. FEV_1 is calculated as

(volume expired in 1 second ÷ forced vital capacity) × 100

An obstructive defect is indicated by $FEV_1 < 70\%$; a restrictive defect, by a forced vital capacity $< 70\%$ of predicted.

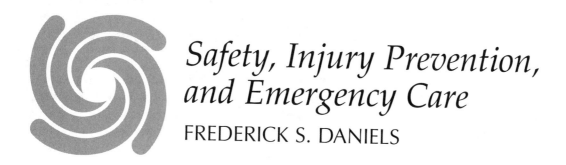

CHAPTER 7

Safety, Injury Prevention, and Emergency Care

FREDERICK S. DANIELS

I. GENERAL CONSIDERATIONS

–All forms of exercise, from clinical testing to supervised exercise, from cardiac rehabilitation to general fitness programs, entail some risk (**Table 7-1**).

–Every clinical exercise physiologist and exercise specialist must understand the risks associated with exercise testing and training, be able to implement preventive measures, and know how to respond in case of injury or medical emergency.

–Every clinical testing and exercise program must have an **emergency response system** in place to respond to injuries and medical emergencies.

Table 7-1. Potential Medical Complications of Exercise

Cardiovascular Complications	Metabolic Complications	Endocrine Complications	Traumatic Injuries
Cardiac arrest	Volume depletion	Amenorrhea	Bruises
Ischemia	Dehydration	Complications in diabetics	Strains and sprains
Angina	Rhabdomyolysis	Hypoglycemia	Muscle and tendon tears and
Myocardial infarction	Renal failure	Hyperglycemia	ruptures
Arrhythmias	Electrolyte disturbances	Retinal hemorrhage	Fractures
Supraventricular tachycardia		Osteoporosis	Contusions and lacerations
Atrial fibrillation	**Thermal Complications**		Bleeding
Ventricular tachycardia	Hyperthermia	**Neurologic Complications**	Crush injuries
Ventricular fibrillation	Heat rash	Dizziness	Blunt trauma
Bradyarrhythmias	Heat cramps	Syncope (fainting)	Internal organ injury
Bundle branch blocks	Heat syncope	Cerebral vascular accident (stroke)	Splenic rupture
AV nodal blocks	Heat exhaustion	Insomnia	Myocardial contusion
Congestive heart failure	Heat stroke		Drowning
Hypertension	Hypothermia	**Musculoskeletal Complications**	Head injuries
Hypotension	Frostbite	Mechanical injuries	Eye injuries
Aneurysm rupture		Back injuries	Death
Underlying medical conditions	**Pulmonary Complications**	Stress fractures	
predisposing to increased	Exercise-induced asthma	Carpal tunnel syndrome	
complications	Bronchospasm	Joint pain/injury	
Hypertrophic cardiomyopathy	Pulmonary embolism	Muscle cramps/spasms	
Coronary artery anomalies	Pulmonary edema	Tendonitis	
Idiopathic left ventricular	Pneumothorax	Exacerbation of musculoskeletal	
hypertrophy	Exercise-induced anaphylaxis	diseases	
Marfan syndrome	Exacerbation of underlying		
Aortic stenosis	pulmonary disease	**Overuse Complications**	
Right ventricular dysplasia		Overuse syndromes	
Congenital heart defects	**Gastrointestinal Complications**	Over-training	
Myocarditis	Vomiting	Over-exercising	
Pericarditis	Cramps	Shin splints	
Amyloidosis	Diarrhea	Plantar fasciitis	
Sarcoidosis			
Long QT syndrome			
Sickle-cell trait			

(From *ACSM's Resource Manual for Guidelines for Exercise Testing and Prescription*, 3rd ed. Baltimore, Williams & Wilkins, 1998, p 489.)

II. EMERGENCY RESPONSE SYSTEM

A. FACILITY

–The facility should be designed to allow safe and effective response to injuries and medical emergencies, with:

1. Handicap accessibility
2. Clear and easy access to emergency exits
3. Wide hallways for stretchers and emergency equipment
4. Proper ventilation, temperature, and humidity controls
5. Nonskid flooring in testing and emergency exit areas
6. Electrical wiring that meets hospital and medical facility code
7. Telephone service

B. EQUIPMENT

1. **Emergency equipment must be:**
   –clearly marked.
   –readily accessible at all times.
   –calibrated and maintained regularly.
2. **Necessary equipment includes the following:**
   –Telephones with telephone numbers of the emergency medical system (EMS) or 911, physicians, cardiac code team, police, and fire
   –First-aid kits
   –First-responder blood-borne pathogen kits
   –Latex gloves
   –Mouthpieces for cardiopulmonary resuscitation (CPR)
   –Resuscitation bags
   –Back board
   –Splints

   –Defibrillator
   –Emergency drugs and materials (i.e., epinephrine, dextrose, blood glucose meter)
3. **Staff** should know how to use and routinely practice using emergency equipment.

C. EMERGENCY PLAN

1. **An emergency plan is mandatory** in all testing and exercise areas
2. **The emergency plan must specify**
   –the specific responsibilities of each staff member.
   –the required equipment.
   –predetermined contacts for emergency response.
   –step-by-step actions to take for each common medical emergency.
3. **All emergency incidents must be documented** with dates, times, actions, people involved, and outcomes.
4. **The plan should be practiced** with announced and unannounced drills on a quarterly basis.

D. PREPARATION OF STAFF

–All staff, including nonclinical staff, should be trained in the emergency plan.

1. **Clinical exercise staff** should have training in the proper handling of medical emergencies.
   –**Mandatory training** includes CPR, basic life support (BLS), and basic first aid.
   –**Recommended training** includes advanced cardiac life support (ACLS) or emergency medical technician (EMT) training.
2. **Nonexercise staff** should have **CPR training.**
3. A **physician** should be present or nearby in every clinical exercise test setting, to assist with or manage emergencies.

III. SAFETY CONSIDERATIONS

A. CONTRAINDICATIONS TO EXERCISE TESTING AND TRAINING

–For certain individuals, the risks for complications during exercise testing and training outweigh the potential benefits.

1. **Identifying a patient's contraindications** to exercise testing and training (Table 6-1) and cardiac rehabilitation (Table 8-1) involves:
   –**Reviewing the medical history**

   –**Assessing cardiac risk**
   –**Evaluating physical examination findings**
   –**Evaluating laboratory test results**
2. A patient with **absolute contraindications** should not undergo exercise testing or training until those conditions are stabilized.
3. A patient with **relative contraindications** may undergo exercise testing and training,

but only after careful analysis of his or her risk-to-benefit ratio.

4. In some cases, clinical exercise testing may still be performed for a patient with contraindications, to guide drug therapy.

B. **SAFETY DURING EXERCISE TESTING AND TRAINING**

1. **Patient safety**

   a. **Monitoring for signs of fatigue and distress**

      –During exercise testing, the clinical exercise specialist monitors the patient's heart rate and rhythm (on an electrocardiogram [ECG]), blood pressure, respirations, and other parameters for signs of fatigue and/or distress.

      (1) **Manifestations of cardiac or pulmonary distress** necessitate stopping the test immediately and possibly initiating the emergency response system (see Chapter 6, Table 6-12).

      (2) **Less severe manifestations** (e.g., lightheadedness, muscular fatigue, intermittent premature ventricular contractions [PVCs], wheezing) may not necessitate immediate test termination.

   b. **Indications for stopping an exercise session** include those listed in Chapter 6, Table 6-2, as well as the following:

      –**Signs of confusion or inability to concentrate**

      –**Dizziness**

      –**Convulsions**

      –**Physical injury**

      –**Nausea**

2. **Staff safety**

   –Safety of the clinical exercise staff can be maximized by following federal Occupational Safety and Health Administration (OSHA) standards, which include the following:

   a. **Wash hands thoroughly** before working with a patient.

   b. **Wear gloves and other protective clothing** (when necessary) when there is any possibility of exposure to blood-borne pathogens.

   c. **Keep cords out of the path** of both staff and patients to eliminate trips and falls.

   d. **Keep long hair and loose clothing from catching on equipment.**

C. **MEDICATIONS AND SAFETY**

   –Various medications can affect a patient's response to exercise testing or training (see Chapter 8, Table 8-6).

IV. GENERAL EMERGENCY RESPONSE GUIDELINES

A. **CONTACTS**

1. **Activating the EMS**

   –This may entail calling a paramedic/ambulance group or an emergency medical team within the facility.

   –**Information to communicate includes:**

   a. **Patient's location**

   b. **Patient's status,** including vital signs

   c. Symptoms and actions that led to the emergency

   d. Actions of the exercise staff in caring for the patient after the onset of symptoms

2. **Communicating with a physician or other appropriate medical professional**

   a. Report the signs and symptoms associated with the emergency, as well as the patient's status before the start of the test.

   b. State current vital signs and symptoms.

   c. Ask for recommendations.

3. **Contacting the patient's family physician**

   –The patient's family physician should be contacted, particularly if a physician is not present at the facility.

   a. Indicate to the family physician that a medical emergency has occurred with one of his or her patients.

   b. Be prepared to report the symptoms associated with the emergency, as well as the patient's status prior to the start of the test.

   c. Present vital signs and present symptoms.

   d. Ask for recommendations.

4. **Contacting the patient's family**

   a. Explain the situation in whatever detail the family needs.

   b. Indicate if the patient has been transported to a hospital or emergency department and how the family can find it.

   c. Assist the family in any other way possible.

B. INITIAL ACTIONS

1. **Initial monitoring** during a medical emergency should include:

   a. **Heart rate** through palpation or ECG

   b. **Heart rhythm** through ECG

   c. **Blood pressure**

   d. **Respirations**

   e. **Physical signs of complications**

     –**Loss of balance**

     –**Convulsions/seizure**

     –**Shivering**

     –**Cold, clammy skin**

     –**Verbal and nonverbal expression of pain**

   f. **Blood glucose level** in a patient with diabetes

2. **First aid procedures** should be initiated as indicated (**Table 7-2**).

3. **After the patient is stabilized,** he or she should be transported to a facility (e.g., hospital, medical center, physician's office) or department (e.g., emergency room or other treatment area) for appropriate treatment.

C. FOLLOW-UP ACTIONS

–After an emergency incident, follow-up with the patient serves several purposes:

1. **It clarifies the patient's current medical status,** aiding understanding of the causes of the emergency.

2. **It provides more information on the consequences of the staff's actions** to help determine whether the response to the emergency was effective.

3. **It allows the staff to finalize the incident report,** with a final analysis of the patient's status (which may not be known for days following the incident).

D. DOCUMENTATION

–Careful documentation of an emergency event provides important information for the safety of the patient, management of the program, and protection of the staff and facility.

–**Information should include:**

1. **Time line of events.**

2. **All people involved,** including witnesses.

3. **Actions of the staff** to resolve the emergency situation.

4. **All communications** with medical personnel, family, and other staff.

5. **Follow-up actions.**

V. RESPONSE TO SPECIFIC EMERGENCIES

–Refer to **Tables 7-2** and **7-3**.

A. CARDIAC ARREST

–**Incidence** is 0.4 in 10,000 clinical exercise tests.

1. **Signs and symptoms**

  –Rapid onset of fatigue

  –Ventricular tachycardia

  –Ventricular fibrillation

  –Bradycardia

2. **Response**

  a. **If the patient is breathing and has a pulse:**

    –Call EMS immediately.

    –Place the patient in the recovery position (i.e., prone with one knee and hip slightly flexed) with the head to one side to avoid airway obstruction. DO NOT attempt this position with patients who have suspected cervical spine injury.

    –Stay with the patient and continue to monitor vital signs.

  b. **If the patient is suspected of not breathing or having a pulse:**

    –Assess breathing and pulse.

    –Call EMS.

    –Perform CPR or use an automatic external defibrillator (AED).

    –Assist medical staff or EMS in caring for the patient.

B. MYOCARDIAL INFARCTION (MI)

–is ischemic myocardial necrosis resulting from an abrupt reduction in blood flow to the myocardium. Reduced blood flow often results from arterial plaque buildup that occludes the coronary arteries.

1. **Signs and symptoms**

  –Visceral pain described as pressure or aching radiating down left arm, chest, back, or jaw

  –Gastrointestinal upset

Table 7-2. Possible Medical Emergencies and Suggested First Aid

Problem	First Aid Procedure
Heat cramps	Replace lost fluids. Increase sodium and potassium lost through excessive sweating.
Heat exhaustion and heat stroke	Move victim to shaded area; have victim lie down with feet elevated above the level of the heart. Remove excess clothing. Cool victim with sips of cool fluid; sprinkle water on him or her and on the facial area; rub ice pack over major vessels in armpits, groin, and neck areas. Victim should seek immediate medical attention and be given intravenous fluids as soon as possible.
Fainting (Syncope)	Leave the victim lying down. Turn on his or her side if vomiting occurs. Maintain an open airway. Loosen any tight clothing. Take blood pressure and pulse if possible. Seek medical attention because it is a potentially life-threatening situation and the cause of fainting must be determined.
Hypoglycemia (symptoms include diaphoresis, pallor, tremor, tachycardia, palpitations, visual disturbances, mental confusion, weakness, lightheadedness, fatigue, headache, memory loss, seizure, or coma)	May become life-threatening. Seek medical attention to treat cause. Give oral glucose solutions such as Kool-aid with sugar, non-diet soft drinks, juice, or milk. If patient is able to ingest solids, gelatin sweetened with sugar, mild chocolate or fruit may be given.
Hyperglycemia (symptoms include dehydration, hypotension, and reflex tachycardia, osmotic diuresis, impaired consciousness, nausea, vomiting, abdominal pain, hyperventilation, odor of acetone on breath)	May be life-threatening if it leads to diabetic ketoacidosis. Seek immediate medical attention. Rehydrate with intravenous normal saline. Correct electrolyte loss (K^+). Insulin.
Sprains/Strains	No weight bearing on affected extremity. Loosen shoes, apply a pillow or blanket-type splint around extremity. Elevate the extremity. Apply bag of crushed ice to the affected area. Seek medical attention if pain or swelling persist.
Simple or compound fractures	Immobilize the extremity. Splint the extremity to prevent further injury to the bone or soft tissue. Use anything at hand as a splint. Do not attempt to reduce any dislocation in the field unless there is danger of losing life or limb. Seek immediate medical attention. Protect the victim from further injury.
Bronchospasm	Maintain open airway. Give bronchodilators via nebulizer if prescribed for patient. Give oxygen by nasal cannula if available.
Hypotension/Shock	Lay the victim down with feet elevated. Maintain open airway. Monitor vital signs (pulse, blood pressure). Call for immediate advanced life support measures because this is a life-threatening emergency that requires intensive monitoring of vital signs, administration of intravenous fluids and drugs to maintain adequate tissue perfusion while evaluation is done as to the cause (i.e., hypovolemia, cardiogenic shock, sepsis).
Bleeding Lacerations Incisions Puncture wounds Abrasions Contusions	Apply direct pressure over the site to stop the bleeding. Protect the wound from contamination and infection. May need to seek medical attention; victim may need stitches, tetanus shot. If bleeding is severe, in addition to direct pressure, elevate the injured part of the body, and if an artery is severed, apply direct pressure over the main artery to the affected limb and seek immediate medical attention.

(With permission from Strauss WE et al. Emergency plans and procedures for an exercise facility. In *ACSM's Resource Manual for Guidelines for Exercise Testing and Prescription,* 2nd ed. Philadelphia, Lea & Febiger, 1993, p 373.)

–Dyspnea

–Shock

–Ventricular fibrillation

–Bradycardia

–Cool, clammy skin

2. **Response**

–Call EMS immediately.

–Assess the patient carefully to determine if an MI is occurring; **prompt diagnosis is critical.**

–Relieve patient distress.

Table 7-3. Acute Responses for Common Injuries/Emergencies

Injury/Emergency	Signs/Symptoms	Acute Care
Closed skin wounds (blisters, corns)	Pain, swelling, infection	Clean with antiseptic soap, apply sterile dressing, antibiotic ointment
Open skin wounds (lacerations, abrasions)	Pain, redness, bleeding, swelling, headache, mild fever	Apply pressure to stop bleeding, clean with soap or sterile saline, apply sterile dressing, refer to physician for stitches/tetanus
Contusions (bruises)	Swelling, localized pain, loss of function if severe	RICES, apply padding if necessary for protection
Strains*		
Grade I	Pain, localized tenderness, tightness	RICES
Grade II	Loss of function, hemorrhage	RICES, refer for physician evaluation if impaired function
Grade III	Palpable defect	Immobilization, RICES, immediate referral to physician
Sprains*		
Grade I	Pain, point tenderness, strength loss, edema	RICES
Grade II	Hemorrhage, measurable laxity	RICES, physician evaluation
Grade III	Palpable or observable defect	Immobilization, RICES, physician evaluation
Fractures		
Stress	Pain, point tenderness	Physician evaluation, rest
Simple	Swelling, disability, pain	Immobilize with splint, physician evaluation, x-rays
Compound	Bleeding, swelling, pain, disability	Immobilize, control bleeding, apply sterile dressing, immediate physician evaluation
Dizziness/Syncope	Disoriented, confused, pale skin color	Determine responsiveness, place supine with legs elevated, administer fluids if conscious, begin emergency breathing or compressions as needed
Hypoglycemia (low blood sugar)	Pale skin color, skin moist and sweaty, tachycardia, hunger, double vision	Administer sugar if conscious; if unconscious, place sugar granules under tongue, if recovery requires more than 1–2 minutes, activate EMS system (12)
Hyperglycemia (high blood sugar)	Confused, nauseous, headache, breath has sweet, fruity odor, thirsty, abdominal pain and vomiting, hyperventilation	Activate EMS, administer fluids if conscious, turn head to side if vomiting
Hypothermia	Shivering but may stop with extreme drops in core temperature, loss of coordination, muscle stiffness, lethargy	Activate EMS and transport to hospital, remove wet clothing, replace with dry, warm clothing
Hyperthermia		
Heat cramps	Involuntary, isolated muscle spasms	Administer fluids, apply direct pressure to spasm and release, massage cramping area with ice
Heat syncope	Weakness, fatigue, hypotension, pale skin, syncope	Move to cool area, place supine with legs elevated, administer fluids if conscious, check blood pressure
Heat exhaustion	Profuse sweating, cold, clammy skin, multiple muscle spasms, headache, nausea, loss of consciousness, dizziness, tachycardia, low blood pressure	Move to cool area, place supine with feet elevated, administer fluids, monitor body temperature, refer for physician evaluation
Heat stroke	Hot, dry skin, but can be sweating, dyspnea, confusion, often unconscious	Activate EMS and transport to hospital immediately, remove clothing, dowse with cool water, wrap in cool wet sheets, administer fluids if conscious
Angina (pain, pressure or tingling in the chest, neck, jaw, arm and/or back)	Pain, sweating, denial of medical problem, nausea, shortness of breath	Stop activity, place in seated or supine position (whichever is most comfortable), activate EMS if pain is not relieved; if unresponsive, check breathing and pulse, begin CPR if necessary
Dyspnea, labored breathing	Hyperventilation, dizziness, wheezing, coughing, loss of coordination	Maintain open airway, administer bronchodilator if prescribed, try pursed lip breathing; if no relief, activate EMS and transport

* Signs and symptoms for each grade include those for the grade below the one listed (i.e., Grade II includes those of Grades I and II; Grade III includes signs and symptoms listed under Grades I, II and III).
RICES = rest, ice, compression, elevation, stabilization

–Assist as needed with administration of thrombolytic agents to reperfuse occluded arteries.

–Administer pain-relief medications as ordered by the physician.

–Stay with the patient and continue to monitor vital signs.

C. HYPERGLYCEMIA

–is an abnormally high blood glucose level (> 200 mg/dl) that can impair function and, if severe, can become an emergency situation (diabetic ketoacidosis).

1. **Signs and symptoms**

   –Confusion

   –Headache

   –Sweet, fruity breath odor

   –Thirst

   –Nausea and vomiting

   –Reflex tachycardia

   –Abdominal pain

   –Hyperventilation

2. **Response**

   –Call EMS.

   –Rehydrate and correct electrolyte loss through fluid administration.

   –Administer insulin.

   –Turn the patient's head to one side if vomiting.

D. TRANSIENT ISCHEMIC ATTACK (TIA)

–TIAs are sudden, brief ischemic attacks usually involving the carotid or vertebral arteries in the neck.

1. **Signs and symptoms**

   –Pain in jaw or neck

   –Slight paralysis of one side (hemiparesis)

   –Difficulty speaking (aphasia)

   –Burning or tingling sensation in extremities

   –Fatigue

2. **Response**

   –Stop exercise immediately.

   –Have the patient sit or lie down.

   –Administer prescribed medication if available.

   –Contact the physician.

   –If pain and other symptoms continue beyond 30 minutes, call EMS.

E. CORONARY THROMBOSIS

–is coronary occlusion by a thrombus (a clot of lipid-rich atherosclerotic plaque). Symptoms are caused by rupture of these plaque deposits within the coronary arteries.

1. **Signs and symptoms**

   –Pain described as pressure or aching radiating down left arm, chest, or back

   –Gastrointestinal upset

   –Dyspnea

   –Shock

   –Ventricular fibrillation

   –Bradycardia

   –Cool, clammy skin

2. **Response**

   –Call EMS immediately.

   –Relieve patient distress.

   –Provide pain relief as prescribed by the physician.

   –Administer thrombolytic agents as ordered by the physician.

   –Stay with the patient and continue monitoring vital signs.

F. INTERNAL CARDIAC DEFIBRILLATOR DISCHARGE

–An internal cardiac defibrillator may dysfunction and discharge when it should not.

1. **Signs and symptoms**

   –Severe, sudden chest pain

   –Dyspnea

   –Muscle contractions in the chest or abdomen associated with discharge

   –Loss of consciousness

   –Ventricular fibrillation

   –Cardiac arrest

2. **Response**

   –Call the EMS and physician immediately.

   –Place the patient in recovery position with the head turned to one side.

   –Stay with the patient and monitor vital signs.

   –If the patient is not breathing or does not have a palpable pulse:

   a. Assess breathing and pulse.

   b. Perform CPR or use an AED, but avoid pressure or contact within the area of defibrillator application.

G. SERIOUS ARRHYTHMIAS

–Various arrhythmias can develop during exercise testing and training. Those considered serious and that require emergency attention include **ventricular fibrillation, ventricular tachycardia, atrial fibrillation, torsades de pointes,** and **bradycardia.**

–The most severe arrhythmias (atrial fibrillation, ventricular fibrillation) **can result in an MI** and require defibrillation to control.

H. HYPOGLYCEMIA

–Actual blood glucose levels that elicit hypoglycemic symptoms are highly individualized; generally, < 50 mg/dl may be problematic.

1. **Signs and symptoms**

   –Tremors

   –Tachycardia

   –Diaphoresis

   –Visual disturbances

   –Confusion

   –Headache

   –Fatigue

   –Lightheadedness

   –Seizures

2. **Response to a hypoglycemic emergency**

   –Contact EMS immediately.

   –Give the patient an **oral glucose solution,** such as orange juice or a nondiet soft drink.

   –Keep the patient comfortable and safe.

I. BRONCHOSPASM

–is obstruction of the airway due to spasm of airway smooth muscle, edema of airway mucosa, increased mucus secretion, or injury.

1. **Signs and symptoms**

   –Dyspnea

   –Hyperventilation

   –Coughing

   –Wheezing

   –Chest tightness

2. **Response**

   –Maintain an open airway.

   –Administer a bronchodilator if prescribed by a physician.

   –Administer oxygen if available.

   –Replace fluids and electrolytes.

   –Keep the patient calm to reduce anxiety.

J. HYPOTENSION/SHOCK

1. **Signs and symptoms**

   –Chills

   –Loss of consciousness

   –Bradycardia

   –Dizziness

   –Confusion

2. **Response**

   –Have the patient lie supine with the feet elevated.

   –Maintain an open airway.

   –Monitor vital signs.

   –Call EMS.

VI. COMMON CATEGORY I MEDICATIONS ADMINISTERED IN MEDICAL EMERGENCIES

A. **EPINEPHRINE** is an endogenous catecholamine that optimizes blood flow to the heart and brain by increasing aortic diastolic pressure and preferentially shunting blood to the internal carotid artery (enhancing cerebral blood flow).

B. **LIDOCAINE** is an antiarrhythmic agent that decreases automaticity in the ventricular myocardium and raises the fibrillation threshold.

C. **OXYGEN** ensures adequate arterial oxygen content and greatly enhances tissue oxygenation.

D. **ATROPINE** is a parasympathetic blocking agent used in the treatment of bradyarrhythmias.

REVIEW TEST

DIRECTIONS: Carefully read all questions and select the BEST single answer.

1. The clinical exercise physiologist shares a responsibility to
   (A) implement measures to stop disease.
   (B) make patients look healthy.
   (C) implement preventive measures to reduce the risk of medical emergencies.
   (D) develop a plan to reduce the physical demands of exercise testing.

2. Which of the following is *not* considered a benefit of the follow-up in an emergency situation?
   (A) It provides information on the patient's current status, which may help determine cause of the emergency.
   (B) It provides statistics that will help justify the emergency response program.
   (C) It allows the staff to finalize the incident report.
   (D) It provides information to determine the consequences of the staff's actions.

3. Which of the following actions involving termination of exercise testing is correct?
   (A) Immediately terminate the test if muscular fatigue occurs.
   (B) Initiate the test termination process when cardiac complications occur.
   (C) Initiate the test termination process when intermittent PVCs are detected on ECG.
   (D) Immediately terminate the test when intermittent PVCs are detected on ECG.

4. Safety procedures for clinical staff help protect them from
   (A) blood-borne pathogens.
   (B) theft.
   (C) violent patients.
   (D) work-related injuries.

5. The treatment modality RICES includes all of the following *except*
   (A) covering.
   (B) ice.
   (C) stabilization.
   (D) rest.

6. Which of the following statements about emergency equipment is *most* important?
   (A) Each piece of equipment should be painted a specific color for easy identification.
   (B) Use of emergency equipment should be practiced routinely.
   (C) Emergency equipment should include pencils, not pens.
   (D) Emergency equipment should be kept clean at all times.

7. Identifying a patient's risk of complications is important. Which of the following is *not* considered a common aspect of the risk identification process?
   (A) Laboratory results
   (B) Assessment of cardiac risk
   (C) Review of medical history
   (D) Assessment of work history

8. Symptoms of hyperglycemia include all of the following *except*
   (A) tremor.
   (B) confusion.
   (C) bradycardia.
   (D) slurred speech.

9. Emergency procedures and safety include
   (A) injury prevention.
   (B) basic principles for exercise training.
   (C) metabolic injuries.
   (D) emergency consequences.

10. Category 1 medications include all of the following *except*
    (A) lidocaine.
    (B) oxygen.
    (C) Xylocaine.
    (D) epinephrine.

11. The emergency response system is
    (A) the combination of the ambulance and the emergency room.
    (B) critical for the staff to be able to respond adequately to an emergency.
    (C) the protocol used to practice safety plans.
    (D) required by most health departments.

12. In developing an emergency plan, program administrators must take into account all of the following factors *except*
    (A) type of flooring.
    (B) type of electrical wiring.
    (C) ventilation, temperature, and humidity.
    (D) types of exercise equipment.

13. Documentation in the context of emergency response commonly refers to
    (A) records of each exercise session.
    (B) records of attendance.
    (C) records of all emergency situations.
    (D) manuals for all emergency equipment.

14. A patient who exhibits tachycardia, diaphoresis, lightheadedness, and visual disturbances may be experiencing
    (A) hypoglycemia.
    (B) congestive heart failure.
    (C) hyperglycemia.
    (D) hypotension.

15. Which of the following is *not* part of an emergency plan?
    (A) The plan should list the schedule of each staff member so they can all be accounted for in an emergency.
    (B) The plan must be written.
    (C) The plan should outline each specific action.
    (D) The staff should be prepared and trained in the plan.

16. The physician's role in an emergency plan is
    (A) not important; most facilities are hospital-based, and the emergency room is nearby.
    (B) not significant, because a physician is not necessary when testing is conducted.
    (C) very important; one of the first steps to be taken during a medical crisis is communication with the physician.
    (D) critical, because the physician must be present and can handle any emergency situation.

17. What is OSHA?
    (A) A state agency that licenses medical facilities
    (B) A federal agency that sets standards for staff and patient safety
    (C) A federal agency that certifies and inspects hospitals
    (D) A state agency that inspects emergency protocols within medical facilities

18. The preparation of professional staff should include training in
    (A) ABLS and ENT.
    (B) CPR and BLS.
    (C) CPR and EMS.
    (D) ACLS and ENT.

19. Which of the following is *not* considered an absolute contraindication to exercise testing?
    (A) Unstable angina
    (B) Psychosis
    (C) Suspected myocarditis
    (D) Moderate valvular heart disease

20. Which of the following manifestations would be an indication for stopping an exercise test?
    (A) Low cholesterol (< 125 mol)
    (B) Diastolic blood pressure > 105 mm Hg
    (C) Intermittent premature ventricular contractions
    (D) Low blood sugar (< 100 mg/dl)

ANSWERS AND EXPLANATIONS

1–C. The clinical exercise physiologist must understand the risks of exercise while realizing the benefits. If the benefits clearly outweigh the risks, preventive measures should be implemented to reduce that risk. The clinical exercise physiologist cannot eradicate or cure disease, but can only work to help prevent or reduce the symptoms of disease. The clinical exercise physiologist is concerned with the patient's health, not appearance.

2–B. The follow-up is an important function following an incident. Justification of a program has no relevance when investigating an incident. The primary concern should be the health status of the patient and the cause of the emergency. The patient's present status is indeed part of the follow-up, because it will provide medical information that can help determine the cause of injury. Also, information from the patient can help piece the specific actions of the incident together. This follow-up information will also help staff members complete their report, because they may learn new and helpful information that should be included in the report. The final report with the follow-up information will assist program administrators in determining the consequences of their actions.

3–C. Intermittent PVCs are not a serious concern, so the tester can begin the test termination process instead of terminating the test immediately. Muscular fatigue and intermittent PVCs do not require immediate termination of the test; initiating the test termination process is appropriate. Cardiac complications are considered very serious and require immediate termination, not merely initiation of the test termination process.

4–A. Because of the importance of infection control, blood-borne pathogens must be a concern for all staff, and OSHA regulations help protect both patients and staff. Theft and violent patients may be concerns, but are not part of any emergency plan. The plan may include injuries in general, but not work-related injuries specifically.

5–A. Covering is not part of RICES; compression is the "C" component.

6–B. Routine practice in using emergency equipment is an important part of the emergency plan, to ensure that staff knows how to use the equipment correctly in an emergency situation. Identification of equipment through tagging, not color, is important. Whether to use pens or pencils is irrelevant, and although equipment should be kept clean, this is not an essential part of emergency equipment protocol.

7–D. Work history is not a relevant part of the identification process. Work history most likely will not provide any meaningful information regarding the risk of medical emergencies. The review of medical history is very important and can identify significant cardiac risk factors. Assessment of laboratory results may indicate signs of potential cardiac or pulmonary risk, which could contraindicate exercise testing. Assessment of cardiac risk is critical to the determination of potential complications and is clearly a part of the identification process.

8–C. Tachycardia, not bradycardia, is a possible sign of hyperglycemia. Elevated blood sugar overloads the endocrine system; tremors, confusion and slurred speech are common responses to this overload.

9–A. Injury prevention is often overlooked, but is an important part of a facility's emergency procedures and safety program. All clinical exercise physiologists should understand how to avoid emergencies. Basic principles for exercise training are important for general day-to-day operations, but not for emergency procedures.

10–C. Xylocaine, though similar to lidocaine, is not an antiarrhythmic agent as lidocaine is, and thus cannot help stabilize the heart in a cardiac crisis. Oxygen is often overlooked as a drug, but helps keep tissues alive. Epinephrine optimizes blood flow to the heart and brain and is an important Category 1 medication.

11–B. The emergency response system is designed to help the staff adequately handle emergencies. The ambulance and emergency room and the protocols used to practice safety procedures may be a part of an emergency response plan, but are not part of the emergency response system. Health departments do not regulate emergency response systems.

12–D. In preparing a facility for emergency situations, program administrators do not need to know what kind of exercise equipment they have. Flooring and electrical wiring are important factors in the risk of accidents. Environmental factors can increase the risk of crises; for example, poor air quality, high temperatures, and high humidity can cause pulmonary difficulties and increase the risk of heat exhaustion.

13–C. Documentation of every aspect of an emergency situation is an important component of any emergency response system. Records of exercise sessions and attendance may be important for standard operations, but are not important for emergency response. Equipment manuals should be on file, but are not considered documentation.

14–A. Common signs and symptoms of hypoglycemia include tachycardia, diaphoresis, lightheadedness, and visual disturbances. Congestive heart failure and hypotension do not produce tachycardia. Hyperglycemia does not produce diaphoresis.

15–A. Accounting for staff in an emergency is not essential. Writing down the plan is essential so that the staff can read it as part of their training, as well as have a document to refer to during an emergency. Delineating specific actions of each staff member in an emergency situation and training the staff in these actions are obviously integral parts of any emergency plan.

16–C. Communication with the physician is very important during a medical crisis, and exercise staff should have a ready means of communicating with a physician in the event of an emergency. A physician should be nearby during any exercise test, but not necessarily in the testing room.

17–B. OSHA is the federal agency that sets safety standards for staff and patients. The NCQA is the federal agency that inspects and certifies hospitals. OSHA is a federal, not a state, agency.

18–B. Cardiopulmonary resuscitation (CPR) and basic life support (BLS) are important certifications in the care of medical emergencies. There is no ABLS certification. EMS and ENT are not appropriate emergency care training for exercise staff.

19–D. Individuals with moderate valvular heart disease are able to function under the stress of exercise, especially if they are under the care of a cardiac specialist and receive permission to undergo an exercise test. Unstable angina may lead to a significant cardiac crisis when exercise is introduced, so it is considered an absolute contraindication with exercise. Psychosis is a significant emotional distress and can lead to difficulties in completing the exercise test, and so is considered an absolute contraindication. Myocarditis is an absolute contraindication of exercise testing, because inflammation of the heart's muscular walls can cause severe cardiac complications with the increased stroke volume and heart rate associated with the stress of exercise.

20–D. Low blood sugar may indicate a lack of glucose for muscle activity. Low blood sugar also leads to hypoglycemia, which can bring lightheadedness, tachycardia, and confusion suggesting that the exercise session be stopped. Low cholesterol should have little or no effect on the exerciser. As long as the diastolic blood pressure does not change significantly (more than 20 mm Hg) during the test, 105 mm Hg is not considered a contraindication to exercise. Intermittent PVCs do not pose a danger to an exerciser, so the test should not be halted.

CHAPTER 8

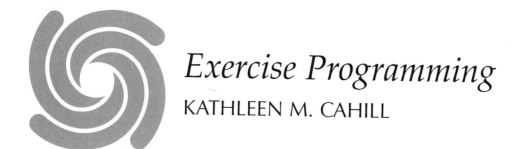

Exercise Programming
KATHLEEN M. CAHILL

I. TYPES OF EXERCISE PROGRAMMING

A. INPATIENT REHABILITATION

1. **Value of early ambulation**

   –Early ambulation stabilizes central and peripheral hemodynamics.

   –Additional medical surveillance during exercise identifies other factors that may influence prognosis.

2. **Indications and contraindications for inpatient rehabilitation**

   –See **Table 8-1**. Indications and contraindications for inpatient rehabilitation for the cardiac population may be used for other patients as well.

3. **Goals of inpatient rehabilitation**

   –To provide orthostatic challenge

   –To prepare the patient to return to work, activities of daily living (ADL), and leisure activities

   –To stabilize the patient's response to low-level activity and to reduce associated anxiety

   –To provide education on the patient's disease state in preparation for discharge to home or a transitional care facility

   –To facilitate entry into outpatient programs

4. **Risk stratification**

   –Each client's risk is stratified according to the hospital's criteria or the suggested stratifications of the American Association of Cardiovascular and Pulmonary Rehabilitation (AACVPR), the American Heart Association (AHA), or the American College of Physicians (ACP). (See Chapter 4, Tables 4-2 and 4-3.)

5. **Exercise guidelines**

   a. **Mode**

      –includes supine and sitting bed activities, self-care activities, and ambulation activities (e.g., stair-climbing, walking, cycling).

   b. **Frequency of activity**

      –can range from 2 to 4 times daily depending on intensity, duration, and the patient's tolerance for activity.

   c. **Intensity**

      –is monitored through heart rate (HR), blood pressure (BP), electrocardiogram (ECG), pulse oximetry, ratings of perceived exertion, and metabolic equivalent (MET) level.

   d. **Duration**

      –is correlated to frequency, intensity, and client tolerance (e.g., 10–20 min).

   e. **Progression for range of motion (ROM)**

      –is from active assistive ROM to active and resistive ROM.

      –An example of ROM progression is as follows: (1) clinician assists patient in performing a straight leg raise (SLR) in bed; (2) patient performs SLR independently; (3) clinician offers manual resistance against the limb while patient performs SLR.

      –A guide for progression of inpatient activities is found in **Table 8-2**.

6. **Normal and abnormal responses to exercise**

   –Physical assessment is a necessary component of each rehabilitative session. Client

Table 8-1. Clinical Indications and Contraindications for Inpatient and Outpatient Cardiac Rehabilitation

Indications

Medically stable post-myocardial infarction

Stable angina

Coronary artery bypass graft surgery

Percutaneous transluminal coronary angioplasty

Compensated congestive heart failure

Cardiomyopathy

Heart or other organ transplantation

Other cardiac surgery including valvular and pacemaker insertion (including implantable cardioverter defibrillator)

Peripheral vascular disease

High-risk cardiovascular disease ineligible for surgical intervention

Sudden cardiac death syndrome

End-stage renal disease

At risk for coronary artery disease, with diagnoses of diabetes mellitus, hyperlipidemia, hypertension, etc.

Other patients who may benefit from structured exercise and/or patient education (based on physician referral and consensus of the rehabilitation team)

Contraindications

Unstable angina

Resting systolic blood pressure of >200 mm Hg or resting diastolic blood pressure of >110 mm Hg should be evaluated on a case-by-case basis

Orthostatic blood pressure drop of >20 mm Hg with symptoms

Critical aortic stenosis (peak systolic pressure gradient of >50 mm Hg with an aortic valve orifice area of <0.75 cm^2 in an average size adult)

Acute systemic illness or fever

Uncontrolled atrial or ventricular arrhythmias

Uncontrolled sinus tachycardia (>120 beats · min^{-1})

Uncompensated congestive heart failure

3° AV block (without pacemaker)

Active pericarditis or myocarditis

Recent embolism

Thrombophlebitis

Resting ST segment displacement (>2 mm)

Uncontrolled diabetes (resting blood glucose of > 400 mg/dL)

Severe orthopedic conditions that would prohibit exercise

Other metabolic conditions, such as acute thyroiditis, hypokalemia or hyperkalemia, hypovolemia, etc.

(From *ACSM's Guidelines for Exercise Testing and Prescription*, 6th ed. Philadelphia, Lippincott Williams & Wilkins, 2000, p 166.)

**Table 8-2. Activity Classification Guide
for Inpatient Activities**

Activity Class I

Sits up in bed with assistance

Does own self-care activities—seated, or may need assistance

Stands at bedside with assistance

Sits up in chair 15 to 30 minutes, 2 to 3 times per day

Activity Class II

Sits up in bed independently

Stands independently

Does self-care activities in bathroom—seated

Walks in room and to bathroom (may need assistance)

Activity Class III

Sits and stands independently

Does own self-care activities in bathroom, seated or standing

Walks in halls with assistance short distances (50 to 100 ft) as tolerated, up to 3 times per day

Activity Class IV

Does own self-care and bathes

Walks in halls short distances (150 to 200 ft) with minimal assistance, 3 to 4 times per day

Activity Class V

Walks in halls independently, moderate distances (250 to 500 ft), 3 to 4 times per day

Activity Class VI

Independent ambulation on unit, 3 to 6 times per day

(From *ACSM's Guidelines for Exercise Testing and Prescription,* 6th ed. Philadelphia, Lippincott Williams & Wilkins, 2000, p 168.)

symptoms, HR, BP, ECG, and oxygen saturation (S_aO_2) are parameters to monitor.

7. **Clinical pathways (critical pathways, care tracks)**

    –Protocols for the client progression through the hospital stay should be followed.

    –A **multidisciplinary approach** is emphasized to ensure positive outcomes.

    –**Clinical practice guidelines** are available through numerous sources, including the U.S. Department of Health and Human Services.

8. **Counseling and referral** to other allied health professionals or hospital education programs assist in patient empowerment and efficient case management.

B. TRANSITIONAL CARE

–With the current emphasis on decreasing the length of hospital stays, additional medical surveillance is now provided through home care, home-based therapy, and transitional care facilities.

1. **Candidates**

    –Status post–acute event clients who require further assessment and monitoring

    –Chronic disease clients with multiple risks

    –Co-morbidity status clients who may require additional care

2. **Facilities**

    –Multidisciplinary care is provided in various types of settings, including:

    a. Nursing homes and skilled nursing facilities

    b. Rehabilitation hospitals (inpatient and outpatient)

    c. The client's home

    d. Clinics or physicians' offices

3. **Individualized goals**

    –Specific outcomes are addressed in depth to promote independent care.

4. **Exercise guidelines and client assessment**

    –Mode, frequency, intensity, duration, and progression are as tolerated by client and prescribed by professionals.

    –Client symptoms, HR, BP, ECG, S_aO_2, and disease-specific criteria (e.g., pulmonary, hematologic) are monitored.

5. **Stepping stone to outpatient care**

    –Available options for outpatient rehabilitation are presented to the client at this time, and the client is encouraged to pursue them.

6. **Transtelephonic monitoring**

    a. **Equipment**

        –Telephone lines are provided for individual or group voice communication and/or ECG transmission.

    b. **Uses**

        –For groups or individuals who are unable to enroll in the typical outpatient program based at a medical facility

        –More common in rural areas

    c. **Design and development of transtelephonic monitoring programs**

        –These programs must include emergency medical system activation and complete standards of operation.

    d. **Limitations**

        –Questionable insurance reimbursement

C. OUTPATIENT/MAINTENANCE CARE

1. Indications and contraindications

–See **Table 8-1.**

2. Limits of intensity

–See Table 8-3.

3. Risk stratification

–See I A 4.

4. Supervision/monitoring needs

–may be delineated through risk stratification. Continue monitoring to detect any deterioration in clinical status.

5. Program design

a. Exercise and education

–These are combined to promote positive health behavior changes. The intent is to return the patient to premorbid activities and to further improve the patient's health status if possible, while at the same time educating the patient and family.

b. Secondary prevention intervention

–consists of modification of all disease risk factors (e.g., heart disease, cancer, metabolic disease, orthopedic problems).

–necessitates involvement of multidisciplinary staff.

6. Guidelines for progression to independent exercise in a safe and effective manner are provided in Table 8-4.

7. Exercise guidelines when graded exercise test (GXT) data are not available

–Patients who have particular symptoms that need to be assessed may have a submaximal test performed by the staff to a level of somewhat hard or hard on the rating of perceived exertion (RPE) scale.

–Proceed with the exercise program under close medical surveillance using necessary equipment appropriate for monitoring the disease state (such as ECG, BP, S_aO_2, blood work).

–Use an activity status questionnaire to derive an appropriate intensity level (e.g., Duke Activity Status Index, Veterans Specific Activity Questionnaire).

 Table 8-3. Signs and Symptoms Below Which an Upper Limit for Exercise Intensity Should be Set[+]

Onset of angina or other symptoms of cardiovascular insufficiency

Plateau or decrease in systolic blood pressure, systolic blood pressure of > 240 mm Hg, or diastolic blood pressure of >110 mm Hg

≥1 mm ST-segment depression, horizontal or downsloping

Radionuclide evidence of left ventricular dysfunction or onset of moderate-to-severe wall motion abnormalities during exertion

Increased frequency of ventricular arrhythmias

Other significant ECG disturbances (e.g., 2° or 3° AV block, atrial fibrillation, supraventricular tachycardia, complex ventricular ecotopy, etc.)

Other signs/symptoms of intolerance to exercise

[+]The peak exercise heart rate should generally be at least 10 beats · min⁻¹ below the heart rate associated with any of the above-referenced criteria. Other variables (e.g., the corresponding systolic blood pressure response and perceived exertion), however, should also be considered when establishing the exercise intensity. (From *ACSM's Guidelines for Exercise Testing and Prescription,* 6th ed. Philadelphia, Lippincott Williams & Wilkins, 2000, p 172.)

 Table 8-4. Guidelines for Progression to Independent Exercise with Minimal or No Supervision

Functional capacity of ≥8 METs or twice the level of occupational demand

Appropriate hemodynamic response to exercise (increase in systolic blood pressure with increasing work load) and recovery

Appropriate ECG response at peak exercise with normal or unchanged conduction, stable or benign arrhythmias, and nondiagnostic ischemic response (i.e., <1 mm ST-segment depression)

Cardiac symptoms stable or absent

Stable and/or controlled baseline heart rate and blood pressure

Adequate management of risk factor intervention strategy and safe exercise participation such that the patient demonstrates independent and effective management of risk factors with favorable changes in those risk factors

Demonstrated knowledge of the disease process, abnormal signs and symptoms, medication use, and side effects

(From *ACSM's Guidelines for Exercise Testing and Prescription,* 6th ed. Philadelphia, Lippincott Williams & Wilkins, 2000, p 174.)

II. STAFFING AND PROGRAM SUPERVISION

A. MULTIDISCIPLINARY MODEL

–Health care professionals from a variety of allied health fields should be integral members of the rehabilitation team. For example, both an exercise physiologist and a registered dietitian will counsel a diabetic patient to help him manage diet and exercise regimens, while a physician and nurse will help manage medications and patient education about the disease. A client with multiple risk factors or co-morbidity can be more efficiently managed by a team of experts from varying disciplines.

B. ROLES OF HEALTH PROFESSIONALS

–The rehabilitation team members may be full-time or part-time employees of the program or independent care providers in the community. The AACVPR provides descriptions of the core competencies of program professionals.

1. **Exercise physiologists** can provide exercise testing, exercise prescription and leadership, and patient counseling and education.

2. **Nurses** who have licensure and ACLS training and certification can provide emergency care and help monitor the patient's clinical status.

3. **Physical therapists, respiratory therapists,** and **occupational therapists** may be able to assist the patient with return to work or ADL.

4. **Physicians** manage each patient and prescribe all rehabilitation programs. They can also serve as medical directors of a program.

5. **Registered dietitians** provide assessment and treatment of all dietary needs.

6. **Social workers/behaviorists** may assess the patient's needs and provide psychosocial care.

C. PROGRAM SUPERVISION

1. The American College of Sports Medicine (ACSM) recommends that supervised exercise programs be under the combined overall guidance of a physician and an ACSM-certified Program Director or Exercise Specialist.

2. **Participants requiring supervision** may include

   –those with functional capacity < 8 METs.

   –those with known disease.

   –those with two or more risk factors.

   –those with signs or symptoms of cardiopulmonary disease.

3. Supervision and staffing recommendations for various populations are available through the ACSM, AACVPR, AHA, and American College of Cardiology (ACC).

4. Insurance companies, organizations offering program certifications, and local agencies also have varying supervision requirements.

III. PATIENT ASSESSMENT

A. MEDICAL HEALTH HISTORY AND RISK FACTOR IDENTIFICATION

–Information is obtained from the client, physician, and hospital discharge summaries (see Chapter 6).

B. RISK STRATIFICATION

1. **ACSM risk stratification for exercise testing**

   –The ACSM provides recommendations for medical clearance, maximal exercise testing, and physician supervision during exercise testing (**Table 8-5**).

2. **Risk stratification categories for cardiac populations**

   –The ACP and AACVPR provide risk stratification criteria for cardiac clients. See Chapter 4, Table 4-3.

   –ACC/AHA Practice Guidelines offer stratification for exercise testing and direction for using these test results in client care strategies.

   –The AHA provides risk stratification criteria for medical clearance, monitoring or supervision, and activity guidelines (see Chapter 4, Table 4-4).

   –Other statewide or hospital risk stratification procedures or protocols for specific diseases provide useful information in client care.

Table 8-5. ACSM Recommendations for (A) Current Medical Examination* and Exercise Testing Prior to Participation and (B) Physician Supervision of Exercise Tests

	Low Risk	Moderate Risk	High Risk
A.			
Moderate exercise[†]	Not necessary[‡]	Not necessary	Recommended
Vigorous exercise[§]	Not necessary	Recommended	Recommended
B.			
Submaximal test	Not necessary	Not necessary	Recommended
Maximal test	Not necessary	Recommended[‖]	Recommended

*Within the past year (see Balady GJ, Chaitman B, Driscoll D, et al. American College of Sports Medicine and American Heart Association Joint Position Statement: Recommendations for cardiovascular screening, staffing, and emergency policies at health/fitness facilities. Med Sci Sports Exerc 30: 1009–1018, 1998).
[†]Absolute moderate exercise is defined as activities that are approximately 3–6 METs or the equivalent of brisk walking at 3 to 4 mph for most healthy adults (13). Nevertheless, a pace of 3 to 4 mph might be considered to be "hard" to "very hard" by some sedentary, older persons. Moderate exercise may alternatively be defined as an intensity well within the individual's capacity, one which can be comfortably sustained for a prolonged period of time (~45 min), which has a gradual initiation and progression, and is generally noncompetitive. If an individual's exercise capacity is known, relative moderate exercise may be defined by the range 40%–60% maximal oxygen uptake.
[‡]The designation of "Not necessary" reflects the notion that a medical examination, exercise test, and physician supervision of exercise testing would not be essential in the preparticipation screening; however, they should not be viewed as inappropriate.
[§]Vigorous exercise is defined as activities of >6 METs. Vigorous exercise may alternatively be defined as exercise intense enough to represent a substantial cardiorespiratory challenge. If an individual's exercise capacity is known, vigorous exercise may be defined as an intensity of >60% maximal oxygen uptake.
[‖]When physician supervision of exercise testing is "Recommended," the physician should be in close proximity and readily available should there be an emergent need.
(From *ACSM's Guidelines for Exercise Testing and Prescription*, 6th ed. Philadelphia, Lippincott Williams & Wilkins, 2000, p 27.)

C. VARIABLES OF CARDIORESPIRATORY ENDURANCE

–See Chapter 2 for definitions of maximal oxygen uptake ($\dot{V}O_{2max}$), HR, BP, respiratory rate, tidal volume, adaptation, and overload.

–Be aware of the various **medications** that affect cardiorespiratory parameters (HR, BP, ECG, and exercise capacity), as outlined in **Table 8-6.**

Table 8-6. Effects of Medications on Heart Rate, Blood Pressure, the Electrocardiogram (ECG), and Exercise Capacity

Medications	Heart Rate	Blood Pressure	ECG	Exercise Capacity
I. β-Blockers (including carvedilol, labetalol)	↓ *(R and E)	↓ (R and E)	↓ HR*(R) ↓ ischemia† (E)	↑ in patients with angina; ↓ or ↔ in patients without angina
II. Nitrates	↑ (R) ↑ or ↔ (E)	↓ (R) ↓ or ↔ (E)	↑ HR (R) ↑ or ↔ HR (E) ↓ ischemia† (E)	↑ in patients with angina; ↔ in patients without angina; ↑ or ↔ in patients with congestive heart failure (CHF)
III. Calcium channel blockers Amlodipine Felodipine Isradipine Nicardipine Nifedipine Nimodipine	↑ or ↔ (R and E)		↑ or ↔ HR (R and E) ↓ ischemia† (E)	↑ in patients with angina; ↔ in patients without angina
Nisoldipine Bepridil Diltiazem Verapamil	↓ (R and E)	↓ (R and E)	↓ HR (R and E) ↓ ischemia† (E)	
IV. Digitalis	↓ in patients with atrial fibrillation and possibly CHF Not significantly altered in patients with sinus rhythm	↔ (R and E)	May produce nonspecific ST-T wave changes (R) May produce ST segment depression (E)	Improved only in patients with atrial fibrillation or in patients with CHF
V. Diuretics	↔ (R and E)	↔ or ↓ (R and E)	↔ or PVCs (R) May cause PVCs and "false positive" test results if hypokalemia occurs May cause PVCs if hypomagnesemia occurs (E)	↔, except possibly in patients with CHF
VI. Vasodilators, nonadrenergic	↑ or ↔ (R and E)	↓ (R and E)	↑ or ↔ HR (R and E)	↔, except ↑ or ↔ in patients with CHF
ACE inhibitors	↔ (R and E)	↓ (R and E)	↔ (R and E)	↔, except ↑ or ↔ in patients with CHF
α-Adrenergic blockers	↔ (R and E)	↓ (R and E)	↔ (R and E)	↔
Antiadrenergic agents without selective blockade	↓ or ↔ (R and E)	↓ (R and E)	↓ or ↔ HR (R and E)	↔
VII. Antiarrhythmic agents	All antiarrhythmic agents may cause new or worsened arrhythmias (proarrhythmic effect)			
Class I Quinidine	↑ or ↔ (R and E)	↓ or ↔ (R)	↑ or ↔ HR (R)	↔
Disopyramide		↔ (E)	May prolong QRS and QT intervals (R) Quinidine may result in "false negative" test results (E)	

Table 8-6. Continued

Medications	Heart Rate	Blood Pressure	ECG	Exercise Capacity
Class I continued Procainamide	↔ (R and E)	↔ (R and E)	May prolong QRS and QT intervals (R) May result in "false positive" test results (E)	↔
Phenytoin Tocainide Mexiletine	↔ (R and E)	↔ (R and E)	↔ (R and E)	↔
Flecainide Moricizine	↔ (R and E)	↔ (R and E)	May prolong QRS and QT intervals (R) ↔ (E)	↔
Propafenone	↓ (R) ↓ or ↔ (E)	↔ (R and E)	↓ HR (R) ↓ or ↔ HR (E)	↔
Class II β-Blockers (see I.)				
Class III Amiodarone	↓ (R and E)	↔ (R and E)	↓ HR (R) ↔ (E)	↔
Class IV Calcium channel blockers (see III.)				
VIII. Bronchodilators	↔ (R and E)	↔ (R and E)	↔ (R and E)	Bronchodilators ↑ exercise capacity in patients limited by bronchospasm
Anticholinergic agents	↑ or ↔ (R and E)	↔	↑ or ↔ HR	
Methylxanthines			May produce PVCs (R and E)	
Sympathomimetic agents	↑ or ↔ (R and E)	↑, ↔, or ↓ (R and E)	↑ or ↔ HR (R and E)	↔
Cromolyn sodium	↔ (R and E)	↔ (R and E)	↔ (R and E)	↔
Corticosteroids	↔ (R and E)	↔ (R and E)	↔ (R and E)	↔
IX. Antihyperlipidemic agents	Clofibrate may provoke arrhythmias, angina in patients with prior myocardial infarction			↔
	Nicotinic acid may ↓ BP			
	All other hyperlipidemic agents have no effect on HR, BP, and ECG			
X. Psychotropic medications				
Minor tranquilizers	May ↓ HR and BP by controlling anxiety; no other effects			
Antidepressants	↑ or ↔ (R and E)	↑ or ↔ (R and E)	Variable (R) May result in "false positive" test results (E)	
Major tranquilizers	↑ or ↔ (R and E)	↑ or ↔ (R and E)	Variable (R) May result in "false positive" or "false negative" test results (E)	
Lithium	↔ (R and E)	↔ (R and E)	May result in T wave changes and arrhythmias (R and E)	

continued

Table 8-6. Continued

Medications	Heart Rate	Blood Pressure	ECG	Exercise Capacity
XI. Nicotine	↑ or ↔ (R and E)	↑ (R and E)	↑ or ↔ HR May provoke ischemia, arrhythmias (R and E)	↔, except ↓ or ↔ in patients with angina
XII. Antihistamines	↔ (R and E)	↔ (R and E)	↔ (R and E)	↔
XIII. Cold medications with sympathomimetic agents	Effects similar to those described in sympathomimetic agents, although magnitude of effects is usually smaller			↔
XIV. Thyroid medications Only levothyroxine	↑ (R and E)	↑ (R and E)	↑ HR May provoke arrhythmias ↑ ischemia (R and E)	↔, unless angina worsened
XV. Alcohol	↔ (R and E)	Chronic use may have role in ↑ BP (R and E)	May provoke arrhythmias (R and E)	↔
XVI. Hypoglycemic agents Insulin and oral agents	↔ (R and E)	↔ (R and E)	↔ (R and E)	↔
XVII. Dipyridamole	↔ (R and E)	↔ (R and E)	↔ (R and E)	↔
XVIII. Anticoagulants	↔ (R and E)	↔ (R and E)	↔ (R and E)	↔
XIX. Antigout medications	↔ (R and E)	↔ (R and E)	↔ (R and E)	↔
XX. Antiplatelet medications	↔ (R and E)	↔ (R and E)	↔ (R and E)	↔
XXI. Pentoxifylline	↔ (R and E)	↔ (R and E)	↔ (R and E)	↑ or ↔ in patients limited by intermittent claudication
XXII. Caffeine	Variable effects depending upon previous use Variable effects on exercise capacity May provoke arrhythmias			
XXIII. Anorexiants/diet pills	↑ or ↔ (R and E)	↑ or ↔ (R and E)	↑ or ↔ HR (R and E)	

Key: ↑ = increase; ↔ = no effect; ↓ =decrease; R = rest; E = exercise; HR = heart rate; PVCs = premature ventricular contractions.
*β-blockers with ISA lower resting HR only slightly.
†May prevent or delay myocardial ischemia (see text).
(From *ACSM's Guidelines for Exercise Testing and Prescription,* 6th ed. Philadelphia, Lippincott Williams & Wilkins, 2000, pp. 277–282.)

IV. PRINCIPLES OF EXERCISE PRESCRIPTION FOR HEALTH AND PHYSICAL FITNESS

A. HEALTH BENEFITS VS PHYSICAL FITNESS

–The amount of exercise needed to achieve health benefits differs from that needed to achieve physical fitness.

1. **Health benefits,** defined as reduced risk of certain chronic diseases, can be achieved through weekly activity caloric expenditure ranging from 700 to 2,000 kcal.

2. **Physical fitness** can be achieved from an exercise prescription (e.g., intensity, frequency, duration) sufficient to improve variables such as $\dot{V}O_{2max}$ and body composition.

B. MODE (TYPE OF ACTIVITY)

–Continuous, rhythmic, aerobic activities involving large muscle groups are used (e.g., walking, jogging, cycling, swimming).

C. FREQUENCY

–is 3 to 5 days per week, preferably alternating days.

D. INTENSITY

1. Intensity is evaluated through:

   –HR, assessed at various pulse locations

   –METs

–RPE scales

–Other parameters, such as ventilatory thresholds, blood lactate thresholds, metabolic values, hemodynamic values (rate pressure product), dyspnea scales, claudication scales, angina scales

2. The client exercises to one of the following limits:

–40% to 85% of heart rate reserve (HRR) or $\dot{V}O_{2max}$ reserve ($\dot{V}O_2R$)

–55% to 90% of HR_{max}

–RPE which correlates with the above-mentioned percentages

E. DURATION

–Each session consists of 20 to 60 minutes of intermittent or continuous aerobic activity, depending on intensity chosen.

F. PROGRESSION

1. **Session progression** involves

–There should be a smooth transition between warm-up through conditioning to cool down, with a progressive increase and decrease in intensity.

2. **Program progression**

–Each client's program consists of various phases of exercise intensity/duration.

   a. **Initial phase**

   –The goal is light, muscular endurance.

–Intensity is 40% to 60% $\dot{V}O_2R$ or HRR, 55% to 75% HR_{max} (lower end of intensity ranges).

–Duration is 12 to 15 minutes, 20 to 30 minutes by the end of the initial phase (continuous or discontinuous).

–Frequency is 2 to 3 times/week on alternating days.

–The length of the initial phase is approximately 4 to 6 weeks, depending on the patient's level of conditioning.

   b. **Improvement phase**

   –Progressive overload is begun to achieve more rapid gains.

   –Intensity is 50% to 85% $\dot{V}O_2R$ or HRR, 65% to 90% HR_{max}.

   –Duration is increased every 2 to 3 weeks until the patient achieves 30 to 40 minutes of continuous exercise.

   –Frequency is 3 to 5 days per week.

   –The length of the improvement phase is approximately 4 to 5 months.

   c. **Maintenance phase**

   –During this phase, the participant's activities are diversified; cross-training may be implemented. The goals for the participant are re-evaluated, and compliance with the program is assessed.

   –The maintenance phase may last approximately 6 months, or it may be ongoing.

V. PROGRAM COMPONENTS OF AEROBIC AND RESISTIVE EXERCISE SESSIONS

A. WARM-UP

–The purpose is to slowly and safely activate the body's responses to exercise, and to increase ROM to prepare joints and muscles for vigorous activity.

1. **Physiological responses** include

–increased HR and stroke volume.

–increased body temperature and muscle temperature.

–increased metabolic activity and respiration.

2. **Components** include

–low-intensity, dynamic activity.

–static stretching to prepare muscles for exercise.

3. **Proper procedure**

–Include both dynamic and static activities. appropriate for the target sport or activity.

–Start slowly and gradually increase intensity.

–Continue for 6 to 15 minutes or longer in colder temperatures.

–Intensity should be sufficient to elevate HR, change breathing, and possibly cause light perspiration.

B. STIMULUS/CONDITIONING

–The purpose is to provide sufficient overload/adaptation.

–Follow the guidelines for basic principles for exercise prescription listed in IV.

–Activities include aerobic modalities supplemented with recreational games.

C. COOL (WARM) DOWN

–The purpose is to gradually bring the body closer to the resting state after the stimulus/conditioning session.

1. **Physiological responses** include

   –decreased respiratory and cardiac activity.

   –decreased lactic acid level.

   –restored cellular metabolic activity.

2. **Components** include

   –low-intensity activities.

   –stretching.

3. **Proper procedure**

   –Continue for 10 to 15 minutes.

   –Decrease intensity gradually to avoid sudden hemodynamic drops and associated symptoms.

   –Stretch muscle groups used for 3 to 5 minutes. (The participant may focus on rehabilitating the injured area.)

   –Rehydrate.

D. **TYPES OF TRAINING PROGRAMS**

   1. **Continuous training**

      –Sustained load and intensity are maintained throughout the stimulus/conditioning session.

      –Examples include walking, hiking, running, and cycling.

   2. **Intermittent (interval) training**

      –Bouts of high-intensity activity are alternated with intervals of rest or lower-intensity activity. These intervals allow higher-intensity training during the activity bouts.

      –Examples include a few minutes of jogging alternated with 1 minute of walking; a few minutes at 100 watts on a bicycle ergometer alternated with 1 minute at 25 watts.

3. **Circuit training**

   –Several stations of activity are performed with a transition or rest period between stations, combining resistance exercises with rhythmic aerobic work.

   –This type of training suits a wide range of populations; it is social and provides variety.

   –Orientation and education are required to reduce the risk of injury with weights.

   –Circuit training should not be the sole program used to improve cardiorespiratory endurance. Greater gains in $\dot{V}O_{2max}$ are seen in sustained endurance training.

E. **EQUIPMENT**

   1. **Resistance training equipment**

      –Free weights (dumbbells, barbells)

      –Isokinetic equipment (e.g., Cybex, Orthotron)

      –Isotonic equipment (e.g., Nautilus, pneumatic)

      –Nontraditional equipment (e.g., elastic bands, tubing, balls, foxtails, soft frisbees, zoom balls)

   2. **Cardiovascular training equipment and modalities**

      –Treadmill, bicycle, rower, stair-climber/bench, multi-extremity ergometer, water resistance tank, classes (e.g., step, slides, aerobics)

   3. **Considerations and precautions**

      –The needs and precautions for each individual program participant must be taken into account when determining which equipment to use. Advantages and precautions for various types of exercise equipment are outlined in **Table 8-7**.

VI. EXERCISE PROGRAM FOR MUSCULAR FITNESS

A. **DEFINITION**

   –**Muscular fitness** is a balance of muscular strength and muscular endurance.

B. **BENEFITS OF RESISTANCE TRAINING**

   –Increased lean body mass

   –Increased bone mass (helpful in preventing osteoporosis)

   –Increased strength of connective tissue

   –Slightly improved cardiorespiratory fitness (when resistance is a component of circuit training)

   –Decreased body fat and lowered BP (when resistance is a component of circuit training)

   –Improved glucose tolerance and lipid profiles (when resistance is a component of circuit training)

   –In elderly clients, improved balance, mobility, and strength to enhance ability to perform ADL

C. **COMPONENTS OF EXERCISE PRESCRIPTION FOR MUSCULAR FITNESS**

   1. **Frequency**

      –2 to 3 days per week

   2. **Duration**

      –Minimum of 1 set, 8 to 15 repetitions per set for general muscular fitness in the healthy adult

Table 8-7. Exercise Equipment and Modalities: Advantages, Precautions, and Considerations

Equipment/Modality	Features/Advantages	Precautions/Considerations
Stair-climbing equipment	Computerized feedback Variety of levels Handrails for balance	Poor biomechanics caused by leaning on handrails may reduce workout and stress lower back. Stepping motion can stress knee joint and ball of foot. Consider specific quad/hams strengthening exercises to assist stability of knee joint. Lowest level on some machines is too intense for deconditioned individuals. Balance may be a concern for older users.
Multi-extremity or combined upper/lower body equipment (skier, stepper)	Good workout for multiple extremities Good options for specificity of training in occupational training (e.g., firefighters, police, mountain climbers)	Requires coordination and balance Lowest level may exceed deconditioned user's ability
Bench (step) aerobic equipment	Variability of impact or intensity Music can be metered from about 120–130 beats/min (30 lifts/min)	Bench height ranges from 4–12 inches; height of bench affects caloric cost of workout. Step patterns that travel up and down, on and off bench can be hard for elderly and may increase risk of injury. Bench that is too high can cause knee injuries. Clients may be prone to overuse if this is their sole mode of exercise training.
Water resistance tank	Allows a variety of non–weight-bearing activities Good for range-of-motion exercises Appropriate for clients with range of fitness levels from severely deconditioned to very fit Water helps "hide" the body from view of others in class	Some clients may be fearful of water. Staff instructors need, at minimum, certification in CPR and water safety; presence of a lifeguard is recommended. Deep-water exercises are more intense and thus appropriate only for advanced fitness level clients or experienced swimmers.
Group aerobics	Group setting provides social environment.	*High-impact vs low-impact:* High-impact aerobics have an unsupported or airborne phase resulting in increased impact force on joints. In low-impact aerobics, one foot is in contact with the ground at all times, so impact forces on the joints are minimal.
Treadmill	Computerized feedback Variety of levels offer precise energy level control. Walking is a comfortable and familiar activity.	Requires balance Weight-bearing activity
Bicycle Ergometer	Non–weight bearing Variety of levels Ideal for those whith poor balance.	Client must be able to maintain workload independently. Early leg fatigue in deconditioned

3. **Intensity**

   –40% to 60% of 1 repetition max (1-RM), with the amount of weight or resistance and repetitions varying, depending on whether the focus is on strength or on endurance. (1-RM is the heaviest weights that can be lifted only once using good form.)

   a. **Rapid muscular strength gains** are produced by higher resistance or weight (80% to 100% 1-RM) and fewer repetitions (6 to 8)

   b. **Muscular endurance** is optimized at lower weights (40% to 60% 1-RM) and more repetitions (8 to 15).

4. Mode

–Static or dynamic contractions are performed on the 8 to 10 major muscle groups chosen (e.g., shoulder/neck, upper back, lower back, abdomen, thighs).

–All contractions are performed with controlled and proper technique, full range of motion, normal breathing pattern, and use of a spotter if necessary.

a. Isometric training (static)

–is often used to rehabilitate an injured area.

–is specific to the joint angle at which it is performed. An example would be "quad sets," wherein the quadriceps muscles are contracted and released while the knee remains in the "straight leg" position.

–Exercises are performed 5 to 10 times per day, 5 days per week.

–Isometric exercises increase intrathoracic pressure, which can elevate BP; therefore, proper breathing and form must be enforced.

b. Isotonic training (dynamic)

–consists of three sets of 8 to 15 repetitions.

–can be concentric (resistance applied during muscle shortening) or eccentric (resistance applied during muscle lengthening).

–Exercises are performed 3 to 5 days per week.

–The number of repetitions and the weight used depend on whether training is focused on strength or on endurance.

–Caution is needed with the eccentric mode to avoid soreness.

c. Isokinetic training (dynamic)

–consists of 2 to 3 sets with 5 to 10 repetitions per set.

–can be concentric or eccentric.

–uses equipment (e.g., Cybex, Orthotron) to maintain constant speed through ROM. Machine speed varies from 24 to 180 degrees/second (low speed helps build strength; high speed, endurance).

–Exercises are performed 3 to 5 days per week.

VII. EXERCISE PROGRAM FOR FLEXIBILITY

A. DEFINITIONS

–**Active ROM** is the range through which a joint can be moved without assistance.

–In **passive ROM,** a joint is moved through a range of motion by an external force (a person or machine) with no voluntary muscular contraction occurring.

–In **active assistive ROM,** a joint is moved through a range of motion with partial assistance from the patient.

B. BENEFITS OF FLEXIBILITY

–Adequate range of motion in all joints allows for optimal musculoskeletal function, increased ADL, and decreased chance of injury.

–Benefits of flexibility include:

1. Reduced muscle tension and increased relaxation
2. Maintained ease of movement
3. Improved coordination through ease of movement
4. Increased ROM
5. Prevention of injury
6. Improved body awareness
7. Improved circulation and gas exchange
8. Decreased muscle viscosity, making contractions easier and smoother
9. Decreased soreness associated with other exercise activities

C. TYPES OF STRETCHING

–**Proprioceptive neuromuscular facilitation (PNF)** is isometric contraction of a muscle followed by relaxation and assisted passive stretch. **Contract-relax** and **hold-relax** are further variations of PNF stretching.

–**Active/assisted stretching** is contraction of a muscle followed by an opposite muscular contraction which moves the body part into the stretch position. The stretch is assisted by another person or device.

–Static stretching refers to a muscle being placed in the stretch position and held for a few seconds.

⊛ **Table 8-8. Precautions for Flexibility Training**

Stretch a joint through limits of normal ROM only

Do not stretch at healed fracture sites for ~8–12 weeks postfracture, after which gentle stretching may be initiated

In individuals with known or suspected osteoporosis, stretch with particular caution (e.g., men older than 80 years old and women over 65 years old, older spinal cord injured individuals).

Avoid aggressive stretching of tissues that have been immobilized (e.g., casted). Tissues become dehydrated and lose tensile strength during immobilization.

Mild soreness should take no longer than 24 hours to resolve after stretching. If more recovery time is necessary, then the stretching force was excessive.

Use active, comfortable ROM to stretch edematous joints or soft tissue.

Do *not* over-stretch weak muscles. Shortening in these muscles may contribute to joint support that muscles can no longer actively provide. Combine strengthen and stretching exercise so that gains in mobility coincide with gains in strength and stability.

Be aware that physical performance may vary from day to day.

Set individual goals.

ROM=range of motion.
(From *ACSM's Resource Manual for Guidelines for Exercise Testing and Prescription*, 3rd ed. Baltimore, Williams & Wilkins, 1998, p 457.)

⊛ **Table 8-9. Contraindications for Flexibility Training**

Motion limited by bony block at a joint interface

Recent unhealed fracture

Infection and acute inflammation, affecting the joint or surrounding tissues

Sharp pain associated with stretch or uncontrolled muscle cramping that occurs when attempting to stretch

Local hematoma as a result of an overstretch injury

If contracture (desired functional shortening) occurs requiring stability to a joint capsule or ligament

If contracture is intentional to improve function particularly in clients with paralysis or severe muscle weakness (e.g., tenodesis of finger flexors to allow grasp in an individual with quadriplegia)

(From *ACSM's Resource Manual for Guidelines for Exercise Testing and Prescription*, 3rd ed. Baltimore, Williams & Wilkins, 1998, p 457.)

D. COMPONENTS OF EXERCISE PRESCRIPTION FOR FLEXIBILITY

1. Mode

–Choose major muscle groups and use one of the above types of stretching techniques. Activities such as yoga or tai chi may also help improve flexibility.

2. Frequency

–Perform stretching exercises 2 to 3 days per week.

3. Duration

–Gradually increase the length of time a stretch is held and the number of times that stretch is performed (e.g., a 10- to 30-second hold repeated 3–4 times).

4. Intensity

–Stretch to a position of mild pull, but not pain.

E. FLEXIBILITY GUIDELINES

1. Precautions for flexibility training are listed in **Table 8-8.**

2. Contraindications for flexibility training are listed in **Table 8-9.**

VIII. CONTRAINDICATIONS TO EXERCISE

–See Table 8-1 as well as Chapter 6 (I B) and Chapter 7 (III A) for situations in which aerobic and resistive exercise should be terminated or not performed.

IX. PATIENT COMPLIANCE AND MOTIVATION

–To improve patient compliance with exercise and diet regimens to reduce risk factors for diseases, one needs to understand behavior change and adult learning. Chapter 5 reviews the components of successful behavior change. Table 8-10 describes strategies for initiating and maintaining patient adherence to an exercise program.

Table 8-10. Behavioral Management Strategies for Initiating and Maintaining Exercise Adherence*

Techniques	Practical Applications/Recommendations
Initiation of Exercise	
Preparation	The exercise professional should establish realistic expectations among new participants. Overly pessimistic or optimistic expectations should be corrected.
Shaping	This strategy is analogous to the physiologic principle of progression. Begin the exercise program at a dosage (intensity, frequency, duration) that is comfortable for the participant, and increase the volume slowly until the optimal level is attained.
Goal-setting	Goals should be individualized and based upon the participant's physiologic and psychosocial status. Goals can be set for both supervised and unsupervised exercise. Short-term goals that are specific, yet flexible, are more effective than longer-term goals.
Reinforcement	Participants should be queried as to what reinforcers (rewards) would work for them. One of the most effective rewards may be praise from program staff that is specific to each individual. Certificates, patches, and attendance charts can also be used as reinforcers.
Stimulus control	Environmental cues or stimuli (e.g., written notes, watch alarms) may be used to remind participants to maintain their exercise commitment. Having a routine time and place for exercise establishes powerful stimulus control.
Contracting	A behavioral contract has been shown to enhance the commitment to exercise. Signing the contract formalizes the agreement and makes it more significant.
Cognitive strategies	Participants should be oriented to the advantages and disadvantages of exercise. Individuals who select their own flexible goals generally demonstrate better adherence as compared with those whose goals are rigidly set by exercise professionals.
Maintenance of Exercise	
Generalization training	Specific steps should be taken to "generalize" the exercise habit from the gymnasium or home setting to other environments (e.g., walk breaks at work, using stairs, gardening, parking the car away from stores).
Social support	The support of family, friends, and coworkers should be sought from the beginning. Finding a compatible exercise partner often serves to enhance exercise adherence.
Self-management	Participants should be encouraged to be their own behavior therapists. They should practice self-reinforcement by focusing on increased self-esteem, enjoyment of the exercise itself, and the anticipated health and fitness benefits.
Relapse prevention training	Exercise professionals should prepare participants for situations that may produce a relapse and ways of coping with them so that a complete relapse is avoided. Relapses should be viewed as inevitable challenges, rather than failures.

*Adapted from Martin JE, Dubbert PM. Behavioral management strategies for improving health and fitness. J Cardiac Rehabil 1984;4:200–208.

X. EXERCISE PROGRAMS FOR SPECIAL POPULATIONS

A. THE HIGH-RISK PATIENT (Table 8-11)

–Exercise training can counteract certain harmful physiological effects of inactivity commonly associated with chronic diseases.

–Ensuring safe, effective training requires good clinical judgment in assessing the individual's condition and in recognizing contraindications to exercise or the need to modify exercise (see Chapter 6).

1. Benefits and implications of exercise

–Complications and death in high-risk patients are generally the result of inadequate quality of care. Enrollment of these patients in rehabilitative exercise and education programs greatly improves outcomes and enhances patient safety.

2. Precautions/contraindications

–High-risk patients can take prophylactic nitroglycerin before beginning an exercise session.

–Use ECG or echocardiographic monitoring for signs of ischemia and decreased cardiac output.

–Avoid exercise in the presence of angina, dyspnea, or extreme fatigue.

–Allow for a very gradual warm up and cool down.

–Avoid exercise in extreme temperatures.

3. Modifications

a. Mode

– Use the stationary bicycle initially, then progress to treadmill, track, and recumbent cycle.

Table 8-11. Definition of High-Risk Client

Left ventricular ejection fraction ≤ 35% of CHF due primarily to diastolic dysfunction

Extremely poor exercise capacity (directly measured VO$_2$ peak less than 14 ml/kg/min)

Evidence of extensive, severe myocardial ischemia during exercise or pharmacological stress testing

Survivor of primary sudden cardiac death without treatment with an implantable cardioverter-defibrillator

Severe unrevascularizable coronary artery disease (left main, severe proximal three-vessel disease)

(From Squires R: *Exercise Prescription for the High-Risk Cardiac Patient*, p 16. Champaign, IL, Human Kinetics, 1998.)

   b. **Intensity**

   –Regulate exercise intensity according to functional capacity (FC) and ischemic threshold from GXT data.

   –To determine FC, use RPE, a percentage of $\dot{V}O_{2max}$, or the HRR methodology.

   –If GXT data are not available, follow the precautions listed above.

   c. **Frequency**

   –Multiple daily sessions 3 to 6 times per week

   d. **Duration**

   –Intermittent to continuous

   e. **Progression**

   –is dependent on intensity and duration.

   f. **Muscular fitness**

   –Use moderate resistance with weight low enough to perform 15 to 20 reps without strain.

B. **THE PATIENT WITH ANGINA/SILENT ISCHEMIA**

   1. **Benefits and implications of exercise**

   –Increased ischemic threshold, or stress level at which angina symptoms occur

   –Decreased myocardial oxygen demand and decreased BP and HR response to submaximal exercise

   –Minimization of risk factors

   2. **Supervision and monitoring**

   –Watch for angina and ischemic ECG changes.

   –Be alert for heart rhythm changes during warm-up and cooldown.

   –Look for BP changes during warm-up and cooldown.

   3. **Precautions/contraindications**

   –Reinforce the proper use of nitroglycerin.

   –Maintain activity below the angina threshold.

   4. **Modifications**

   a. **Intensity**

   –Using GXT data, note the level (workload, HR, RPE, BP) at which symptoms and ischemia occur.

   –Set HR at ≥ 10 beats · min^{-1} *below* the ischemic threshold.

   –Decrease intensity if the angina rating is ≥ +2 on the 1–4 angina scale. Stop exercise to administer nitroglycerin if angina ≥ +3.

   –The AHA Exercise Standards present additional intensity guidelines.

   b. **Frequency**

   –3 to 7 times per week

   c. **Duration**

   –Longer, more gradual warm-up and cooldown

   –20 to 60 minutes per session

   d. **Progression**

   –The patient progresses to independent home exercise or to a less supervised/monitored setting based on the results of GXT.

   (1) If ST segment depression is < 1.5 mm and the patient is asymptomatic, the intensity can be set at 70%–85% HR$_{max}$.

   (2) If the patient is symptomatic or if ST segment depression is ≥ 2 mm at HR > 135, the intensity can be set at 70%–85% of HR at onset of 1.5 mm ST depression or angina.

   e. **Muscular fitness**

   –Use light resistance; avoid isometric strain and Valsalva's maneuver.

C. **THE PATIENT WITH CONGESTIVE HEART FAILURE**

   1. **Benefits and implications of exercise**

   –Peripheral enhancements, such as skeletal muscle metabolism, with consequent improved exercise capacity at given submaximal workload

   –Decreased symptoms, mortality, and hospital readmission rates

   –Improved quality of life and functional capacity

   2. **Supervision and monitoring**

   –Observe the patient for tolerance to exercise training.

–Observe for significant weight gain (> 4 lb) over 1 or 2 days (a sign of fluid retention).

–Stop the exercise if the patient shows BP changes or a sudden change in symptoms indicating decompensation.

–Perform ECG if the patient evidences new dysrhythmias or a change in dysrhythmias, especially in those with a history of ventricular tachycardia or cardiac arrest.

3. **Precautions/contraindications**

–Monitor ECG for arrhythmias, often caused by abnormal electrolytes (e.g., diuretics decrease potassium).

–Monitor BP for hypotension or failure of systolic BP to increase with increasing work, especially for a patient taking a combination of a vasodilator, an angiotensin-converting enzyme inhibitor, and a diuretic.

–Observe for excessive dyspnea at rest.

–Ensure prolonged warm-up and cooldown.

–Avoid isometric activities.

4. **Modifications**

   a. **Intensity**

   –Use moderate intensity, or RPE 11 to 14. RPE and dyspnea scales are preferred over target HR.

   –The intensity should remain below a level that would result in wall motion abnormalities, below the point at which the ejection fraction decreases, or below a pulmonary wedge pressure of 20 mm Hg, or the ventilatory threshold.

   –A range of 40% to 75% $\dot{V}O_{2max}$ may be suggested.

   b. **Duration**

   –Intermittent exercise (e.g., 22 min exercise/1 to 2 min rest) may be necessary as the patient's tolerance improves.

   –Exercises can be of longer duration and lower intensity for patients who cannot tolerate higher intensity training.

   c. **Muscular fitness**

   –Avoid isometric resistance training.

   –Have the patient perform more repetitions with less weight (circuit training works well).

D. **THE PATIENT WITH MYOCARDIAL INFARCTION, CORONARY ARTERY BYPASS GRAFT (CABG), OR VALVE SURGERY**

   1. **Benefits and implications of exercise**

–Decreased myocardial oxygen demand, with consequent decreased angina at a given submaximal workload

–Minimization of risk factors

–Decreased HR, BP, and myocardial oxygen demand at any given resistance from strength training

2. **Supervision and monitoring**

   a. **Inpatient programs**

   –Inpatient programs can assist the clinician in identifying **post-MI patients** who are at risk for exercise-related complications (**Table 8-12**). They can also be helpful to the physician and other multidisciplinary team members by providing classification guidelines for inpatient activities (see Table 8-2).

   (1) ECG monitoring of inpatients is necessary because of the acuity of the cardiac event and limited data on exercise tolerance.

   (2) Monitor symptoms, RPE, HR, BP, and exercise tolerance.

   (3) Monitor percutaneous transluminal coronary angioplasty (PTCA) patients for signs of early restenosis (symptoms, ECG changes, hemodynamic abnormalities).

   (4) Monitor the mitral valve repair patient for atrial dysrhythmias.

   b. **Outpatient programs**

   (1) ECG-monitor the outpatient as workload increases.

 Table 8-12. Complicating Factors After Myocardial Infarction

Low-risk patients

No complicating factors by day 4

Moderate-risk patients

Poor ventricular function (EF of <30%), or

Significant myocardial ischemia with low-level activity (2–3 METs) beyond day 4

High-risk patients

Continued myocardial ischemia

Left ventricular failure

Episode of shock

Serious arrhythmias

(From *ACSM's Guidelines for Exercise Testing and Prescription*, 6th ed. Philadelphia, Lippincott Williams & Wilkins, 2000, p 167.)

(2) The efficiency of the patient's medical management can be improved through supervision, as a result of the detection of problems that may arise during ADL.

3. **Precautions/contraindications**

   a. Avoid extreme tension on upper body to avoid injuring the surgical wound, which requires 4 to 8 weeks to heal completely.

      –For postsurgical patients, focus on a gentle, progressive ROM program for the upper body.

      –Observe the patient for infection or discomfort along incisions.

   b. Monitor the patient for signs and symptoms such as chest pain, dizziness, and dysrhythmias. Provide feedback to the physician if any of these signs and symptoms are observed.

   c. Avoid high-intensity exercise during early recovery.

   d. Monitor the patient for complications from other diseases such as diabetes.

   e. Patients with valvular diseases are generally limited by symptoms. Increasing symptoms may indicate the need for valve replacement surgery.

   f. Prohibit vigorous activity in a patient who has severe valvular stenosis.

   g. Be alert for anxiety or denial of angina in a patient who has undergone PTCA.

   h. Monitor for anemia in a patient who has undergone CABG.

4. **Modifications**

   a. **Mode**

      –Use large muscle group activities or equipment that adjusts in 1-MET increments.

   b. **Intensity**

      (1) The upper limits of activity for inpatients is physician-directed. (Suggested upper limit of post-MI HR is < 120 bpm, or HR_{rest} + 20 bpm; suggested upper limit of post-surgery HR is HR_{rest} + 30 bpm.)

      (2) GXT 2 weeks after discharge

      –40% to 50% $\dot{V}O_2$ reserve for initial outpatient

      –60% to 80% $\dot{V}O_2$ reserve as outpatient progresses

      (3) RPE

      –11 to 13 inpatient or early outpatient

      –12 to 15 outpatient

   c. **Frequency**

      –is multiple times daily for inpatients, progressing to once daily for 3 to 5 days per week for outpatients.

   d. **Duration**

      –varies from 5 to 10 minutes of intermittent activity, to 60 minutes of continuous activity

   e. **Progression**

      –Inpatient activity should progress to levels equivalent to the client's home ADL before discharge.

      –Symptom-limited GXT after discharge assists in prescribing the appropriate level of exercise that will optimize the client's progression through the rehabilitation period.

   f. **Muscular fitness for outpatients**

      –Have patient exercise at 40% to 50% of 1-RM, avoiding Valsalva, 2 to 3 times per week, 1 to 3 sets, 10 to 15 repetitions. Flexibility exercises are to be performed 2 to 3 times per week.

      –A patient who has undergone CABG can work on ROM initially until the sternum has healed.

      –Follow ACSM guidelines for outpatient resistance training (**Table 8-13**).

 Table 8-13. Resistance Training (RT) for Cardiac Populations

Contraindications for RT

See Table 8-1.

Left ventricular outflow obstruction (e.g., hypertrophic cardiomyopathy with obstruction)

Recent history of CHF that has not been evaluated and effectively treated

Uncontrolled hypertension (values of SBP ≥ 160 mmHg and/or DBP ≥ 105 mmHg apply to resistance training)

Moderate to good left ventricular function

Exercise capacity > 5 METs without angina or ischemia

Progression of RT

Two to three weeks post-MI or post-surgery, patient can begin a progressive program of ROM, low-level resistance bands, or very light handweights (1–3 lb).

Four to six weeks post-MI, patient can begin use of weight machines.

Post-surgery, patient should wait 3 months before beginning moderate to heavy resistance (the sternum must be healed and stable).

E. THE HEART TRANSPLANT PATIENT

1. Benefits and implications of exercise

–Improved cardiovascular and muscular fitness and enhanced quality of life

2. Precautions/Contraindications

a. Resting tachycardia

b. Reduced peak HR and delayed recovery of HR

c. Hypertension (from immunosuppressive medications)

d. Early onset of anaerobiosis due to limited aerobic capacity

e. Delayed HR and stroke volume (SV) response

f. Diminished maximal functional capacity due to low cardiac output

g. Asymptomatic angina due to denervation

h. Signs of rejection in cardiac biopsy scores (patient's tolerance to exercise will decrease during rejection)

i. Two separate P waves seen on ECG

j. Limited ROM until sternum is healed, as with surgical patients

k. Calf muscle cramping

l. Left ventricular assist device

–Patients awaiting heart transplant who have a left ventricular assist device may have difficulty with hip flexion or may have abdominal discomfort from the device. This population also requires extensive patient education about the operation of the device.

3. Modifications

a. Intensity

–RPE 11 to 15 (primary measurement tool for intensity)

–As tolerated by symptoms

–60% to 70% maximal METs

–50% to 75% $\dot{V}O_{2max}$

–Ventilatory threshold

b. Frequency

–4 to 6 days per week

c. Duration

–Prolonged warm-up/cooldown

d. Muscular fitness

–Low to moderate intensity

–2 days per week, 15 to 20 minutes per resistance session. (A client on long-term corticosteroid therapy may have increased risk of fracture.)

F. THE PATIENT WITH AN AUTOMATIC IMPLANTABLE CARDIOVERTER DEFIBRILLATOR (AICD) OR A PACEMAKER

1. Benefits and implications of exercise

–Improved HR response to exercise

–Relieved symptoms associated with impaired HR

2. Precautions and monitoring

–Caution the patient to avoid intensive upper body stretching or intense lifting early after pacer insertion, and to avoid lifting arms over head for 2 to 3 weeks while lead placement and surgical incisions are healing.

–Know the type and function of the pacemaker or the activation rate of the AICD (Table 8-14).

–Monitor HR closely during exercise to ensure that it does not reach the level that will activate the AICD and shock the patient.

3. Modifications

–GXT data are needed to assess rate response, BP, symptoms, and RPE. Results of metabolic testing may be needed where accurate functional assessment is necessary.

a. Intensity

–Use RPE and METs from GXT.

(1) Rate-responsive pacer

–12 beats per minute (bpm) below the upper tracking rate

(2) Target HR

–Below ischemic threshold and arrhythmia or AICD activation threshold

(3) 50% to 85% of HR reserve

b. Frequency

–4 to 7 times per week

c. Muscular fitness

–Exercise should be low to moderate intensity.

–Limited ROM is possible after insertion.

G. THE PATIENT WITH PULMONARY DISEASE

1. Benefits and implications of exercise

–Increased functional capacity and enhanced ability to perform ADL, avoiding the downward spiral of deconditioning associated with dyspnea and inactivity

–Increased comfort with sensations of breathlessness

Table 8-14. International Five-Letter Code Pacemakers

1st position letter: Chamber paced	2nd position letter: Chamber sensed	3rd position letter: Mode of response to sensed event	4th position letter: Degree of programmability	5th position letter: Antitachycardia mechanism
V	V	I	P	B
A	A	T	M	N
D	D	D		S
				E
	O	O	O	O
S	S			

1st position letter:
V = Ventricle
A = Atrium
D = Both chambers (atrium and ventricle)
S = Either chamber (used by manufacturers)

2nd position letter:
V = Ventricle
A = Atrium
D = Both chambers (atrium and ventricle)
O = Neither chamber
S = Either chamber (used by manufacturers)

3th position letter:
I = Inhibited
T = Triggered
D = Either (inhibited or triggered)
O = None

4th position letter:
P = Programmable (1 or 2 parameters)
M = Multiprogrammable (3 or more parameters)
O = Nonprogrammable

5th position letter:
B = Burst pacing
N = Normal rate competition
S = Scanning with critically timed stimuli
E = External device required to activate mechanism
O = No antitachycardia mechanism

Examples of Codes:
AAI = Atrial-inhibited pacing mode
AAT = Atrial-triggered pacing mode
AOO = Atrial asynchronous pacing mode
DAD = Dual-chamber atrial sensed pacing mode
DAT = Dual-chamber atrial sensed, triggered pacing mode
DDD = Dual-chamber pacing mode
DDI = A-V sequential dual-chamber inhibited pacing mode
DDT = Dual-chamber triggered pacing mode
DDT/I = Dual-chamber atrial-triggered, ventricular-inhibited pacing mode
DOO = Dual-chamber asynchronous pacing mode
DVI = A-V sequential ventricular-inhibited pacing mode
VAT = Atrial-synchronized ventricular pacing mode
VDD = Atrial-synchronized ventricular-inhibited pacing mode
VOO = Ventricular asynchronous pacing mode
VVI = Ventricular-inhibited pacing mode
VVT = Ventricular-triggered pacing mode

2. **Supervision**

–The multidisciplinary staff should include a respiratory therapist to direct breathing retraining, chest, or oxygen therapy.

3. **Breathing retraining**

a. **Diaphragmatic and pursed-lip breathing** (along with pulse oxygen for feedback) is done to help control respiratory muscles, maintain breathing patterns, and limit anxiety, thus improving gas exchange.

b. **Paced breathing** is taught to help coordinate breathing with performance of ADL.

c. **Respiratory muscle training** is implemented to increase respiratory muscle strength and endurance; one form is resistive inspiratory muscle training (RIMT), which is implemented as follows:

–25% to 35% of maximal inspiratory pressure measured at the mouth (functional residual capacity)

–4 to 5 times per week

–One 30-minute session or two 15-minute sessions

d. **Flow-resistive training** is done, in which the patient breathes through a progressively smaller opening.

e. **Threshold loading training** is done, using a preset inspiratory pressure usually at the same fraction of maximal inspiratory pressure.

f. **Isocapneic hyperventilation** is taught.

g. **Supplemental oxygen** is required to prevent oxygen desaturation in the patient who is breathing room air if the patient's S_aO_2 is < 88% at rest or ≤ 90% during exercise.

h. **Continuous positive airway pressure (CPAP)** may be considered for some clients during exercise training to increase exercise duration and/or decrease breathlessness.

4. **Precautions/contraindications**

a. In some patients there may be limitations to exercise because of mechanical ventilatory constraints or compromised gas exchange.

b. Assess the patient for comorbidity and implement related disease state modifications.

c. In many programs, patients who smoke are required to stop smoking before beginning the program.

d. **Patients with obstructive disease**

   –Flow obstruction in patients with certain disorders (e.g., asthma, cystic fibrosis, interstitial lung disease, chronic bronchitis, emphysema) may limit exercise capacity.

   (1) Program modifications for patients with **asthma** are listed in **Table 8-15.**

   (2) Program modifications for patients with **cystic fibrosis** are listed in **Table 8-16.**

   (3) In patients with **interstitial lung disease,** exercise intensity is dependent on adequate oxygenation and the patient's dyspnea level. Modify exercise as tolerated in relation to these factors.

e. **Patients with restrictive disease**

   –Patients whose lung volumes are restricted owing to disease or damage to the lungs (e.g., lupus, injury, pulmonary edema, tuberculosis, lung cancer) may have exercise limitations.

5. **Modifications**

   a. **Intensity**

      –Intensity should be as tolerated; the main focus is to encourage adherence and a positive experience with exercise.

      –The patient should exercise to 50% of $\dot{V}O_{2max}$.

      –Intensity is determined from a maximal GXT; HR is set at or above the anaerobic threshold.

      –Oxygen saturation is maintained at > 90%.

      –AACVPR guidelines for the bicycle ergometer are 85% of peak workload from the bicycle test.

      –RPE scales may be used to determine exercise intensity.

      –Breathing scales may be used to determine exercise intensity; a rating of 3 (on a scale of 1 to 10) is equal to 50% $\dot{V}O_2$. See **Table 8-17.**

      –Visual scales may also be used.

   b. **Duration**

      –Longer (30 to 90 minutes) with decreased intensity

Table 8-15. Program Modifications for Patients with Asthma

Age-specific patient/family training

Recognition of triggers

Peak flow monitoring

Role of medical therapy

Exercise training

Self-management plan

Importance of exercise warm-up and cooldown

Premedication prior to exercise to prevent exercise-induced bronchospasm

Dietary intake and evaluation for patients on chronic systemic steroids

(Reprinted from American Association of Cardiovascular and Pulmonary Rehabilitation. *Guidelines for Pulmonary Rehabilitation,* 2nd ed, p 99. Champaign, IL, Human Kinetics, 1998.)

Table 8-16. Program Modifications and Options for Patients with Cystic Fibrosis

Age-specific patient/family training

Nutritional evaluation and counseling

Strength and endurance training

Sodium and chloride replacement when exercising in the heat

Controlled cough technique

Postural drainage therapy

Lung transplantation

(Reprinted from American Association of Cardiovascular and Pulmonary Rehabilitation. *Guidelines for Pulmonary Rehabilitation,* 2nd ed, p 103. Champaign, IL, Human Kinetics, 1998.)

Table 8-17. Dyspnea Scale

Nothing	0
Very, very slight	0.5
Very slight	1
Slight	2
Moderate	3
Somewhat severe	4
Severe	5
	6
Very severe	7
	8
	9
Very, very severe	10

c. **Muscular fitness**

–Focus on improving muscular strength (particularly upper body) to improve ability to perform ADL.

–Coordinate breathing with upper extremity resistance (exhale with exertional phase of motion).

H. THE DIABETIC PATIENT

1. **Benefits and implications of exercise**

   a. **Type 1 diabetes mellitus** (pancreatic deficiency of insulin secretion)

      –Improved insulin sensitivity

      –Increased glucose uptake by working muscles

      –Improved blood lipid profile

      –For obese clients, assists in maintenance of lean body mass and reduction of body fat

   b. **Type 2 diabetes mellitus** (a combination of inadequate secretion of insulin and resistance to insulin action)

      –Improved overall glucose tolerance and insulin response to oral medications

      –Improved blood lipid profile

      –Reduced blood glucose and glycosylated hemoglobin levels

2. **Supervision, monitoring, and precautions**

   –Reinforce the importance of proper footwear and foot care.

   –Ensure adequate hydration. (Dehydration can affect glucose levels.)

   –Monitor for signs of hyperglycemia and hypoglycemia by means of daily glucose checks.

   –Instruct the client to wear a medical alert ID.

   –If the client's blood glucose level is < 100 mg/dl, the client should eat a carbohydrate-rich food, then glucose should be remeasured before beginning exercise.

   –Insulin should not be injected into an exercising muscle. If it is injected, exercise should be delayed for 1 hour postinjection.

   –The client should always exercise with a partner.

   –The client must understand the signs and symptoms of hypoglycemia and hyperglycemia.

   –Exercise should be avoided during times of peak insulin activity. To prevent exercise-induced hypoglycemia, the insulin dose may be decreased, or carbohydrate intake may be increased before exercise.

   –The client needs regular assessment of glucose and glycosylated hemoglobin level, medication dosages, and dietary records.

3. **Contraindications**

   a. Blood glucose > 300 mg/dl

   b. Blood glucose > 240 mg/dl with ketones

   c. Untreated high-risk proliferative retinopathy (or recent therapy for retinopathy)

      –The client should avoid strenuous high-intensity activities and avoid lowering or jarring the head.

   d. Recent significant retinal hemorrhage

   e. Uncontrolled kidney failure

   f. Severe autonomic neuropathy

      –Resting HR > 100 bpm

      –Drop in systolic BP > 20 mm Hg when moving from sitting to standing (could cause a dangerous fall in systolic BP during exercise)

      –Signs of dehydration or thermoregulatory problems

   g. Acute illness, infection, or fever

   h. Peripheral neuropathy

      –Treadmill, walking, jogging, and step exercise are contraindicated for clients with loss of protective sensation in the feet; recommend swimming or cycling instead.

4. **Pre-exercise and postexercise guidelines**

   –Insulin requirements and adjustments should be monitored closely and charted in a log.

   –Diet requirements and adjustments are also documented in the log.

   –Blood glucose should be monitored before, during, and after exercise.

   –Perform ketone monitoring before exercise.

5. **Modifications**

   a. **Mode**

      –Use non–weight-bearing activities.

      –For type 1 diabetics, avoid activities that carry a high risk for foot trauma.

   b. **Intensity**

      –50% to 90% HR_{max}, 50% to 85% $\dot{V}O_{2max}$

      –RPE use is strongly recommended.

   c. **Frequency**

      –Clients with type 1 diabetes should exercise daily to maintain consistent blood glucose control.

–Clients with type 2 diabetes who are concerned with weight control should exercise 5 to 7 days per week.

–Late evening exercise should be avoided because of the risk of nocturnal hypoglycemia.

d. **Muscular fitness**

–Clients with diabetes should avoid high-intensity isometrics, use less weight, and increase repetitions to 10 to 15.

I. THE PATIENT WITH PERIPHERAL VASCULAR DISEASE

1. **Benefits and implications of exercise**

–Redistribution of and increased blood flow to legs

–Increased tolerance for walking; improved claudication tolerance and improved gait

–Reduced blood viscosity

–Improved muscle cell metabolism

2. **Precautions/contraindications**

–Hemorheologic medications decrease blood viscosity. Observe for interactions with other medications.

–Monitor for signs of cardiovascular complications. (Clients with peripheral arterial disease are likely to have cardiac disease.)

–Assess for musculoskeletal problems.

–The onset of claudication may be short in patients who are on beta-blockers.

3. **Modifications**

a. **Mode**

–Walking

b. **Intensity**

–Intermittent with symptom-limited work (to 3 or 4 on claudication scale, **Table 8-18**) and rest periods

–40% to 70% $\dot{V}O_{2max}$

c. **Frequency**

–Numerous times per day, 5 days per week

d. **Duration**

–20 minutes twice daily to 60 minutes daily for 3 months

e. **Progression**

–Progress until the walking bouts total 35 minutes of a 50-minute walking session exclusive of warm-up and cooldown.

 Table 8-18. Subjective Grading Scale for PVD Pain

Grade 1 Definite discomfort or pain, but only of initial or modest levels (established, but minimal)

Grade 2 Moderate discomfort or pain from which the patient's attention can be diverted, for example by conversation

Grade 3 Intense pain (short of grade 4) from which the patient's attention cannot be diverted

Grade 4 Excruciating and unbearable pain

PVD = peripheral vascular disease.
(From *ACSM's Guidelines for Exercise Testing and Prescription,* 6th ed. Philadelphia, Lippincott Williams & Wilkins, 2000, p 209.)

J. THE HYPERTENSIVE PATIENT

–Hypertension is generally defined as systolic blood pressure (SBP) ≥ 140 and/or diastolic blood pressure (DBP) ≥ 90 mm Hg. It is classified as essential, primary, or idiopathic.

1. **Benefits and implications of aerobic exercise**

–Reduced BP (Exercise has been advocated as therapy for hypertension.)

–Reduced severity of hypertension and subsequent reduction of antihypertensive medication dosage.

2. **Monitoring**

–ECG often shows left ventricular hypertrophy with strain; it may reveal false-positive ST changes.

–ECG may show arrhythmias caused by diuretic therapy and consequent potassium loss.

3. **Precautions/contraindications**

–Exercise is contraindicated in a client with resting SBP > 200 mm Hg or DBP > 115 mm Hg.

–High-intensity and isometric exercise should be avoided.

–Clients with mild to moderate hypertension experience higher SBP and cardiac output increase with exercise than do normotensive clients.

–Clients with severe hypertension (> 180/110 mm Hg) may drop cardiac output owing to decreased stroke volume, and may maintain high SBP and/or DBP owing to high peripheral resistance; thus, these clients should not begin an exercise program until cleared to do so by a physician.

–Nutritional counseling for control of weight, potassium, sodium, and magnesium may be indicated. (For example, diuretics may reduce potassium and lead to arrhythmias.)

–Smoking cessation and limitation of alcohol intake should be advocated.

–Clients taking vasodilators may need a longer cooldown period to prevent venous pooling.

–Clients with hypertension may also have other co-morbidities that need to be considered in designing an effective exercise program.

4. **Modifications**

   a. **Intensity**

      –Low-intensity exercise is acceptable, especially for clients with markedly elevated BP.

      –Use RPE instead of HR for a client taking medication that limits cardiac output (e.g., beta blockers, calcium antagonists). Refer to Table 8-6.

   b. **Frequency**

      –4 to 7 times per week

   c. **Duration**

      –is 30 to 60 minutes at a lower intensity.

      –Use a longer cooldown for those on medications that decrease total peripheral resistance (e.g., vasodilators).

   d. **Relaxation techniques** and **biofeedback** can be helpful.

   e. **Muscular fitness**

      –Use low resistance and a high number of repetitions (20).

      –Resistance training should be one component of the exercise program (i.e., the client should not use resistance training as the primary form of exercise).

K. **OTHER PATIENT POPULATIONS**

1. **The client with an orthopedic disorder**

   a. **The client with osteoarthritis: special considerations**

      –Back pain from spondylosis and spinal stenosis

      –Decreased ROM and weight-bearing ability

   b. **The client with rheumatoid arthritis**

      (1) **Special considerations**

         –Loss of ROM

         –Ulnar deviation and loss of grip strength

         –Foot instability, leading to gait abnormalities

         –Neurological symptoms indicative of subluxation (metatarsal heads and cervical spine)

   (2) **Modifications**

      (a) **Mode**

         –Choose smooth, non–weight-bearing activities; avoid jarring or jumping.

         –Choose an appropriate activity according to the joints affected.

         –For swimming or other water exercise, maintain pool water temperature at 83° to 88°F.

         –Proper footwear must always be worn for support and protection.

      (b) **Intensity**

         –is determined by pain level.

         –There should be no vigorous exercise for swollen, inflamed joints.

   c. **The client with osteoporosis**

      (1) **Benefits of exercise**

         –Increased bone mineral density

         –Conservation of bone mass from strength training

         –Maintenance of bone mass or decreased rate of bone loss in older adults, which helps prevent osteoporosis and fractures

      (2) **Special considerations**

         –Instruct the client to avoid forward flexion of the spine.

         –Control the client's environment to reduce the risk of falling.

         –Encourage nutritional counseling for calcium, vitamin D, and food–drug interactions.

         –Stress current calcium intake recommendations for men and women.

      (3) **Muscular strength**

         –Have client exercise to 50% to 75% 1 RM, using fewer repetitions (6 to 8), at least 2 times per week.

2. **The client with a neuromuscular disease**

   –Neuromuscular disease is commonly accompanied by respiratory impairment resulting in dyspnea, bronchial secretions, and respiratory muscle weakness

   –Table 8-19 lists specific program modifications for these clients.

   a. **The client with stroke**

      (1) **Special considerations**

         –Closely monitor the ECG because of increased risk for coronary artery disease (CAD).

Table 8-19. Program Modifications for Patients with Neuromuscular and Neurologic Conditions

Age-specific patient/family training

Treatment of underlying disorders

Assessment of severity of disease

Psychological support for patient and family

Strength training

Ambulation and cycle exercise for early disease states

Interval training

Orthotics

Postural drainage therapy

Proper body positioning

Suctioning

Mechanical ventilation

(Reprinted from American Association of Cardiovascular and Pulmonary Rehabilitation. *Guidelines for Pulmonary Rehabilitation,* 2nd ed, p 102. Champaign, IL, Human Kinetics, 1998.)

–Monitor for signs of peripheral arterial disease and modify the exercise program as needed (see X I).

(2) Modification of equipment

–To accommodate joint problems such as arthritis or loss of motor control of a limb, special braces or fastening to a bike pedal or an arm ergometer may be required.

(3) Duration of exercise is decreased and **frequency** increased because of the neuromuscular limitations (e.g., 15 minutes of stationary bike riding 2×/day vs. 30 minutes 1×/day).

(4) Intensity is based on 40% to 70% HR$_{max}$.

(5) Balance and coordination exercises should be performed daily.

b. **The client with muscular dystrophy**

–The main goals for clients with muscular dystrophy are to maintain muscular endurance and strength for as long as possible and to prevent contractures.

(1) Frequency

–Daily increase with decreasing duration of each session

(2) Intensity

–Low intensity as tolerated, but can try 40% to 85% HRR

(3) Duration

–The client should exercise until fatigued or cramping; dystrophic muscles don't tolerate high intensity levels.

(4) Special considerations

–Modify equipment as needed.

–Ensure safety of all exercises.

c. **The client with multiple sclerosis or polio**

–Exercise yields only short-term functional ability in muscular strength and endurance and in aerobic endurance.

(1) Special considerations

–Numerous client symptoms require modifications such as special strapping and support on exercise equipment.

–Impaired coordination and balance result from muscle weakness, paralysis, and spasticity.

–Heat intolerance may be a problem.

–Attenuated BP response to exercise may occur.

–The client who has cognitive deficit or memory problems will need verbal and written cues for exercise.

–A client with braces or an orthotic device may experience pain and extreme weakness in the braced limbs.

–Maintain hydration; muscles in a state of disuse can become dehydrated.

(2) Mode

–Use a variety of modes if muscle weakness in lower extremities causes early fatigue.

–Non–weight-bearing modes are recommended for those with balance, coordination, paralysis, or orthopedic problems.

(3) Strength training should be done on nonendurance or aerobic days.

(4) Flexibility training should be performed daily and before any aerobic or strength training.

(5) Duration should be decreased and **frequency** increased.

(6) Exercise prescription

–Be prepared to modify the program daily to adapt to the client's numerous and ever-changing symptoms.

–Focus on maintaining strength, endurance, and flexibility rather than on improvement.

3. **The client with a renal disorder**
   a. **Benefits of exercise**
      –Increased time to exhaustion
      –Improved BP
   b. **Intensity**
      –50% to 90% HR_{max}
      –50% to 85% $\dot{V}O_{2max}$
      –RPE scales
   c. **Frequency**
      –4 to 7 days per week
   d. **Duration**
      –20 to 60 minutes
   e. **Progression**
      –Very gradual
   f. **Resistance**
      –Avoid high resistance; use low weight, high repetitions.
   g. **Special considerations and precautions**
      –Diabetes is common in clients on dialysis.
      –The client may tend to become easily fatigued.
      –A client on hemodialysis can exercise before or during the dialysis treatment.
      –BP should not be assessed in an arm with an arteriovenous fistula.
      –The client may be anemic; hematocrit should be 30% to 35%.
      –A client receiving peritoneal dialysis should exercise only after the abdomen is empty of fluid.
      –Long-term dialysis may cause renal bone disease; care should be taken to prevent spontaneous tendon ruptures.

4. **The obese client**
   –Focus on combining an exercise program (increased caloric expenditure) with dietary modifications (decreased caloric intake).
   a. **Classifications and associated risks**
      (1) Body fat
      –There is an increased risk of various diseases when body fat is > 25% for men and > 32% for women.
      (2) Height/weight tables
      –There is an increased risk of disease at > 20% above ideal weight.
      (3) Waist circumference
      –Waist circumference of > 102 cm in men and > 88 cm in women indicates increased risk of disease.

(4) Body mass index (BMI)
–There is an increased risk of disease at a BMI of 25 kg/m^2 and above.
–Obesity is defined as a BMI of $\geq$ 30 kg/m^2.

(5) Waist-to-hip ratio
–is defined as the circumference of the waist divided by the circumference of the hip. Health risk increases as the waist-to-hip ratio increases. Focus has shifted from waist-to-hip ratio to waist circumference alone as a measure of abdominal obesity.

(6) Other obesity classifications
–Phenotype
–Hyperplastic or hypertrophic cell morphology

   b. **Benefits of exercise**
      –Weight reduction
      –Body fat reduction
      –Reduced risk of coronary artery disease and other chronic diseases
      –Enhanced ability to perform ADL
   c. **Frequency**
      –5 to 7 days per week
   d. **Duration**
      –Duration is increased (rather than intensity) to maximize caloric expenditure.
   e. **Mode**
      –Low-impact, large-muscle activities, water activities, or non-weight-bearing activities are best.
      –Increase the intensity of ADL (e.g., use stairs rather than elevator; do garden/yard work or active house chores instead of watching television; park car far from entry door; walk to store instead of driving).
      –**Resistance training** is an extremely useful component of the exercise prescription.
   f. **Intensity**
      –Promote daily caloric expenditure of $\geq$ 300 kcal.
   g. **Precautions**
      –Orthopedic injuries
      –Increased risk of hyperthermia
      –Possible need for modified equipment (e.g., wider seats, larger scales)

REVIEW TEST

DIRECTIONS: Carefully read all questions and select the BEST single answer.

1. Which of the following is *not* an appropriate treatment activity for inpatient rehabilitation of a client on day 2 post-CABG surgery?
   (A) Limit activities as tolerated to the development of self-care activities, ROM for extremities, and low-resistance activities.
   (B) Limit upper body activities to biceps curls, horizontal arm adduction, and overhead press using 5-pound weights while sitting on the side of the bed.
   (C) Progress all activities performed from supine to sitting to standing.
   (D) Measure vital signs, symptoms, RPE, fatigue, skin color, and ECG before, during, and after treatments to assess activity tolerance.

2. Which of the following situations indicates progression to independent and unsupervised exercise for a post-CABG surgery client in an outpatient program?
   (A) The client exhibits mild cardiac symptoms of angina occurring intermittently during exercise and some at home while reading.
   (B) The client has a functional capacity of > 8 METs with appropriate hemodynamic responses to this level of exercise.
   (C) The client is noncompliant with smoking cessation and weight loss intervention programs.
   (D) The client is unable to palpate HR, deliver RPEs, or maintain steady workload intensity during activity.

3. Which of the following issues would you include in discharge education instructions for a client with congestive heart failure to avoid potential emergency situations related to his condition at home?
   (A) Record body weight daily and report weight gains to a physician.
   (B) Note signs and symptoms such as dyspnea or intolerance to ADL and report them to a physician.
   (C) Do not palpate the pulse during daily activities or periods of lightheadedness, as an irregular pulse is normal and occurs at various times during the day.
   (D) Both A and B

4. Initial training sessions for a person with severe COPD most likely would *not* include
   (A) continuous cycling activity at 70% of $\dot{V}O_{2max}$ for 30 minutes.
   (B) the use of dyspnea scales, RPE scales, and pursed-lip breathing instruction.
   (C) intermittent bouts of activity on a variety of modalities (i.e., exercise followed by short rest).
   (D) encouraging the client to achieve an intensity at or above the anaerobic threshold.

5. Symptoms of claudication include
   (A) cramping, burning, and tightness in the calf muscle usually triggered by activity and relieved with rest.
   (B) acute, sharp pain in the foot on palpation at rest.
   (C) crepitus in the knee during cycling.
   (D) pitting ankle edema at a rating of 3+.

6. Treatment for claudication during exercise includes all of the following *except*
   (A) daily exercise sessions.
   (B) intensity of activity to maximal tolerable pain with intermittent rest periods.
   (C) cardiorespiratory building activities that are non–weight-bearing if the plan is to work on longer duration and higher intensity to elicit a cardiorespiratory training effect.
   (D) stopping activity at the onset of claudication discomfort to avoid further vascular damage from ischemia.

7. A client with angina exhibits symptoms and 1-mm down-sloping ST-segment depression at a HR of 129 bpm on his exercise test. His peak exercise target HR should be set at
   (A) 128 bpm
   (B) 109 to 119 bpm
   (C) 129 bpm
   (D) 125 to 128 bpm

8. Special precautions for clients with hypertension include all of the following *except*
   (A) avoiding muscle strengthening exercises that involve low resistance.
   (B) avoiding activities that involve Valsalva's maneuver.
   (C) monitoring a client taking diuretics for arrhythmias.
   (D) avoiding exercise if resting systolic BP is > 200 mm Hg or diastolic BP is > 115 mm Hg.

9. According to the most recent National Institutes of Health's Clinical *Guidelines for the Identification, Evaluation and Treatment of Overweight and Obesity in Adults,* recommendations for practical clinical assessment include
   (A) determining total body fat through the body mass index (BMI) to assess obesity.
   (B) determining the degree of abdominal fat and health risk through waist circumference.
   (C) using the waist-to-hip ratio (WHR) as the only definition of obesity and lean muscle mass.
   (D) Both A and B.

10. A client with type 1 diabetes mellitus checks her fasting morning glucose level on her whole blood glucose meter (fingerstick method), and it is 253 mg/dl (14 mmol/L). A urine test is positive for ketones before her exercise session. What action should you take?
    (A) Allow her to exercise as long as her glucose is not >300 mg/dl (17 mmol/L).
    (B) Not allow her to exercise this session and notify her physician of the findings.
    (C) Give her an extra carbohydrate snack and wait 5 minutes before beginning exercise.
    (D) Readjust her insulin regimen for the remainder of the day to compensate for the high morning glucose level.

11. A 62-year-old obese factory worker complains of pain in his right shoulder on arm abduction; decreased ROM and strength are noted on evaluation. You notice that he is beginning to use accessory muscles to substitute movements and to compensate. These symptoms may indicate
    (A) a referred pain from a herniated lumbar disc.
    (B) rotator cuff strain or impingement.
    (C) angina.
    (D) advanced stages of multiple sclerosis.

12. All of the following are special considerations in prescribing exercise for the client with arthritis *except*
    (A) the possible need to splint painful joints for protection.
    (B) periods of acute inflammation result in decreased pain and joint stiffness.
    (C) the possibility of gait abnormalities as compensation for pain or stiffness.
    (D) the need to avoid exercise of warm, swollen joints.

13. What common medication taken by clients with end-stage renal disease requires careful management for those undergoing hemodialysis?
    (A) Antihypertensive medication
    (B) Lithium
    (C) Cholestyramine
    (D) Cromolyn sodium

14. Which of the following is an appropriate exercise for diabetic clients with loss of protective sensation in the extremities?
    (A) Prolonged walking
    (B) Jogging
    (C) Step class exercise
    (D) Swimming

15. A client taking a calcium channel blocker will most likely exhibit which of the following responses during exercise?
    (A) Hypertensive response
    (B) Increased ischemia
    (C) Improved anginal thresholds
    (D) Severe hypotension

16. During the cooldown phase of an exercise session, clients should be encouraged to
    (A) rehydrate.
    (B) decrease the intensity of activity quickly, to decrease cardiac afterload.
    (C) limit the cooldown period to 5 minutes.
    (D) increase the number of isometric activities.

17. Muscular endurance training is best accomplished by
    (A) performing 4 to 6 repetitions per set.
    (B) using high resistance.
    (C) incorporating high repetitions.
    (D) performing isometric exercises only.

18. Transitional care exercise and rehabilitation programs are *not* appropriate for
    (A) clients with functionally limiting chronic disease.
    (B) clients with comorbid disease states.
    (C) asymptomatic clients with a functional capacity of 10 METs.
    (D) clients at 1 week post-CABG surgery.

19. Many clients have VVI mode programmed pacemakers. Which of the following is true regarding exercise programming with VVI pacemakers?
    (A) Persons with VVI pacemakers may be chronotropically (HR) competent with exercise but require longer warm-up and gradual increase in intensity during the initial exercise portion of their session.
    (B) Persons who are chronotropically competent are tachycardic at rest and should not exercise at low intensities.
    (C) BP response is not a good marker of intensity effort in those with VVI pacemakers and need not be evaluated during an exercise session.
    (D) Persons with VVI pacemakers must avoid exercise on the bicycle ergometer due to the location of the ventricular lead wire and potential for displacement.

20. Controlling pool water temperature (83° to 88° F), avoiding jarring and weight-bearing activities, and avoiding movement in swollen, inflamed joints are special considerations for exercise in
    (A) clients who are post-atherectomy.
    (B) angina clients.
    (C) clients with osteoporosis.
    (D) arthritic clients.

21. Which of the following is a resistive lung disease?
    (A) Asthma
    (B) Tuberculosis
    (C) Cystic fibrosis
    (D) Emphysema

22. A specific benefit of regular exercise for patients with angina is
    (A) improved ischemic threshold at which angina symptoms occur.
    (B) increased myocardial oxygen demand at the same submaximal levels.
    (C) eradication of all symptoms.
    (D) elevated blood pressure.

23. Which of the following is *not* a benefit of increased flexibility?
    (A) Increased muscle viscosity, allowing easier and smoother contractions
    (B) Reduced muscle tension and increased relaxation
    (C) Improved coordination by allowing greater ease of movement
    (D) Increased range of motion

ANSWERS AND EXPLANATIONS

1–B. Strenuous and resistive upper body exercises and activity may cause injury to the sternum immediately after CABG surgery. Such exercises should be avoided until the sternum and chest incisions have healed.

2–B. Progression to more independent self-managed programs is encouraged for those who have a good functional capacity, exhibit appropriate hemodynamic and ECG responses to exercise and recovery, are asymptomatic, have stable resting HR and BP, manage risk factor intervention strategies safely and effectively, demonstrate knowledge of the disease process, and are compliant with their program.

3–D. Symptoms of worsening heart failure (leg edema, activity intolerance, dyspnea, orthopnea, paroxysmal dyspnea) must be explained to clients. A weight gain of 3 to 5 pounds since the last appointment should be reported. During symptoms of lightheadedness or chest discomfort, palpating the pulse provides helpful information if the heartbeat suddenly becomes irregular during these episodes. The development of an arrhythmia should be reported to the physician.

4–A. A client with severe chronic obstructive pulmonary disease who is just beginning an exercise program would not be able to tolerate vigorously intense exercise for prolonged periods due to limitations such as dyspnea, muscle weakness, and cardiovascular deconditioning as a result of previous inactivity.

5–A. Sharp, palpable pain over an area typically indicates fasciitis or tendonitis. Crepitus in the knee is indicative of inflammation, arthritis, and other joint structural problems. Ankle edema is indicative of poor venous return in conditions such as right heart failure, and is not an indication of an atherosclerotic artery.

6–D. Clients with claudication are encouraged to exercise at an intensity that causes intense pain (grade III) or unbearable pain (grade IV). This is followed by a full recovery rest period.

7–B. Peak exercise HR is set at 10 to 20 bpm below the ischemic level (which was symptomatic down-sloping ST depression at 129 bpm).

8–A. Low-resistance muscle-strengthening exercises can be performed by those diagnosed with hypertension if they follow appropriate lifting techniques and avoid Valsalva's maneuver. In addition, hemodynamic parameters (HR and BP) and medications should be controlled.

9–D. BMI can be used to classify overweight and obesity levels. In addition, waist circumference has been found to be a better marker of abdominal fat content than WHR.

10–B. Whole blood glucose values are generally 10% to 15% lower than plasma glucose levels. Type 1 diabetics should avoid exercise when ketones are present at a glucose level > 240 mg/dl (14 mmol/L), or if glucose levels exceed 300 mg/dl (17 mmol/L) regardless of whether ketosis is present. Carbohydrate snacks are taken only when glucose levels are too low to help maintain proper glycemic control during exercise. Only a physician can prescribe changes in medication regimen.

11–B. The subdeltoid bursa, supraspinatus muscle, and nerves become impinged between the coracoid and acromion process with shoulder abduction. The resulting pain leads to decreased ROM, disuse, and muscle atrophy. Such impingement of the rotator cuff is common in assembly line workers who perform repetitive overhead tasks.

12–B. During periods of acute arthritic inflammation, affected joints will be painful, stiff, hot, and swollen. These joints should not be exercised and may need to be protected to allow the client to perform other motor tasks.

13–A. The hemodialysis process interacts with antihypertensive medications and lowers the drug level, causing a potentially severe hypertensive response. To avoid such a reaction, clients may skip their hypertension medication on dialysis days.

14–D. Prolonged walking, jogging, and step classes are high- impact or weight-bearing activities that can lead to sores, ulcers, or fractures in those with loss of sensation in the feet (peripheral neuropathy).

15–C. Clients with angina who are taking calcium channel blockers will improve their exercise capacity response to exercise regimens.

16–A. A longer cooldown period of 10 to 15 minutes (or longer for certain disease states) and a gradual decrease in intensity will provide a smoother recovery period and avoid sudden adverse hemodynamic responses and associated symptoms.

17–C. Muscular endurance (the ability to sustain prolonged muscular contractions) is best accomplished by using lighter weights and performing more repetitions per set.

18–C. Transitional or home care rehabilitation can be provided through nursing homes, rehabilitation hospitals, or clinics to those needing supervised care for exercise or ADL.

19–A. Chronotropically competent VVI clients are often bradycardic at rest but have good atrioventricular conduction. Gradual increases in activity are recommended to allow the sinus node time to respond. BP should be monitored during exercise to help assess intensity levels.

20–D. Clients with arthritis should avoid exercising joints that are acutely inflamed and will benefit from non–weight-bearing pool exercises in warm water. Clients with cardiac diagnoses are not limited to non–weight-bearing activities and do not have inflamed joints as a result of their disease. Clients with osteoporosis benefit from exercise that decreases the rate of bone loss.

21–B. Obstructive lung diseases are "flow" obstructions, including asthma, cystic fibrosis, interstitial lung disease, chronic bronchitis, and emphysema. Restrictive lung diseases are those involving restricted lung capacity due to disease or damage of the lungs, including lupus, pulmonary edema, tuberculosis, and lung cancer.

22–A. The ischemic threshold is predictable in stable angina patients. A benefit of regular exercise for patients with angina is an improved ischemic threshold at which angina symptoms occur. In addition, myocardial oxygen demand decreases, as do blood pressure and the heart rate response to submaximal exercise.

23–A. There are numerous benefits of increased flexibility including reduced muscle tension and increased relaxation, increased ease of movement, improved coordination, increased range of motion; improved body awareness, improved capability for circulation and air exchange, decreased muscle viscosity, causing contractions to be easier and smoother, and decreased soreness associated with other exercise activities.

CHAPTER 9

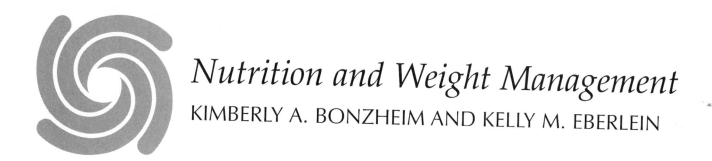

Nutrition and Weight Management
KIMBERLY A. BONZHEIM AND KELLY M. EBERLEIN

I. ESSENTIAL NUTRIENTS

A. FAT

1. Fat is stored in adipose tissue and provides energy; insulates and protects vital organs; transports the fat-soluble vitamins A, D, E, and K; and provides essential fatty acids, linoleic acids, and linolenic acids.

   –**Essential fatty acids** are required for growth, for healthy skin, and for producing elements of the immune system.

2. The primary fats in food and in the body are **triglycerides** and **cholesterol.**

   a. **Triglycerides** are composed of three fatty acids and a glycerol molecule. They are classified as either saturated or unsaturated fats.

      (1) Saturated fatty acids come primarily from animal sources (exceptions are palm oil, coconut oil and cocoa butter) and form triglycerides that are solid at room temperature.

      (2) Unsaturated fatty acids (in monounsaturated and polyunsaturated forms) come from vegetable sources and form triglycerides that are liquid at room temperature.

      –**Serum triglycerides** are derived from ingested fats and from fats that the body produces from other energy sources, such as carbohydrates and alcohol.

      –A **high serum triglyceride level** (> 200 mg/dl) is a risk factor for heart disease, because it decreases the oxygen-carrying capacity of blood.

   –**Strategies to lower serum triglyceride level** include maintaining optimum body weight, exercising regularly, limiting intake of saturated fats and alcohol, and substituting complex carbohydrates for simple sugars.

   b. **Cholesterol** is a waxy, fat-like substance found in foods of animal origin.

      –Cholesterol is necessary for cell membranes and performs numerous essential anatomical and physiological functions.

      –The liver produces sufficient amounts of cholesterol to meet the body's requirements without the need for dietary consumption.

      –Monitoring cholesterol and fat intake— particularly saturated fat, which has the greatest impact on blood cholesterol—is important to help prevent coronary artery disease.

3. **Lipoproteins,** produced by the liver and intestinal mucosa, transport cholesterol and triglycerides through the blood.

   a. **Very low-density lipoproteins** (VLDLs) are major carriers of triglycerides.

   b. **Low-density lipoproteins** (LDLs) are composed primarily of cholesterol and may be deposited in the arterial walls, contributing to the development of atherosclerosis.

   c. **High-density lipoproteins** (HDLs) carry cholesterol away from the arterial walls to the liver for catabolism and excretion, and interfere with the binding of LDL cholesterol to cell membranes.

4. **Ideal cholesterol and lipoprotein levels** to reduce the risk of atherosclerosis have been defined by the **National Cholesterol Education Program.**

   a. **Total cholesterol:** < 200 mg/dl

   b. **LDL cholesterol:** < 130 mg/dl for individuals without known heart disease, and < 100 mg/dl for those with heart disease

   c. **HDL cholesterol:** > 35 mg/dl; > 60 mg/dl is considered a negative risk factor for coronary artery disease.

B. **CARBOHYDRATES**

   –provide energy, vitamins, minerals, fiber, and protein, all of which contribute to a balanced diet.

   –There are two types of carbohydrates: simple and complex.

   1. **Simple carbohydrates** (sugars)—glucose, fructose, sucrose (table sugar), and lactose (milk sugar)—are found in such foods as candy, soft drinks, milk, and fruits.

   2. **Complex carbohydrates** (starches) are composed of chains of simple sugars and are found in pasta, bread, cereal, rice, fruits, and vegetables.

      –**Fiber,** the nondigestible portion of complex carbohydrates, is found only in plant foods and may play a role in the prevention and treatment of diabetes, cancer, cardiovascular disease, and obesity.

      a. **Soluble fiber** dissolves in water and is found in citrus fruits, apples, grains, legumes, and peas. It has been linked to decreasing cholesterol and offering protection against coronary artery disease.

      b. **Insoluble fiber,** contained in whole-grain products and vegetables, absorbs water in the large intestine and produces soft stools that pass quickly through the intestinal tract. It is theorized that this process reduces the time that potential carcinogens are in contact with intestinal cells, decreasing the risk of colon cancer.

C. **PROTEIN**

   –provides energy and the **amino acids** needed for building brain cells, muscle tissue, blood, and skin; for repairing tissues; and for creating antibodies, enzymes, and many necessary hormones.

   –**Eight of the 20 amino acids are essential** and cannot be synthesized in adequate amounts by the body.

   1. **Complete proteins**

      –Proteins from animal and soy sources are generally considered complete, or high quality, because they contain all eight essential amino acids.

   2. **Incomplete proteins**

      –Plant proteins are lower-quality, or incomplete, because each is missing one or more essential amino acids. Therefore, vegetarians must consume a variety of plant proteins to ensure intake of all essential amino acids.

D. **VITAMINS**

   –facilitate metabolic reactions, blood coagulation, vision, and cellular protection.

   –are not manufactured by the body and thus must be ingested in the diet or in supplements.

   –Primary functions, dietary sources, and recommended dietary allowances (RDAs) for vitamins are listed in **Table 9-1.**

   1. **Classification**

      –Vitamins are classified as fat-soluble or water-soluble.

      a. **Fat-soluble vitamins** (A, D, E, and K) are **stored in fatty tissues.** In excess, these vitamins are **potentially toxic** because they can be stored and accumulate.

      b. **Water-soluble vitamins** (C, thiamin, riboflavin, niacin, B6, folacin, B12, biotin, and pantothenic acid) are **not stored in body tissues,** and **must be ingested regularly** to maintain recommended levels.

   2. **Vitamin toxicity**

      a. **Vitamin A toxicity**

         –Vitamin A ingested from plant sources is less bioavailable and cannot build up to toxic levels.

         –Excessive vitamin A ingested from animal sources can cause headaches, vomiting, and liver damage, and has been linked to birth defects and miscarriage.

      b. **Vitamin D toxicity**

         –may occur in young children who spend their summer months outdoors, drink plenty of milk, and take vitamin D supplements.

         –Signs and symptoms include loss of appetite, headache, excessive thirst, and irritability.

Table 9-1. Function, Source and Recommended Dietary Allowances (RDA) for Vitamins

Vitamin	Main Function	Good Sources	RDA (ADULT)
A	Maintenance of skin, bone, growth, vision, and teeth	Eggs, cheese, margarine, milk, carrots, broccoli, squash, and spinach	m: 1000 µg f: 800 µg
D	Bone growth and maintenance of bones	Milk, egg yolk, tuna, and salmon (sunlight)	m: 5 µg f: 5 µg
E	Antioxidant	Vegetable oils, whole-grain cereal, bread, dried beans, & green leafy vegetables	m: 10 mg f: 8 mg
K	Blood clotting	Cabbage, green leafy vegetables, milk	m: 80 µg f: 65 µg
Thiamine (B_1)	Energy-releasing reactions	Pork, ham, oysters, breads, cereals, pasta, green peas	m: 1.5 mg f: 1.1 mg
Riboflavin (B_2)	Energy-releasing reactions	Milk, meat, cereals, pasta, mushrooms, dark green vegetables	m: 1.7 mg f: 1.3 mg
Niacin	Energy-releasing reactions	Poultry, meat, tuna, cereal, pasta, bread, nuts, legumes	m: 19 mg f: 15 mg
Pyridoxine (B_6)	Metabolism of fats & proteins & formation of red blood cells	Cereals, bread, spinach, avocados, green beans, bananas	m: 2.0 mg f: 1.6 mg
Cobalamin (B_{12})	Formation of red blood cells & functioning of nervous system	Meat, fish, eggs, milk	m: 2.0 µg f: 2.0 µg
Folacin	Assists in forming proteins & in formation of red blood cells	Dark green leafy vegetables, wheat germ, oranges, bananas	m: 200 µg f: 180 µg
Pantothenic acid	Metabolism of proteins, CHO, & fats, formation of hormones	Bread, cereals, nuts, eggs & dark green vegetables	ESADDI = 7–9 mg
Biotin	Formation of fatty acids & energy-releasing reactions	Egg yolk, leafy green vegetables	ESADDI = 30–100 µg
C	Maintenance of bones, teeth, blood vessels, & collagen: antioxidant	Citrus fruits, tomatoes, strawberries, melons, green peppers, potatoes	m: 60 mg f: 60 mg

m = male; f = female; ESADDI = Estimated Safe and Adequate Daily Dietary Intake
(With permission from the National Resource Council: *Recommended Dietary Allowances,* 10th ed. Washington, DC, National Academy of Sciences, 1989.)

—Increased calcium loss from the bones into the bloodstream, excretory system, and tissues can lead to irreversible organ damage and even death.

c. **Vitamin E toxicity** may cause muscle weakness, fatigue, and nausea and can also interfere with blood clotting.

d. **Niacin (B3) toxicity**

—is marked by flushing, headache, and itching.

—High doses of niacin to decrease cholesterol and triglycerides should be administered under medical supervision.

e. **Pantothenic acid (B5) toxicity** is rare, but may cause diarrhea and water retention.

f. **Vitamin B6 toxicity** is associated with nerve damage.

g. **Vitamin C toxicity** can cause diarrhea, nausea, and headache.

3. **Vitamin supplements**

—should not be used to compensate for poor dietary habits.

—may be advisable during pregnancy or lactation or when food intake is erratic.

E. **MINERALS**

1. **Functions of minerals** include creating and maintaining bones and teeth, facilitating various body functions, and serving as essential components of certain body fluids. Major functions, food sources, and RDAs for minerals are listed in **Table 9-2**.

2. **Fifteen essential minerals** have been identified.

—The **major minerals** include calcium, phosphorous, potassium, sodium, chloride, magnesium, and sulfur.

—The **trace minerals** are iron, iodine, zinc, chromium, selenium, fluoride, molybdenum, copper, and manganese.

Table 9-2. Function, Source and Recommended Dietary Allowances (RDA) for Minerals

Mineral	Main Function	Good Sources	RDA (ADULT)
Calcium	Formation of bones, teeth, maintenance of nerve impulses, blood clotting	Cheese, sardines, dark green vegetables, vegetables, clams, milk	m: 800 mg f: 800 mg
Phosphorus	Formation of bones & teeth, acid-base balance	Milk, cheese, meat, fish, poultry, nuts, grains	m: 800 mg f: 800 mg
Magnesium	Activation of enzymes and protein synthesis	Nuts, meat, milk, whole-grain cereal, green leafy vegetables	m: 350 mg f: 280 mg
Sodium	Acid-base balance, body water balance, nerve function	Most foods	min. = 500 mg
Potassium	Acid-base balance, body water balance, nerve function	Meat, milk, many fruits, cereals, vegetables, legumes	min. = 2000 mg
Chloride	Gastric juice formation & acid-base balance	Table salt, seafood, milk, meat, eggs	
Iron	Component of hemoglobin & enzymes	Meats, legumes, eggs, grains, dark green vegetables	m: 10 mg f: 15 mg
Zinc	Component of many enzymes	Milk, shellfish, & wheat bran	m: 15 mg f: 12 mg
Iodine	Component of thyroid hormone	Fish, dairy products, vegetables, iodized salt	m: 150 mg f: 150 mg
Copper	Component of enzymes, delivers iron from storage	Shellfish, grains, cherries, legumes, poultry, oysters, nuts	ESADDI = 1.5–3 mg
Manganese	Component of enzymes, fat synthesis	Greens, blueberries, grains, legumes, fruit	ESADDI = 2–5 mg
Fluoride	Maintenance of bones and teeth	Water, seafood, rice, soybeans, spinach, onions, and lettuce	ESADDI = 1.5–4 mg
Chromium	Glucose and energy metabolism	Fats, meats, clams, cereals	ESADDI = 50–200 µg
Selenium	Functions with vitamin E antioxidant	Fish, poultry, meats, grains, milk, vegetables	m: 70 µg f: 55 µg
Molybdenum	Component of enzymes	Legumes, cereals, dark green leafy vegetables	ESADDI = 70–250 µg

m = male; f = female; ESADDI = Estimated Safe and Adequate Daily Dietary Intake
(With permission from the National Resource Council: *Recommended Dietary Allowances,* 10th ed. Washington, DC, National Academy of Sciences, 1989.)

3. **Supplementation** of certain minerals (e.g., calcium, iron) is usually not necessary but may be recommended for some clients.

   a. **Calcium supplements**

   –Calcium supplementation is commonly recommended in women **to help prevent osteoporosis.**

   –The RDA for women under age 25 and postmenopausal women is increased to 1,200 mg from the 800 mg recommended for all other persons.

   –Calcium carbonate and calcium citrate are acceptable supplement choices.

   –**Excessive calcium** intake may inhibit the absorption of other nutrients and increase the risk of kidney damage.

   b. **Iron supplements**

   –Iron supplementation may be recommended for athletes and women who are iron deficient.

   –In pregnant women, the RDA increases to 30 mg from the 15 mg recommended for all other women.

   –Iron from supplements is not as readily absorbed as that from food sources; taking supplements with meats or vitamin C–rich foods can improve absorption.

   –Iron supplementation should not exceed the RDA, unless prescribed, to avoid **iron toxicity,** which can cause liver damage and heart disease.

F. ANTIOXIDANTS

–are substances that limit the formation of free radicals or neutralize them before they can damage body tissues.

–include some forms of vitamin A, vitamin C, vitamin E, selenium, and carotenoids.

–**Carotenoids** (plant pigments that occur in vegetable, fungi and some crustacea) are not vitamins, but the body does convert some of them to vitamins, and most have antioxidant properties.

–In some studies, test subjects who ate high amounts of antioxidant-containing foods were determined to have a decreased risk of heart attack or stroke.

–Recommendations specify eating a variety of foods high in antioxidants (fruits, vegetables, nuts, and grains), because these substances work in concert and benefits may not be realized with large doses of an isolated antioxidant vitamin or mineral.

G. FLUIDS

–Water serves as a solvent for chemical reactions, transports nutrients to cells, provides a medium for excretion of waste products, acts as a lubricant between cells, and assists in temperature regulation.

–A person can live for up to 30 days without food, but for only a few days without water.

H. ENERGY YIELD OF NUTRIENTS

–During metabolism, three of the four classes of organic nutrients—carbohydrates, fat, and protein—provide energy for the body to use.

–Vitamins, minerals, and water do not yield energy in the human body.

–The energy-yielding nutrients are vital to life; without continual replenishment of expended energy, death would soon occur.

–As these nutrients break down, they release energy—some released as heat, some transferred into other compounds that compose the structures of body cells, and some used as fuel for the body's activities.

–The energy released is measured in **calories.**

1. One gram of carbohydrate equals 4 calories.
2. One gram of protein equals 4 calories.
3. One gram of fat equals 9 calories.
4. One gram of alcohol equals 7 calories.

II. DIETARY STANDARDS

A. DIETARY GUIDELINES FOR AMERICANS

–Set by the Food and Nutrition Board of the National Research Council in 1995, these are general guidelines for improving health (**Table 9-3**).

1. **Fat intake should be less than 30% of total calories,** of which saturated fat should be no more than 10%, and cholesterol should be limited to 300 mg/day.
2. **Protein** consumption should be approximately 15% of total calories.
3. **Carbohydrate** intake should be approximately 55% of total calories, with only about 15% from simple carbohydrates.

B. RECOMMENDED DIETARY ALLOWANCES (RDA)

–are determined by the National Research Council of the National Academy of Sciences to represent the levels of essential nutrients considered adequate to meet the needs of most healthy people.

–An RDA has been established only for those nutrients for which adequate data are available. A range of **estimated safe and adequate daily dietary intake** (ESADDI) has been identified for those nutrients where insufficient data are available to set specific recommendations (see Tables 9-1 and 9-2).

1. The **RDA for caloric intake** is set at the mean intake of the normal weight population, and should be adjusted for activity level.
2. The **RDA for protein** is based on body weight (0.8 g of protein/kg of body weight), with increased amounts required during growth, pregnancy, and lactation and in physically active persons.
3. **RDAs for fats and carbohydrates** have not been established, because these nutrients can be synthesized and are not considered essential.
4. **RDAs for selected vitamins and minerals** are listed in Tables 9-1 and 9-2.

Table 9-3. The Dietary Guidelines for Americans

Eat a variety of foods.

Balance the food you eat with physical activity. Maintain or improve your weight.

Choose a diet with plenty of grain products, vegetables and fruits.

Choose a diet low in fat, saturated fat and cholesterol.

Choose a diet moderate in sugars.

Choose a diet moderate in salt and sodium.

If you drink alcoholic beverages, do so in moderation.

(From U.S. Dept. of Agriculture: *Dietary Guidelines for Americans.* Washington, DC, U.S. Dept. of Health and Human Services, 1995.)

C. FOOD GUIDE PYRAMID

–was created by the U.S. Department of Agriculture. It classifies food on the basis of nutrient content and the recommended frequency of consumption (**Figure 9-1**)

A Guide to Daily Food Choices

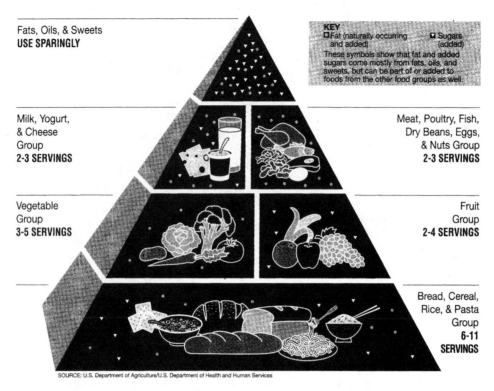

FIGURE 9-1 Food guide pyramid (Source: U.S. Department of Agriculture)

III. BODY COMPOSITION AND HEALTH

A. TWO COMPONENTS OF BODY COMPOSITION

–The two components of body composition are fat-free mass, also called lean body weight, and percent fat.

1. **Fat-free mass (FFM)** is assumed to be relatively constant and to have a density of 1.1 g/ml at 37°C, a water content of 72%–74%, and a potassium content of 60–70 mmol/kg in men and 50–60 mmol/kg in women.

2. **Percent fat** refers to the percentage of body weight that is fat; its measurement is based on the fact that body weight comprises FFM and fat weight.

B. MEASUREMENT OF BODY COMPOSITION

–Body composition can be measured on elemental (atomic), chemical, cellular, and tissue/system levels.

1. **Models for characterizing human body composition** have been developed using different levels of analysis. A common feature of all useful models is that the **sum of the** components (FFM and fat) closely approximates body weight.

–**Molecular models** generally are accessible with current technology and are used in most validation studies of field methods.

–**Laboratory models,** including total body water (TBW), total body potassium, and hydrodensitometry, are the most common models used for estimating fat and FFM. These models can produce erroneous findings when the client's actual body composition differs from that assumed by the model.

2. **Methods of determining body composition**

–Selection of an appropriate method is based on the relative precision, reliability, and accuracy of available methods; the availability of appropriate equations; and cost considerations.

   a. **Anthropometric measurements (see Chapter 6)**

   –The reliability and validity of anthropometric methods are affected by the skill of the measurer, the equipment used, the client's body type, and the prediction equation used.

Table 9-4. Adult Intervention Guidelines Based on Body Mass Index (BMI)

BMI (kg/m²)		Guidelines
19–34 years	> 35 years	
< 25	< 27	Normal; refer to waist-to-hip ratio
25–27	—	Intervention indicated if there is a family history of presence of heart disease, type II diabetes, hypercholesterolemia, or hypertension
> 27	> 27	Intervention indicated even in the absence of another risk factor

(From *ACSM's Resource Manual for Guidelines for Exercise Testing and Prescription,* 3rd ed. Baltimore, Williams & Wilkins, 1998, p 571.)

(1) Skinfold measurements generally give accurate estimates of percent fat and FFM, because they directly measure subcutaneous fat.

(2) Circumference measurements reflect both fat and muscle, and thus do not provide accurate estimates of percent fat and FFM in the general population; they are most useful in obese and athletic persons.

–One circumference measurement, **waist-to-hip ratio** (WHR), determined by dividing waist circumference by hip circumference, is useful in assessing disease risk.

(3) Body mass index (BMI) is calculated from weight (in kg) divided by height (in m²). **Table 9-4** presents recommendations for intervention in adults based on BMI.

–BMI is a poor predictor of percent body fat, and often misclassifies an individual as obese who has above-average muscularity and skeletal mass rather than excess fat.

–BMI can be misleading in the elderly and children, in whom the muscle and bone-to-height relationship changes regularly.

b. Bioelectrical impedance analysis (BIA)

–is a rapid, noninvasive, and relatively inexpensive method for estimating fat and FFM.

–Total body impedance at the constant frequency of 50 kHz primarily reflects the volumes of water (intracellular and extracellular fluid) and muscle compartments comprising the FFM.

–Accuracy is affected by instrumentation, subject factors, technician skill, and the prediction equation used to estimate FFM.

–Factors such as eating, drinking, and exercising must be controlled, because

hydration status is an important source of error in resistance measurement.

3. Prediction equations

a. Prediction equations are either population-specific or generalized.

–**Population-specific equations** are derived for specific homogeneous populations (e.g., elderly African-Americans), and are useful only for the intended populations.

–**Generalized equations** can be applied to individuals who differ greatly in physical characteristics, age, sex, race, and other characteristics.

b. Various factors need to be considered when selecting an equation:

–To whom is the equation applicable?

–Was an appropriate reference method used to develop the equation?

–Was a representative sample of the population studied?

–How were the predictor variables measured?

–Was the equation cross-validated in another sample of the same population?

c. Useful equations give estimates of percent fat or FFM that are significantly correlated ($R \geq 0.80$) with criterion measurements.

C. STANDARDS OF BODY COMPOSITION

–A typical body fat standard is $\leq 15\%$ for young adult men and $\leq 25\%$ for young adult women; the usefulness of this standard in other groups has not been established.

–Body fat standards of $\leq 25\%$ in males and $\leq 30\%$ in females have been proposed for persons age 6–18 years.

–The National Institutes for Health has suggested that a BMI > 27 indicates obesity and BMI > 30 indicates morbid obesity.

–The Expert Panel on Healthy Weight recommends that adults maintain a BMI < 25, and that those with a BMI > 25 work to achieve a healthier weight.

D. HEALTH IMPLICATIONS OF BODY COMPOSITION PATTERNS

1. **The pattern of obesity,** or the distribution of adipose tissue in the body, has health implications.

   a. **Gynoid obesity,** body fat accumulation around the hips and lower abdomen, occurs most often in women.

   b. **Android obesity** describes fat accumulation over the chest and arms (upper body) rather then over the lower trunk; most common in men, it is associated with greater morbidity and mortality than gynoid obesity.

2. A WHR > 0.95 for men and > 0.85 for women is considered a significant **risk factor for cardiovascular disease (Table 9-5).**

3. Epidemiological studies indicate that a BMI of 21–22 is associated with the lowest risk for cardiovascular disease.

⑤ Table 9-5. Waist-To-Hip Circumference Ratio (WHR) Standards for Men and Women

	Age	Risk Low	Moderate	High	Very High
Men	20–29	< 0.83	0.83–0.88	0.89–0.94	> 0.94
	30–39	< 0.84	0.84–0.91	0.92–0.96	> 0.96
	40–49	< 0.88	0.88–0.95	0.96–1.00	> 1.00
	50–59	< 0.90	0.90–0.96	0.97–1.02	> 1.02
	60–69	< 0.91	0.91–0.98	0.99–1.03	> 1.03
Women	20–29	< 0.71	0.71–0.77	0.78–0.82	> 0.82
	30–39	< 0.72	0.72–0.78	0.79–0.84	> 0.84
	40–49	< 0.73	0.73–0.79	0.80–0.87	> 0.87
	50–59	< 0.74	0.74–0.81	0.82–0.88	> 0.88
	60–69	< 0.76	0.76–0.83	0.84–0.90	> 0.90

(With permission from Heyward VH, Stolarcyzk LM: *Applied Body Composition Assessment.* Champaign, IL, Human Kinetics, 1996, p 82.)

IV. BLOOD LIPID MODIFICATION

A. EFFECTS OF DIET THERAPY

1. **Restriction of dietary fat, saturated fat, and cholesterol intake can help reduce blood cholesterol and triglyceride levels.**

   –Lowering cholesterol, particularly LDLs, decreases the risk of atherosclerotic events (e.g., heart attack, stroke, bypass surgery).

   –Lowering blood lipid levels may stabilize arterial plaques and reduce the risk of subsequent fissuring and resulting thrombus or vessel occlusion.

   –Large population studies suggest that each 1% reduction in blood cholesterol level brings a 2%–3% reduction in the incidence of cardiovascular events.

2. The **National Cholesterol Education Program** defines **guidelines for treating abnormal cholesterol values (Table 9-6).**

3. The **American Heart Association** provides **diet recommendations** for counseling clients (Table 9-7).

4. **Various dietary factors are known to positively influence blood lipid levels.**

   a. Eating 2 oz/day of **oat bran** is recommended because of oat bran's **soluble fiber** content.

   b. **Replacing animal sources of protein with soy protein** has been shown to lower blood cholesterol.

   c. A large dose of **omega-3 fatty acids** does not decrease cholesterol, but acts directly on blood vessels and the heart muscle to reduce the likelihood of heart disease.

   d. **Folic acid** is given to decrease high blood **homocysteine** levels.

      –High levels of homocysteine have been shown to be an independent risk factor for premature coronary artery disease. Accumulation of homocysteine in the blood has a toxic effect on the endothelium and stimulates the proliferation of smooth muscle within the vessels. In general, good nutrition, including foods high in folic acid and vitamin B6, may lower homocysteine.

5. Table 9-8 summarizes an optimal diet for improving blood lipids.

Table 9-6. Target Lipid Levels in Adults Over 19 Years of Age and Adolescents

Category	Total Cholesterol (mg/dl)	LDL Cholesterol (mg /dl)	HDL Cholesterol (mg /dl)
Without documented CVD 20+ yrs of age	< 200	< 130	> 35*
With documented CVD 20+ yrs of age	< 200	< 100	> 35*
Youth 13–19 yrs of age	< 170	< 100	No recommendation

*It is the opinion of the authors that HDL should be > 45 mg/dl in females with or without CVD. An HDL > 60 mg/dl is considered a negative risk factor. (From *ACSM's Resource Manual for Guidelines and Prescription,* 3rd ed. Baltimore, Williams & Wilkins, 1998, p 296.)

Table 9-7. American Heart Association Dietary Therapy Recommendations for Treating Abnormal Lipids

Step	% Fat Cals	% Sat Fat Cals	% Protein	% Carbohydrates	Mg/Day Cholesterol
I	< 30	10	15	55	300 or less
II	< 25	8	15	60	200–250 or less
III	< 20	< 7	15	65	100–150 or less

With permission from American Heart Association. Recommendations for Treatment of Hyperlipidemia in Adults. *Am Heart J* 69:1065A–1084A, 1984.

B. EFFECTS OF AEROBIC EXERCISE
(50%–85% $\dot{V}O_{2max}$ for 3.5–7 days/week)

1. **HDL cholesterol normally can be increased** through regular exercise training (expenditure of 1,000–1,200 kcal/week minimum to 2,000–3,500 kcal/week optimum); **Table 9-9** provides guidelines.

2. **Reducing triglyceride level** requires approximately 45 minutes of intensive exercise daily.

3. The effects of exercise on **total cholesterol** and **LDL cholesterol** are more controversial; these lipoproteins usually change only in response to caloric restriction and weight loss.

C. THE EFFECTS OF RESISTANCE TRAINING on lipid levels are not clear.

 Table 9-8. Optimal Diet for Improving Blood Lipids

Dietary Component	Recommendation
Total Calories	Adequate to support nutritional needs but low enough (not < 1500 calories) to allow a 10% loss of weight if indicated
Total Fat Intake	20% of calories or less
Saturated Fat Intake	7% of calories or less
Cholesterol Intake	100–150 mg/day or less
Fiber Intake	25–40 g/day
Soluble Fiber Intake	10–15 g/day
Protein	15% of calories (0.50–0.55 g/lb bdw in active persons) with an increase in vegetable and decrease in animal protein
Carbohydrate	65% of calories (55% complex)

bdw = body weight
(From *ACSM's Resource Manual for Guidelines for Exercise Testing and Prescription,* 3rd ed. Baltimore, Williams & Wilkins, 1988, p 298.)

 Table 9-9. Target Aerobic Exercise Guidelines for Improving Lipids

Intensity:	50%–80% $\dot{V}O_{2max}$
Frequency:	3.5–7 days/wk
Duration:	30–60 min/session
Minimum:	1000–1200 kcal/wk
Optimum:	2000–3500 kcal/wk
Time:	9–12 months
% responding:	90% HDL, 70% TG

These guidelines may require modifications for sedentary, obese individuals and patients with chronic disease such as diabetes, high blood pressure, and coronary heart disease. For more information on special populations, see *ACSM Guidelines for Exercise Testing and Prescription,* 6th ed (Baltimore, Lippincott Williams & Wilkins, 2000).
HDL = high-density lipoprotein; TG = triglycerides
(Adapted from *ACSM's Resource Manual for Guidelines for Exercise Testing and Prescription,* 3rd ed. Baltimore, Williams & Wilkins, 1998, p 299, Table 35.3.)

D. CHOLESTEROL-LOWERING MEDICATIONS (e.g., HMG-COA reductase inhibitors) may be prescribed if diet and exercise do not lower lipid levels **(Table 9-10).**

Table 9-10. Lipid-Lowering Agents and Their Expected Effect

Drug	TC	LDL-C	HDL-C	TG
Bile-acid resins	↓20%	↓20–25%	↑35%	Neutral or ↑
Nicotinic acid	↓25%	↓25%	↑15–30%	↓20–50%
Fibric acid derivatives	↓10–20%	↓5–25%	↑10–30%	↓20–60%
Probucol	↓25%	↓10–15%	↓20–30%	Neutral
Reductase inhibitors	↓15–30%	↓20–35%	↑2–12%	↓10–25%

TC = total cholesterol, LDL-C = low-density lipoprotein cholesterol, HDL-C = high-density lipoprotein cholesterol, TG = triglycerides, ↓ = decreases, ↑ = increases.
(Adapted from Farmer JA, Gotto AM J: Lipid abnormalities—Management. In *Atherosclerosis and Coronary Artery Disease.* Edited by Fuster V, Ross R, Topel EJ. Philadelphia, Lippincott-Raven, 1996.)

V. WEIGHT CONTROL

A. WEIGHT LOSS GOALS

–Weight loss of 1–2 lb/week (after the first 1–2 weeks) is considered safe; greater weight loss should not be undertaken without medical supervision.

–Persons with a BMI > 25 should decrease their index by two BMI units, then maintain that weight loss for 6 months before undertaking further weight loss.

B. CALORIC NEEDS

1. Planning a weight loss program begins with **determining the client's current caloric requirements,** based on daily caloric intake and caloric expenditure. Guidelines for caloric intake include the following:

   –Daily intake of 1,200–1,500 calories for women and 1,800–2,000 calories for men are common recommendations.

   –A moderately calorie-restricted program is 1,200 kcal/day or more; 1,200 calories is believed to be the minimum level at which the recommended amounts of essential nutrients can be obtained without supplementation.

   –In a very-low-calorie diet (800–1,200 kcal/day), supplementation is necessary to meet the minimum requirements for essential nutrients.

2. The **estimated daily caloric requirement minus 500 kcal/day** (achieved through diet, exercise, or exercise and diet combined) promotes a **negative energy balance** and resulting weight loss.

C. WEIGHT LOSS STRATEGIES

1. **Making dietary changes only**

   –Significant weight loss can be achieved by reducing intake by 500 or more kcal/day.

   However, compliance with such strict calorie modification is difficult for most people.

   –A danger of severe calorie restriction is an insufficient intake of essential nutrients.

2. **Increasing physical activity only**

   –Weight loss solely through physical activity would require an expenditure of 500 kcal/day. However, this caloric expenditure may be difficult for many individuals, who may not be able to tolerate the frequency, duration, or intensity of exercise needed to achieve this level.

   –Maintaining weight loss may be difficult with this strategy.

3. **Modifying both diet and physical activity**

   –A typical strategy involves reducing intake by 250 kcal/day and increasing energy expenditure by 250 kcal/day, or some other combination of decreased intake and increased expenditure equal to a loss of 500 kcal/day.

   –This combination method is most likely to help individuals achieve a slow, gradual weight loss that is easier to maintain, because of the gradual changes in lifestyle needed to achieve the weight loss.

D. INAPPROPRIATE STRATEGIES FOR WEIGHT LOSS

1. **Too-rapid weight loss,** generally defined as greater than 3 lb/week for women and 3–5 lb/week for men, may be unsafe and also difficult to maintain; the likelihood of gaining back the lost weight is high.

2. **Dehydration** through saunas, body wraps, and sweat suits can provide only temporary weight loss or circumference decrease.

   –Reductions are due to a loss of body water in a particular area, not a reduction in fat; weight and circumference measurements will return to baseline once the body is rehydrated.

–In some cases, dehydration and the body's inability to cool itself can lead to a reduction in effective circulating blood volume and a drop in blood pressure.

3. **Spot reduction,** through such devices as vibrating belts or electric stimulators, is not an effective weight loss method.

VI. DISORDERS RELATED TO NUTRITION AND EXERCISE

A. THE FEMALE ATHLETE TRIAD

–describes a set of medical conditions that can occur in women who are very physically active and who believe that low body weight will enhance their appearance or physical performance. It is a potentially life-threatening syndrome marked by inadequate food (energy) intake to meet metabolic demands, followed by amenorrhea and finally osteoporosis.

1. **Disordered eating,** the problem that triggers the other two components of the triad, may range from slight restriction of food intake, to occasional binging and purging, to bulimia and anorexia nervosa.

   –**Bulimia** is a cycle of food restriction or fasting followed by overeating or binging followed by purging.

   –**Anorexia nervosa** is an extreme restrictive eating behavior in which an individual continues to starve and feel fat despite being 15% or more below ideal body weight.

2. **Amenorrhea** (absence of menstruation) can result from excessive exercise and decreased food intake.

3. **Osteoporosis** (loss of bone mineral density) can result from chronically low levels of ovarian hormones. The amount of bone loss is correlated with the severity and length of menstrual irregularity, nutritional status, and the amount of skeletal loading during activity.

4. **Treatment** may involve a daily calcium intake of 1,500 mg, oral contraceptives or hormone replacement, and increasing intake by 250–350 kcal/day and/or reducing exercise training by 10%–20%.

5. **Prevention** focuses on instruction and counseling to reinforce:

   –Health and well-being

   –Positive self-image

E. WEIGHT GAIN STRATEGIES

–To increase weight, energy intake must exceed energy output. Basic energy needs must be met, plus an additional 500–1,000 kcal/day. Additional calories may be provided in various ways, including eating extra portions of usual foods at regular meals, eating more calorie-dense foods, and eating more between-meal snacks.

–Realistic fitness goals

–Sensible body composition

B. DISORDERS RELATED TO INADEQUATE HYDRATION

1. **Heat stress**

   –results from a combination of environmental conditions, metabolic rate, and clothing that restricts the body's ability to cool itself.

   –If a balance between all sources of heat gain and heat loss is not achieved, then the risk for excessive core temperature increases.

   –The major avenue for heat loss is evaporative cooling through evaporation of sweat from the skin's surface.

2. **Heat-related disorders**

   –occur when the normal responses to heat stress (elevated core temperature, increased heart rate, and water loss due to sweating) go unchecked. **Table 9-11** lists the heat-related disorders along with their symptoms, signs, and first aid.

3. **Prevention**

   –**Adequate fluid intake** before, during, and after exercise or strenuous activity can help prevent heat stress and heat disorders. Recommendations include:

   a. 16 oz of water or a nonfat, noncarbonated beverage, such as a sports drink, 2 hours before exercise or activity

   b. 8–12 oz of fluid ½ hour before exercise or activity

   c. 4–8 oz of fluid every 15–20 minutes during exercise or activity

   d. Additional fluids to replace those lost (16–36 oz) after exercise or activity

4. **Other protective measures** to prevent heat disorders are listed in **Table 9-12**.

Table 9-11. Heat-Related Disorders: Symptoms, Signs, and First Aid

	Symptoms	Signs	First Aid
Heat cramps	Painful muscle cramps, especially in abdominal or fatigued muscles	Incapacitating pain in voluntary muscles	Rest in cool environment Drink salted water (0.5% salt solution) Massage muscles
Heat syncope	Blurred vision (gray-out) Brief fainting (black-out)	Brief fainting or near-fainting behavior	Lie on back in cool environment Drink water
Dehydration	No early symptoms Fatigue/weakness Dry mouth	Loss of work capacity Increased response time	Fluid and salt replacement
Heat exhaustion	Fatigue Weakness Blurred vision Dizziness Headache	High pulse rate Profuse sweating Low blood pressure Insecure gait Pale face Collapse Body temperature normal to slightly increased	Lie down flat on back in cool environment Drink water Loosen clothing
Heat stroke	Chills Restlessness Irritability	Red face Euphoria Shivering Disorientation Erratic behavior Collapse Unconsciousness Convulsions Body temperature $\geq 40°C$ (104°F)	Immediate, aggressive, effective cooling Transport to hospital

(Adapted from *ACSM's Resource Manual for Guidelines for Exercise Testing and Prescription*, 3rd ed. Baltimore, Williams & Wilkins, 1998, p 208, Table 24.1.)

Table 9-12. Personal Protective Practices to Reduce Risk for Heat Disorder

Seek relief from heat stress exposure with sensation of extreme discomfort, lightheadedness, nausea, headache, loss of coordination, or weakness.

Maintain adequate hydration by drinking small amounts of water, sports drinks, diluted citrus-flavored drinks, diluted iced tea, etc. at frequent intervals. (A weight loss of 2% of body weight in 1 day is evidence of dehydration.)

Maintain a healthy lifestyle through sound diet, adequate sleep, and avoiding drug abuse.

Avoid heat stress exposure and exercise during acute illness (eg, fever, nausea, vomiting, diarrhea).

Seek medical advice if diagnosed with a chronic disease (disease or treatment may reduce heat tolerance).

Reduce expectations if no recent exercise in warm or hot environments.

(From *ACSM's Resource Manual for Guidelines for Exercise Testing and Prescription*, 3rd ed. Baltimore, Williams & Wilkins, 1998, p 211.)

REVIEW TEST

DIRECTIONS: Carefully read all questions and select the BEST single answer.

1. When counseling a patient with a low-density lipoprotein cholesterol level of 142 mg/dl, your emphasis would be on
   (A) diet.
   (B) exercise.
   (C) hormone replacement therapy.
   (D) weight training.

2. How much energy is contained in 1 gram of fat?
   (A) 4 calories
   (B) 9 watts
   (C) 9 calories
   (D) 7 watts

3. Which of the following nutrients is the most likely to elevate blood cholesterol?
   (A) Polyunsaturated fat
   (B) Cholesterol
   (C) Saturated fat
   (D) Monounsaturated fat

4. Recommendations to lower high blood homocysteine levels include consuming more
   (A) oranges.
   (B) nuts.
   (C) soy.
   (D) whole grains.

5. Which of the following medical conditions is *not* part of the female athlete triad?
   (A) Disordered eating
   (B) Osteoporosis
   (C) Amenorrhea
   (D) Anemia

6. Symptoms of heat stress associated with dehydration include all of the following *except*
   (A) lightheadedness.
   (B) headache.
   (C) chest pressure.
   (D) loss of coordination.

7. For any athlete, the primary nutrient requiring replacement before, during, and after exercise is
   (A) sodium.
   (B) water.
   (C) carbohydrate.
   (D) protein.

8. Examples of foods high in saturated fats include all of the following *except*
   (A) red meat.
   (B) cookies made with palm oil.
   (C) pasta tossed with olive oil.
   (D) four-cheese pizza.

9. Studies have found that persons who eat high amounts of antioxidant-containing foods have a reduced risk of heart attack and stroke, in part because these foods contain
   (A) vitamin E.
   (B) vitamin B6.
   (C) iron.
   (D) zinc.

10. Which of the following body mass indices indicates obesity?
    (A) 28 kg/m²
    (B) 32 kg/m²
    (C) 24 kg/m²
    (D) 16 kg/m²

11. Fat accumulation over the chest and arms (upper body) that occurs most often in men describes which type of obesity?
    (A) Gynoid obesity
    (B) Android obesity
    (C) Morbid obesity
    (D) Testosterone obesity

12. What is the most effective way to modify body composition?
    (A) Diet
    (B) Dehydration
    (C) Exercise
    (D) Diet and exercise together

13. What is the generally accepted calorie deficit needed to promote a 1 lb/wk weight loss?
    (A) 3,500 calories
    (B) 4,000 calories
    (C) 2,000 calories
    (D) 5,000 calories

14. At what daily caloric intake is it difficult to obtain the minimum recommended amounts of essential nutrients without supplementation?
    (A) < 1,200 kcal/day
    (B) 1,200–1,400 kcal/day
    (C) 1,400–1,600 kcal/day
    (D) 1,600–1,800 kcal/day

15. Which of the following body mass indices is associated with the lowest risk for cardiovascular disease?
    (A) 27 kg/m²
    (B) 30 kg/m²
    (C) 21 kg/m²
    (D) 25 kg/m²

16. What is calculated as weight (in kg) divided by height (in m²) and is considered a poor predictor of percent body fat in most individuals?
    (A) Fat-free mass
    (B) Body mass index
    (C) Bioelectrical impedance analysis
    (D) Skinfold measurements

17. Which is the eating disorder marked by an overwhelming fear of becoming fat, a distorted body image, and the inability to eat?
    (A) Bulimia
    (B) Anorexia nervosa
    (C) Chronic dieting
    (D) Yo-yo dieting

ANSWERS AND EXPLANATIONS

1–A. The restriction of dietary fat, saturated fat, and cholesterol reduces low-density lipoprotein (LDL) cholesterol. Changes in LDL cholesterol with exercise occur indirectly because they are associated with caloric restriction and weight loss. Hormone replacement therapy can decrease LDL cholesterol by approximately 10 mg/dl; however, this therapy is appropriate only for postmenopausal women and is used in concert with a low-fat diet. The effects of weight training on blood lipids are unclear.

2–C. The amount of energy in 1 gram of fat is 9 calories. Energy in food is measured in calories, not watts.

3–C. A high intake of saturated fat will tend to increase blood cholesterol even more than high intakes of cholesterol or other types of fat. Using polyunsaturated and monounsaturated fats in place of saturated fats will favorably affect lipid values.

4–A. Recommendations to reduce the risk of premature coronary artery disease by reducing elevated homocysteine levels include increasing the consumption of folic acid, which is found in oranges.

5–D. Disordered eating is the first problem in the female athlete triad that can lead to absence of

menstruation (amenorrhea) and premature bone loss (osteoporosis). Anemia (low iron) is not considered part of the triad.

6–C. Lightheadedness, headache, and loss of coordination are all warning symptoms of heat stress. Chest pressure is not a typical symptom.

7–B. Water must be replaced before, during, and after exercise. The other nutrients can be replaced in a meal or snack after exercise, unless exercise is prolonged more than 1 hour.

8–C. Olive oil is high in monounsaturated fat, unlike the others, which include animal products or tropical oils that are high in saturated fat.

9–A. The antioxidants include some forms of vitamin A, vitamin C, vitamin E, carotenoids, and selenium. Eating more fruits and vegetables, whole grains, and nuts will increase the intake of antioxidants. Antioxidants work in teams, and the benefits may not be realized with large doses of an isolated antioxidant vitamin or mineral.

10–A. A body mass index (BMI) of > 27 kg/m² indicates obesity. A BMI of > 30 kg/m² indicates morbid obesity. A BMI of < 25 kg/m² is recommended by the Expert Panel on Healthy Weight for adults.

11–B. Android obesity is defined as fat accumulation over the chest and arms rather than the lower trunk, and occurs most often in men. Gynoid obesity is fat accumulation around the hips and lower abdomen, occurring most often in women. Morbid obesity does not describe where the fat is accumulated, but rather describes the degree of obesity. There is no such term as testosterone obesity.

12–D. Modifying both diet and physical activity is recommended. Reducing intake by approximately 250 kcal/day and increasing energy expenditure by 250 kcal/day results in a loss of 500 kcal/day. This will help individuals achieve the best results. With diet or exercise alone, it is often too difficult to maintain the needed 500-kcal/day deficit. Dehydration accomplishes only temporary weight loss or circumference decrease; weight or circumference measurements will return to baseline once the body is rehydrated.

13–A. A 3,500-calorie deficit per week (500 kcal/day deficit) generally promotes weight loss of 1 lb/week in most individuals. A 2,000-calorie deficit is too little, and deficits of 4,000 and 5,000 calories will most likely result in weight loss greater than 1 lb/week.

14–A. At 1,200 calories and below, it is difficult to obtain the minimum recommended amounts of essential nutrients without supplementation. At higher caloric intake with a varied diet, it should not be difficult to meet the recommended amounts of essential nutrients.

15–C. Epidemiological research indicates that a body mass index (BMI) of 21–22 kg/m² is associated with the lowest risk of cardiovascular disease. A BMI of > 27 kg/m² indicates obesity, and a BMI of > 30 kg/m² indicates morbid obesity. A BMI of < 25 kg/m² is recommended by the Expert Panel on Healthy Weight.

16–B. Body mass index (BMI) is calculated as weight in kg divided by height in m², and is often a poor predictor of percent body fat. The composition and density of the fat-free mass (FFM) is similar and constant in all individuals. Bioelectrical impedance analysis is a rapid, noninvasive, and relatively inexpensive method for estimating percent fat and FFM.

17–B. Anorexia nervosa is an eating disorder marked by an overwhelming fear of becoming fat, a distorted body image, and the inability to eat. Bulimics binge on food, then try to get rid of it quickly by inducing vomiting or taking laxatives and diuretics. Chronic dieting (yo-yo dieting) is a continuous cycle of weight loss and weight gain using various commercial diets.

CHAPTER 10

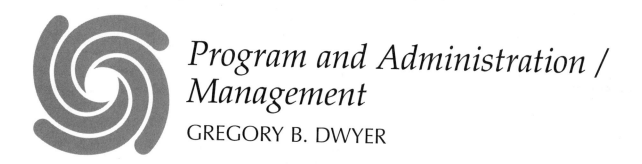

Program and Administration / Management
GREGORY B. DWYER

I. ASPECTS OF PROGRAM ADMINISTRATION/MANAGEMENT

–The program director/manager ensures that the program meets the often-changing standards and practices for clinical exercise rehabilitation services.

–The program director/manager needs knowledge of modern management principles.

–Coordination of many interrelated components and services is involved (**Figure 10-1**).

–The input of the institution's medical director into program development and implementation is crucial and must be solicited by the program director/manager.

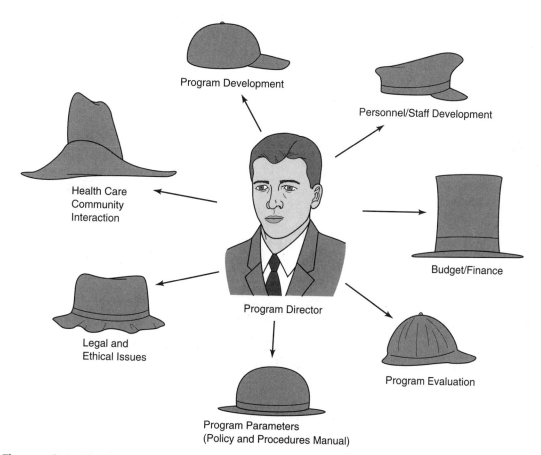

Program Development

Personnel/Staff Development

Health Care
Community
Interaction

Budget/Finance

Program Director

Legal and
Ethical Issues

Program Evaluation

Program Parameters
(Policy and Procedures Manual)

FIGURE 10-1 The many hats a program director/manager must wear in managing a clinical exercise rehabilitation program.

Table 10-1. Sample Mission Statements

Example 1

The mission of the Maintenance Cardiac Rehabilitation Component (MCRC) of the _____ complements the Mission Statements of the _____ and _____ . Specifically, the mission of the MCRC has several facets and targeted groups for intervention. One group that the MCRC addresses through its services are the undergraduate and graduate students of _____ through its opportunities in research, service, and academic training in the rehabilitation of individuals with chronic diseases. The other important targeted group for the MCRC are those members of the community who have Coronary Artery Disease and other chronic diseases, as defined by the participant inclusion criteria of the MCRC. The MCRC provides educational, research and service opportunities for those individuals with Coronary Artery Disease in health and physical fitness assessment, exercise prescription and exercise programming components as well as in other lifestyle management areas (e.g., smoking, nutrition, etc.).

Example 2

The mission of the _____ program is to provide in equal partnership with referring physicians, high quality, safe, and affordable preventive and rehabilitative health care to persons at risk for or with known cardiovascular disease.

The goals of the _____ program are identified below:

- Enhance the patient's quality of life.

- Increase the patient's functional capacity.

- Decrease the patient's risk of future cardiovascular complications.

- Increase the patient and family member's knowledge of cardiovascular disease and ways to reduce the risk of future cardiovascular complications.

The various programs of _____ are identified below:

The various services of _____ are identified below:

II. PROGRAM DOCUMENTATION

A. THE MISSION STATEMENT

–is a simple **statement of the program's main purposes or goals** (Table 10-1).

–forms the foundation of program planning, implementation, and evaluation.

–should be clearly worded, compatible with the parent organization's or institution's mission statement, and regularly reviewed and updated to reflect program changes.

–A central aspect of continuous quality improvement (CQI) is the evaluation of how a program is meeting its goals as specified in the mission statement.

B. THE POLICY AND PROCEDURES (P&P) MANUAL

–provides documentation and dissemination of the program's specific policies and procedures.

–should contain everything about a program from the organizational structure to the maintenance schedule for the facility and equipment.

–should be readily accessible to all staff members.

–is revised as the policies or procedures of a program are modified, and as such should be viewed as a document in progress.

–must be reviewed from a legal perspective, written in close collaboration with the program's medical directorship, and approved by the parent organization.

–should be consistent with the ever-changing standards and practices of applicable national, regional, and local organizations.

III. ORGANIZATIONAL STRUCTURE AND STAFFING

–A major challenge facing a program director/manager is to integrate the proper mix of staff into the program to provide the depth of knowledge and expertise needed.

–A program's organizational structure and staffing mix are closely tied to the budgetary process and outcome assessment.

A. DELINEATION OF ROLES

–Considerations for role assignment include individual staff expertise, staffing levels and mix, medicolegal issues, and certification/licensure.

–Important factors in the delineation of roles are the needs of the clients served, the

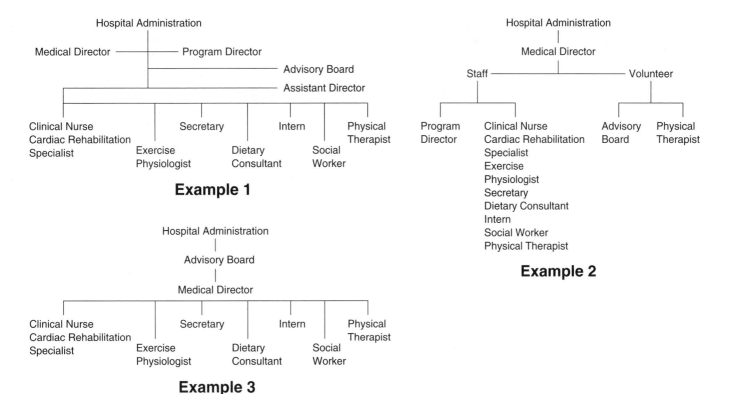

FIGURE 10-2 Organizational grids used for management of cardiopulmonary rehabilitation programs. (Redrawn with permission from Berra K, Hall LK: Administration of cardiac rehabilitation outpatient programs. In *Heart Disease and Rehabilitation.* Edited by Pollock ML, Schmidt DH. Champaign, IL, Human Kinetics, 1995, p 188.)

program's mission statement, and the organizational structure.

–As a program grows and changes, the delineation of roles must be reviewed and altered as needed.

B. JOB DESCRIPTIONS

–Each staff position needs a specific, written job description that clearly details the **duties, responsibilities, and evaluation criteria** for the position.

–The job descriptions for all positions in the organization should be part of the P&P manual.

–The job description provides criteria to evaluate for purposes of the employee performance review.

–An effective job description is tailored to the specific needs and goals of the individual program.

–Because all possible duties and responsibilities cannot be detailed in a job description, some degree of flexibility and adaptability must also be built into each job description.

C. ORGANIZATIONAL FLOWCHART

–A program's organizational flowchart specifies the **hierarchy of decision making responsibility**

and **lines of communication** in the program (**Figure 10-2**).

–The chart should clearly reflect the program's mission statement, goals, staffing mix, and other important aspects of the program.

–The organizational chart should be readily accessible to all staff and be part of the P&P manual.

D. STAFF COMPETENCY AND DEVELOPMENT

–Maintaining staff competency is a major responsibility of the program director/manager.

1. **Continuous professional development** is important for staff competency.

    –The program director/manager must guide staff in seeking out professional development opportunities.

    –A typical staff is multidisciplinary, possibly including nurses, exercise physiologists, respiratory therapists, and other health professionals. The various staff members will have varying professional development needs and opportunities.

    –Staff meetings focused on professional development issues can be aimed at a particular group of staff (e.g., operation of a new exercise machine) or can encompass the entire staff (e.g., client service issues).

–In-service staff meetings are an excellent forum for professional development programs.

2. **Good communication** among staff members is an essential component of overall staff competency

   –Strategies to foster staff communication include:

   a. **Following lines of communication** depicted on the program's organizational chart

   b. **Holding regular staff meetings,** both formal and informal and both with the entire staff and with selected staff members involved in a particular project or issue

3. **Certification and licensure** of various staff members is another aspect of staff competency.

–Whereas credentialing is relatively standardized for some staff (i.e., physical therapists), it is less standardized for other positions (e.g., exercise physiology).

–A current issue related to staff certification is the impact of the ACSM's recently launched Registry for Clinical Exercise Physiologists (RCEP). It remains to be seen how influential the RCEP will be to overall staff certification.

E. **PROGRAM CERTIFICATION**

–The move toward certification of clinical exercise programs, led by the American Association of Cardiovascular and Pulmonary Rehabilitation, is relatively recent. The overall impact that program certification may have on the field is unknown. Eventually, program certification might impact reimbursement from insurance companies.

IV. PROGRAM DEVELOPMENT (Figure 10-3)

A. NEEDS ASSESSMENT

–involves gathering data to use in program planning.

–includes a thorough market analysis for financial considerations and an analysis of staffing and facility needs.

–is often a creative tool developed in-house to meet the program's specific needs; thus, generalizing the results may be difficult.

B. PROGRAM PLANNING

1. **Scope of program services**

   –The scope of the program services depends on various factors, including the needs of potential clients, the expertise of the staff in certain areas, and the market demand for particular services.

   a. The **needs of clients** change with innovations in clinical exercise; thus, program directors/managers need to be aware of the research literature and health care trends, and modify program offerings based on this information.

   b. The **expertise of the staff** or of consultants available to the staff necessarily will shape program offerings.

   c. An identified **market demand** is strong justification for offering a particular program or service, because it increases the likelihood of acceptance and financial success.

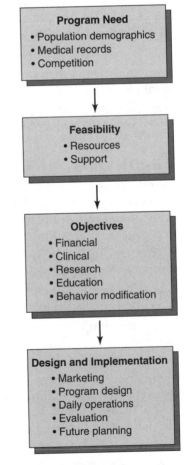

FIGURE 10-3 Steps in planning cardiac rehabilitation. (Redrawn with permission from Fardy PS, Yanowitz FG: *Cardiac Rehabilitation, Adult Fitness, and Exercise Testing.* Baltimore, Williams & Wilkins, 1995, p 280.)

2. **Financial and budgetary considerations**

   a. **Program revenue (income)** generally comes from two sources:

      (1) **Direct billing** for services, either to an individual client or to the client's health insurance carrier

      (2) A **contract for services** for a specific client group with a managed care organization

   b. **Expenses** of various types are defined in accounting.

      (1) **Capital expenses** are those used for the purchase of equipment, buildings, and other tangible assets of the program.

      (2) **Fixed expenses** are those that are typically unchanged from month to month, such as full-time salaries, rent, and utilities.

      (3) **Variable expenses** are not as predictable in that they may vary based on various factors; examples include disposable supplies and part-time salaries.

   c. **Profit and loss analyses**

      –The choice of the profit-and-loss model for a particular program is based on such factors as financial expectations and mission statement (e.g., for-profit versus not-for-profit program).

      –**Two basic forms of profit and loss analyses** are the break-even analysis and the profitability analysis.

      (1) Basically, a **break-even analysis** is designed around the function of the program such that the revenue generated is enough to pay for the expenses incurred, or the business venture is not-for-profit.

      (2) A **profitability analysis** is an attempt to forecast future profits for the program based on potential revenue generation as well as on predicted fixed and variable expenses.

   d. A **sample budget** for a clinical exercise program is given in **Table 10-2**.

C. **PROGRAM IMPLEMENTATION**

   1. **Program components**

      a. **Client care plan**

         –The foundation for any clinical exercise program, the client care plan provides a **specific plan for rehabilitation and criteria for outcome assessment.**

         –The client care plan should be comprehensive, individualized, documented, reviewed and followed by the entire staff, and modified and evaluated regularly.

         –The client care plan should be reflected in, or be part of, periodic progress reports to the client's health care team.

      b. **Risk stratification (pre-participation screening)**

         –can be modeled after published criteria, including those from the ACSM, American Association of Cardiovascular and Pulmonary Rehabilitation, and American College of Physicians (see Chapter 6).

         –can be useful for participant entry criteria, exercise testing guidelines, and ECG monitoring and supervision guidelines.

         –may be tied to insurance reimbursement.

      c. **Other program components that will need to be addressed**

         (1) Participant referral criteria

         (2) Participant inclusion/exclusion criteria

         (3) General exercise prescription guidelines

         (4) Home exercise plans

         (5) Medical supervision guidelines, including participant/staff ratios, and ECG and other medical monitoring needs

         (6) Weight training guidelines

         (7) Intensive risk factor monitoring/counseling guidelines

         (8) Periodic participant progress reports

         (9) Communication with the client's health care team

         (10) Emergency plans as well as physician referral procedures post-emergency

         (11) Graduation procedures and guidelines from various program components or phases

         (12) Guidelines for referral to other services or providers (e.g., psychological counseling)

         (13) Program data analyses and outcome assessment

         (14) Continuing client education

   2. **Interaction with the medical community**

      –Because a client's participation in a clinical exercise rehabilitation program generally

Table 10-2. Sample Budget for a Clinical Exercise Program

	Existing Clients	Monthly	New	Average Fee	CXLS	Total	Total $
Enrollment Projections							
Jan	700	45	0	150	0	750	42,120
Feb	750	45	75	150	23	803	44,320
March	803	45	75	150	24	853	46,640
Apr	853	45	65	150	26	893	47,380
May	893	45	55	150	27	921	47,620
June	921	45	50	150	28	943	48,110
July	943	45	50	150	28	965	49,100
Aug	965	45	50	150	29	986	50,060
Sept	986	45	60	150	30	1,017	52,480
Oct	1,017	45	65	150	30	1,051	54,580
Nov	1,051	45	70	150	32	1,090	56,850
Dec	1,090	45	50	150	33	1,107	55,540
							594,840

TOTAL MEMBER REVENUE:

OTHER REVENUE:	
Smoking Cesation	1,200
Massage	16,200
Guest Fees	35,000
1–1 training	32,400
Weight Management	12,000
Pro-Shop	1,200
Rest	3,000
Wellness Programs	1,200
Misc	10,000
Total Other Revenue	112,200
MEMBER REVENUE	594,840
OTHER REVENUE	112,200
TOTAL REVENUE	707,040

PAYROLL PROJECTIONS

General Manager	35,000
Sales 1	35,000
Administrator	20,000
Fitness Director	26,000
FT Fitness 1	22,000
FT Fitness 2	20,000
PT Fitness	21,840
Receptionist	25,000
Aerobics	18,000
Nutrition	9,500
Cleaning	24,000
Bonus	8,000
Total Payroll	264,340
TAXES	34,364
BENEFITS	18,240
TOTAL SALARIES	316,944

EXPENSE PROJECTIONS

TOTAL OPERATING EXPENSES:	
SALARIES TAX & BENEFITS	316,944
MARKETING	48,000
MAINTENANCE/REPAIR	
HVAC	1,500
Equipment	2,400
Exterminating	1,200
Other	500
TOTAL MAINTENANCE	5,600
OPERATING SUPPLIES	
Cleaning Supplies	1,200
Locker Room	3,000
Other Supplies	1,500
Towels	2,000
TOTAL SUPPLIES	7,700
OTHER EXPENSES	
Printing	3,600
Postage	3,000
Travel Seminars	2,000
Uniforms	6,000
Misc	1,000
Programs	500
Office Supplies	600
Telephone	7,200
TOTAL OTHER EXPENSES	10,800
TOTAL FIXED EXPENSES:	
Cam	24,000
Debt	10,000
Insurance	18,000
Leasing	8,400
Management Fees	48,000
Rent	70,705
Utilities	
Elec	36,000
Gas	4,800
Water	2,000
TOTAL UTILITIES	42,800
TOTAL FIXED	264,705
TOTAL EXPENSES	653,749
NET PROFIT/(LOSS)	53,299

(With permission from McCarthy J: Fund allocation has become critical. *Club Business International.* 1990.)

depends on referral from a physician, the program director/manager (and medical director) should foster a good working relationship with the local medical community. This relationship can be fostered by **soliciting input** from physicians (and other health professionals, as applicable) on planning and implementation, and by **maintaining regular communication** through consultation and progress reports. A program may even consider **establishing a medical advisory board** to ensure good communication with the medical community.

3. **Legal and ethical considerations**

   a. **Risk assessment and management**

      –The program director/manager needs to recognize all potential risk exposures in the program and make the staff aware of these risks.

      –Identified risks need to be minimized through appropriate means, such as procedures for dealing with malfunctioning equipment and for dealing with client injuries.

   b. **Standards of care**

      –Applicable standards of care must be the basis of the program's policies and procedures.

      –An example of an applicable standard of care is the sixth edition of the *ACSM's Guidelines for Exercise Testing and Prescription* (GETP), which may be used when performing various tasks in a clinical exercise rehabilitation program such as exercise testing.

      –A program affiliated with a hospital or other care facility must adhere to the standard of care set by the institution.

      –A program that includes nurses, respiratory therapists, and other health care professionals must take into account the standards of care for all involved professions.

   c. **Confidentiality**

      –All client and staff records are considered confidential and are kept secure by the program director/manager.

      –Individuals who do not have a legitimate, program-related need to see data should not have access to the data.

   d. **Emergency plans and procedures**

      –A plan for responding to emergency events should be outlined in the P&P manual (see Chapter 7). This **emergency response plan** must be well defined and well known to all staff members.

      –**Emergency drills** should be carried out on a regular basis (at least quarterly), involve all staff members, and be documented. To increase the effectiveness of drills, scenarios that reflect common or "most likely" emergency situations can be developed and practiced.

   e. **Accident/injury reporting**

      –A process must be developed for the timely reporting of any and all accidents or injuries that may result from participation in a clinical exercise rehabilitation program.

      –The accident/injury reporting process should be specified in the P&P manual.

      –The form used to document accidents and injuries and the responses to these events must be kept in a secure location.

D. **PROGRAM EVALUATION**

   –Careful evaluation of a program's effectiveness is an essential extension of program development and implementation.

   –**Subjective evaluation** is accomplished through **surveys** of program participants, program staff, referring physicians, and any others involved.

   –**Objective evaluation** can be based on **client outcomes** as outlined in the plan of care. Standardized tools can be used for outcome assessment; an example is the American Association of Cardiovascular and Pulmonary Rehabilitation (AACVPR)'s outcome assessment and program resources manual.

   –**Continuous quality improvement (CQI),** also known as quality assurance, is a systematic process of evaluation and implementation designed to maximize program effectiveness.

   –A program's evaluation criteria and process should be outlined in the P&P manual.

   –As an aspect of overall program evaluation, the program director/manager needs to take into account **trends in health care** and assess how well the program is adapting to these trends.

REVIEW TEST

DIRECTIONS: Carefully read all questions and select the BEST single answer.

1. In a budget for a clinical exercise rehabilitation program, all of the following are examples of variable expenses *except*
   (A) ECG electrodes.
   (B) temporary wages.
   (C) rental fees for the facility space.
   (D) consultant fees.

2. Which of the following statements about a clinical exercise rehabilitation program's mission statement is *not* correct?
   (A) Perhaps the most important feature of the mission statement is its clarity or understandability.
   (B) The mission statement should elucidate the program's goals.
   (C) There should be a different mission statement for each program or perhaps even a different mission statement for each component of a program.
   (D) A program's mission statement is generally fixed.

3. A program's policy and procedures manual should *not*
   (A) be stored away for safekeeping.
   (B) be revised as the program's policies and/or procedures are modified.
   (C) be viewed as a document in progress.
   (D) contain program information ranging from the organizational structure to the facility's maintenance schedule.

4. A comprehensive patient care plan is necessary for effective program management because it
   (A) is required by federal law.
   (B) provides a "road map" for interventions.
   (C) is a requirement for insurance reimbursement.
   (D) provides raw data for analysis in continuous quality improvement or outcomes assessment.

5. The process of risk stratification is often used for the criteria for clinical exercise rehabilitation program admission. Which of the following statements about risk stratification is *not* correct?
   (A) Risk stratification can be modeled after the criteria published by the American Association of Cardiovascular and Pulmonary Rehabilitation.
   (B) Risk stratification can be useful for participant entry criteria, exercise testing guidelines, ECG monitoring, and supervision guidelines.
   (C) Risk stratification can be tied to insurance reimbursement.
   (D) Risk stratification is often used to determine the intensity of prescribed exercise.

6. Which of the following statements about confidentiality is *not* true?
   (A) All records must be kept by the program director/manager under lock and key.
   (B) Data must be available to all individuals who need to see it.
   (C) Data should be kept on file for at least 1 year before being discarded.
   (D) Sensitive information, such as participant's name, needs to be protected.

7. Which of the following statements about injury reporting is *not* correct?
   (A) A process for injury reporting, backed up with a form, should be developed.
   (B) The process that is to be used and the accompanying forms must be part of the policy and procedures manual.
   (C) Injury reporting forms must be kept under lock and key just like data records.
   (D) A physician should sign every injury report form filed.

8. One important aspect of staff competency is ensuring that staff members are well trained and kept up to date. Which of the following organizations has recently launched the Registry for Clinical Exercise Physiologists?
   (A) AACVPR
   (B) ACP
   (C) AHA
   (D) ACSM

9. Informed consent is best described as
   (A) a legal form.
   (B) a process that is backed up by a form.
   (C) something only a lawyer can provide to an exercise program.
   (D) being an informed consumer to ensure that one undertakes the proper exercise program.

10. Which of the following elements is *not* part of an emergency plan for a clinical exercise program?
    (A) Annual practice sessions involving all staff
    (B) Emergency plan that constantly refers to national established guidelines such as ACLS without addressing unique features of the program
    (C) Emergency drills carried out on a regular basis and documented
    (D) Scenarios developed to increase the applicability of the emergency plan practice sessions

11. Which of the following is a fixed expense?
    (A) Office supplies
    (B) Salaries
    (C) Utilities, such as telephone
    (D) Laboratory charge backs for blood work

12. Which type of financial analysis would be appropriate for a not-for-profit program that wishes to determine the amount of revenue from program fees needed so that no other sources of revenue are needed to meet program expenses?
    (A) Break-down analysis
    (B) Break-even analysis
    (C) Profitability analysis
    (D) Margin analysis

13. Continuous quality improvement (CQI) is a systematic process of program evaluation that involves all of the following steps *except*
    (A) data analysis.
    (B) goals assessment.
    (C) outcomes assessment.
    (D) budget assessment.

14. Outcome assessment evaluates a program's effectiveness. Which of the following statements about outcome assessment is *not* true?
    (A) The client care plan for each individual participant is not used in this process.
    (B) Data that are subjective or anecdotal in nature can be used in the assessment.
    (C) Periodic progress reports are valuable and should stimulate the need to collect objective data to support any subjective findings.
    (D) Standardized tools should be used for outcome assessment.

15. According to the American Association of Cardiovascular and Pulmonary Rehabilitation (AACVPR), elements of successful adult education include all the following *except*
    (A) goal setting.
    (B) rewards.
    (C) contracts.
    (D) knowledge testing.

16. Which one of the following statements concerning a needs assessment is *not* true?
    (A) The needs and/or program assessment is a useful tool for gathering data and support for program implementation.
    (B) The needs and/or program assessment often must be a creative tool developed in-house to meet the program's specific needs.
    (C) Given that the needs assessment may be developed in-house without the benefit of external validity, generalizing the results may be difficult.
    (D) Program planning is an essential step before needs assessment.

17. A comprehensive clinical exercise rehabilitation program
    (A) is based on historical features of program administration.
    (B) adapts to trends in program services.
    (C) is limited in scope and practice.
    (D) is the same for the entire client population served.

ANSWERS AND EXPLANATIONS

1–C. Rent is typically an agreed-upon cost and thus is a fixed, as opposed to a variable expense. Variable expenses vary based on program use; examples would include supplies (e.g., ECG electrodes) and any part-time or temporary wages.

2–D. The mission statement should be reviewed and revised as often as is necessary as a program changes in character. Thus, the mission statement is fixed but rather is a dynamic component of the policy and procedures manual.

3–A. The policy and procedures manual must be available to all staff and thus kept in a readily accessible location, not filed away. Also, the policy and procedures manual is meant to be referred to and revised as needed.

4–B. A patient care plan is a thoughtfully produced document that plans for effective, individualized interventions. It should be used often in planning for any and all interventions.

5–D. Risk stratification is rarely, if ever, used to determine the intensity of prescribed exercise. However, risk stratification can be an important tool for patient inclusion/exclusion criteria; it can be used for insurance reimbursement as well.

6–C. There is no accepted minimum or maximum amount of time that data should be stored. However, it is clear that data must be stored in a confidential (lock-and-key) manner; discretion must be used when sharing data.

7–D. Legal advice suggests that the injury report form does not necessarily require a physician's signature. However, a process for injury reporting needs to be consistently followed and described in the policy and procedures manual.

8–D. The American College of Sports Medicine launched the RCEP or Registry of Clinical Exercise Physiologists in 2000. The overall impact of this registry is hard to predict at present.

9–B. Informed consent is a process, backed up by a form, that among other things describes the risks and benefits of participation in certain activities, such as an exercise test. It is suggested that a legal expert be consulted regarding any informed consent procedures.

10–A. Practice sessions involving all staff members should be held at least quarterly. These sessions should be documented and may be most effective if scenarios are "played out" to mimic real emergencies.

11–B. Staff salaries usually are a fixed expense not subject to change based on variable factors such as number of program participants. However, as program use increases, so do expenses such as blood work charge-backs, telephone expenses,

and office supplies. These expenses are thus known as variable expenses.

12–B. A break-even analysis is ideal for not-for-profit organizations that wish to understand how to best meet all of their expenses, including payroll. The for-profit sector will use a profitability analysis to determine how much, if any, money can be earned in a period of time.

13–D. Budget assessment is not necessarily a part of the CQI process, although it is a valuable step in program evaluation. CQI is generally an outcomes assessment based on the program's goals, using data analysis of various measures.

14–A. The client care plan is a vital component of outcomes assessment. Outcomes assessment is driven by goals established for each client or patient.

15–D. According to the AACVPR, adult education can involve many techniques to foster education and behavior change including goal setting, contracts, rewards, and support. However, there is little justification for knowledge-based testing for promoting behavioral change.

16–D. Needs assessment should be done *before* the program planning and implementation phases, to provide data on which to base these steps. However, needs assessment is not a one-time measure. Successful programs perform frequent formal or informal needs assessments as they grow.

17–B. The justification for a clinical exercise rehabilitation program is based on its ability to adapt to changing operating practices and procedures for rehabilitation services. Thus, while history is important and interesting, flexibility is needed to adapt to an ever-changing health-care model.

CHAPTER 11

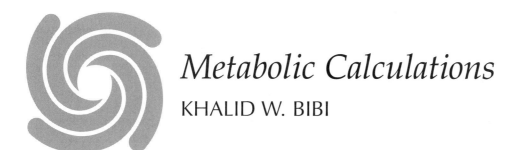

Metabolic Calculations

KHALID W. BIBI

I. OVERVIEW

A. RATIONALE FOR USE OF THE ACSM METABOLIC FORMULAE

–Fundamental to the application of proper exercise testing or prescription is the ability to measure or estimate energy expenditure.

1. **Direct measurement of $\dot{V}O_2$ is impractical.**

   –Actual oxygen consumption ($\dot{V}O_2$), using open-circuit spirometry, provides the health professional with the best measure of the energy cost of physical activity. Oxygen uptake values obtained during maximal exercise ($\dot{V}O_{2\,max}$) are commonly used as the index of cardiopulmonary fitness. Unfortunately, accurate $\dot{V}O_2$ measurement is arduous and costly.

2. **$\dot{V}O_2$ can be estimated using the ACSM metabolic formulae.**

   –The American College of Sports Medicine (ACSM) introduced the ACSM metabolic formulae to provide clinical practitioners with a practical method to estimate the oxygen cost of the most common exercises. **Practical uses for the ACSM metabolic formulae are as follows:**

   a. Estimating the rate of oxygen uptake during exercise allows for an **estimate of the energy expenditure and hence caloric consumption** from fat associated with exercise.

   b. An estimate of the rate of oxygen uptake during maximal exercise ($\dot{V}O_{2\,max}$) indicates the maximal capacity for aerobic work, allowing for **fitness categorization, and inter- and intra-subject comparisons.** See Appendix D in the *ACSM's Guidelines for Exercise Testing*

   and Prescription, 6th edition, for more information about $\dot{V}O_{2\,max}$ estimation.

   c. Calculating the appropriate exercise intensity (**work rate**) needed to elicit the desired oxygen consumption will allow the health professional **to develop more accurate exercise prescriptions.**

B. WHAT TO EXPECT REGARDING METABOLIC CALCULATIONS QUESTIONS ON THE ACSM WRITTEN EXAM

1. Expect from **6 to 10 metabolic calculation questions** on the examination. A few of these questions will be simple, requiring straightforward algebraic calculations. Some may be classified as moderately difficult, requiring simple mathematical substitution. One or two questions may be classified as difficult, requiring additional mathematical manipulation.

2. A copy of the ACSM metabolic formulae (**Table 11-1**) is included in the written examination packet. You should be familiar with these formulae before you take the exam.

3. The **unit conversion factors** and the **energy equivalency factors** will not be provided with the examination. **Commit these numbers to memory.**

4. The written examination might contain metabolic calculation questions that will not require the use of the metabolic equations. However, a good understanding of energy expenditure and energy equivalency will be needed to obtain the correct answer.

Table 11-1. Summary of Metabolic Calculations

Walking
$\dot{V}O_2 = (0.1 \cdot S) + (1.8 \cdot S \cdot G) + 3.5$

Treadmill and Outdoor Running
$\dot{V}O_2 = (0.2 \cdot S) + (0.9 \cdot S \cdot G) + 3.5$

Leg Ergometry
$\dot{V}O_2 = (10.8 \cdot W \cdot M^{-1}) + 7$

Arm Ergometry
$\dot{V}O_2 = (18 \cdot W \cdot M^{-1}) + 3.5$

Stepping
$\dot{V}O_2 = (0.2 \cdot f) + (1.33 \cdot 1.8 \cdot H \cdot f) + 3.5$

*Where $\dot{V}O_2$ is gross oxygen consumption in ml · kg^{-1} · min^{-1}; S is speed in m · min^{-1}; M is body mass in kg; G is the percent grade expressed as a fraction; W is power in watts; f is stepping frequency in min^{-1}; H is step height in meters.
Note: These equations are presented in conventional units following each mode of exercise, simplifying the calculations.
(From *ACSM's Guidelines for Exercise Testing and Prescription*, 6th ed. Philadelphia, Lippincott Williams & Williams, 2000, p 303.)

C. EXPRESSIONS OF ENERGY

–Energy expenditure in humans can be expressed in many terms. Converting from one expression to another is simple. Be familiar with the following terms:

1. **Absolute oxygen consumption**

   –This is the volume of oxygen consumed by the whole person, expressed in liters per minute (L · min^{-1}) or milliliters per minute (ml · min^{-1}).

   a. **Resting absolute oxygen consumption** for a 70-kg person is approximately 0.245 L · min^{-1}.

   b. In highly trained subjects, **maximal absolute oxygen consumption** as high as 4.9 L · min^{-1} may be expected.

   c. Absolute oxygen consumption is useful because it allows for an easy **estimation of caloric expenditure.** Each liter of O_2 consumed expends 5 kilocalories (5 kcal), or 20.9 kilojoules (20.9 kJ).

2. **Relative oxygen consumption**

   –This is the measure of **oxygen consumption relative to body weight,** measured in ml · kg^{-1} · min^{-1}—in other words, the **volume of oxygen consumed by the cells of each kilogram of body weight every minute.**

   a. **For the purpose of the ACSM examination,** a given mass of lean body tissue requires the same amount of O_2 at rest, and at any given work rate, irrespective of gender, race, age, and level of fitness. The **resting relative oxygen consumption is always assumed to be 3.5 ml · kg^{-1} · min^{-1}.**

   b. In highly trained aerobic athletes, a maximal relative oxygen consumption ($\dot{V}O_{2\,max}$) as high as 75–80 ml · kg^{-1} · min^{-1} may be expected.

   c. **Relative $\dot{V}O_2$** is commonly used to compare oxygen consumption of individuals who vary in size and weight. Because $\dot{V}O_{2\,max}$ is also used as an index of cardiopulmonary fitness, **a higher value is indicative of greater aerobic fitness.**

   d. All ACSM formulae provide $\dot{V}O_2$ values in gross relative terms.

3. **Metabolic Equivalents (METs)**

   –Physicians and clinicians commonly use the term **MET** as an expression of **energy expenditure or exercise intensity.** One MET is equivalent to the relative oxygen consumption at rest. Therefore, **1 MET = 3.5 ml · kg^{-1} · min^{-1}.**

   a. **METs are calculated by dividing the relative oxygen consumption by 3.5.** For example, an individual consuming 35 ml · kg^{-1} · min^{-1} during steady-state exercise is exercising at 10 METs.

   b. A MET is a useful expression because it allows for an easy **comparison of the amount of oxygen uptake during exercise with that at rest.**

4. **Calorie**

   –This expression of energy intake and expenditure is commonly used to quantify the **amount of energy derived from consumed foods** as well as the **amount of energy expended at rest and during physical activity** (see Chapter 9 for more information about this topic).

5. **Fat stores**

   –The human body stores the majority of excess energy intake in adipose tissue as fat.

   –It takes **3500 calories** to make and store **1 pound of body fat.**

   –Stated in reverse, **1 pound of fat can provide the body with 3500 calories**—the amount of energy needed to fuel the activity needed to **run about 35 miles!**

6. **Net vs. gross $\dot{V}O_2$**

   –**Humans require about 3.5 ml · kg^{-1} · min^{-1} (1 MET)** of oxygen at rest. This amount of oxygen uptake is **vital for the survival of the body's tissues and systems.**

   –**Physical activity elevates oxygen consumption** above resting oxygen requirements.

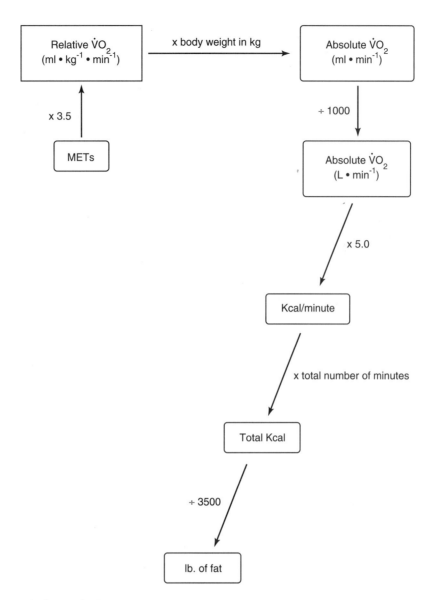

FIGURE 11-1 The energy equivalency chart.

a. **Net $\dot{V}O_2$** is the difference between the oxygen consumption value for exercise and the resting value. Net $\dot{V}O_2$ is used to assess the caloric cost of exercise.

b. **Gross $\dot{V}O_2$** is the sum of the oxygen cost of physical activity and the resting component.

c. Hence,

net $\dot{V}O_2$ = gross oxygen uptake – resting oxygen uptake

d. Net and gross oxygen uptake **can be expressed in relative or absolute terms.**

e. The **ACSM metabolic formulae** in *ACSM's Guidelines for Exercise Testing and Prescription,* 6th edition, and those described in this chapter, were designed to provide you with **gross values.**

The ability to convert from one energy expression to another is fundamental. Do not proceed to the next section of this chapter until you master this task.

- Converting an expression merely requires the multiplication or division of that expression by a constant. For example, to convert from METs to relative oxygen consumption, multiply the MET value by 3.5. Conversely, to convert from relative oxygen consumption to METs, divide by 3.5. *Commit these constants to memory.*
- **Figure 11-1, the Energy Equivalency Chart,** will help you to remember these conversions.
- **Figure 11-2** is a **practice sheet.** Duplicate this sheet and practice completing it from memory. Then answer the following questions.

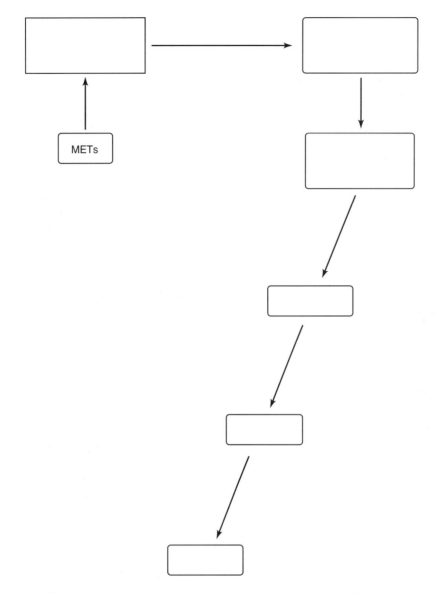

FIGURE 11-2 The energy equivalency chart practice sheet.

🌀 PRACTICE QUESTIONS: CONVERTING ENERGY EXPRESSIONS

1. What is the MET equivalent to 8.75 ml · kg^{-1} · min^{-1}?

2. What is the absolute oxygen consumption equivalent to 10 METs for a 155-pound male?

3. What is the equivalent total caloric expenditure of 2.5 pounds of fat?

4. A 70-kg male expends 7.5 kcal · min^{-1} while exercising. What is the equivalent MET value?

5. How many pounds of fat will a 50-kg woman lose after 4 weeks of training if she exercises at a frequency of three days per week, a duration of 45 minutes per session, and an energy expenditure of 6.5 kcal · min^{-1}? Assume that there are no modifications in her eating habits during the 4 weeks of training.

6. Using the ACSM walking formula, you calculate a gross $\dot{V}O_2$ of 13.0 ml · kg^{-1} · min^{-1}. What is the net oxygen uptake?

SOLUTIONS

1. To convert from ml · kg^{-1} · min^{-1} to METs, divide 8.75 by 3.5. The correct answer is **2.5 METs.**

2. To convert from METs to $\dot{V}O_2$ in absolute terms, first multiply the MET value by 3.5 to convert METs to $\dot{V}O_2$ in relative terms (ml · kg^{-1} · min^{-1}), then multiply the product (35 ml · kg^{-1} · min^{-1}) by body weight in kg (155 pounds ÷ 2.2 = 70.5 kg). The correct answers are **2467.5 ml · min^{-1}** or **2.47 L · min^{-1}.**

METABOLIC CALCULATIONS **171**

3. To convert from pounds of fat to total kcal, multiply the fat weight (in pounds) by 3500. The correct answer is **8750 kcal.**

4. To convert from kcal · min^{-1} to METs:

   a. First, convert the value to absolute $\dot{V}O_2$ in L · min^{-1}:

   $$7.5\ kcal \cdot min^{-1} \div 5.0 = 1.5\ L \cdot min^{-1}$$

   b. Then to absolute $\dot{V}O_2$ in ml · min^{-1}:

   $$1.5\ L.min^{-1} \times 1000 = 1500\ ml.min^{-1}$$

   c. Then to relative $\dot{V}O_2$:

   $$1500\ ml \cdot min^{-1} \div 70\ kg = 21.43\ ml \cdot kg^{-1} \cdot min^{-1}$$

   d. Then to METs:

   $$21.43\ ml \cdot kg^{-1} \cdot min^{-1} \div 3.5 = 6.12\ METs$$

5. The first step to solving this conversion question is to calculate the total number of minutes spent exercising during the 4 weeks.

   a. Because she trained for 45 minutes per session, three times per week, she accumulated a total of 540 minutes of exercise during the 4 weeks:

   $$45\ minutes\ /\ session \cdot 3\ sessions\ /\ week \cdot 4\ weeks = 540\ minutes$$

   b. The second step is to calculate the total number of calories expended during exercise throughout the 4 weeks (540 minutes) of training:

   $$6.5\ kcal \cdot min^{-1} \cdot 540\ minutes\ of\ exercise = 3510\ kcal$$

   c. Finally, find the fat weight equivalent to the expended calories:

   $$3510\ kcal \div 3500 = 1.003\ pounds\ of\ fat\ or\ approximately\ 1\ pound\ of\ fat.$$

6. Because gross $\dot{V}O_2$ = net $\dot{V}O_2$ + resting $\dot{V}O_2$, then net $\dot{V}O_2$ = gross $\dot{V}O_2$ − resting $\dot{V}O_2$:

$$Net\ \dot{V}O_2 = 13.0\ ml \cdot kg^{-1} \cdot min^{-1} - 3.5\ ml \cdot kg^{-1} \cdot min^{-1}$$

$$Net\ \dot{V}O_2 = 9.5\ ml \cdot kg^{-1} \cdot min^{-1}$$

D. OTHER CONVERSION FACTORS

–You must also commit to memory some other important conversions. Practice writing out the conversions in **Table 11-2** from memory.

Table 11-2. Conversion Factors

To convert from:	to:	do this:
Centimeters (cm)	Meters (M)	÷ by 100
Inches (in)	Meters (M)	× by 0.0254
Inches (in)	Centimeters (cm)	× by 2.54
kg · m · min^{-1}	Watts (W)	÷ by 6.0
Liters (L)	Milliliters (ml)	× by 1000
Miles per hour (mph)	Meters per minute (m · min^{-1})	× by 26.8
Minutes per mile	Miles per hour (mph)	÷ by 60
Pounds (lbs)	Kilograms (kg)	÷ by 2.2
Revolutions per minute (RPM) on a	Meters per minute (m · min^{-1})	
Monark arm ergometer		× by 2.4
Monark leg ergometer		× by 6
Tunturi or BodyGuard cycle ergometer		× by 3

PRACTICE QUESTIONS: OTHER CONVERSION FACTORS

Convert the following values to the desired units:

1. 1.5 meters to cm

2. 59.1 inches to meters

3. 70 kg to pounds

4. 6.0 mph to meters per minute

5. 50 RPM on the Monark™ leg ergometer to meters per minute

SOLUTIONS

1. 1.5 meters · 100 = **150 cm**

2. 59.1 inches · 0.0254 = **1.5 meters**

3. 70 kg · 2.2 = **154 pounds**

4. 6.0 mph · 26.8 = **160.8 m · min^{-1}**

5. 50 RPM · 6 = **300 m · min^{-1}**

II. THE ACSM METABOLIC FORMULAE

–All ACSM formulae yield gross oxygen uptake in relative terms.

A. WALKING AND RUNNING FORMULAE
(Figure 11-3)

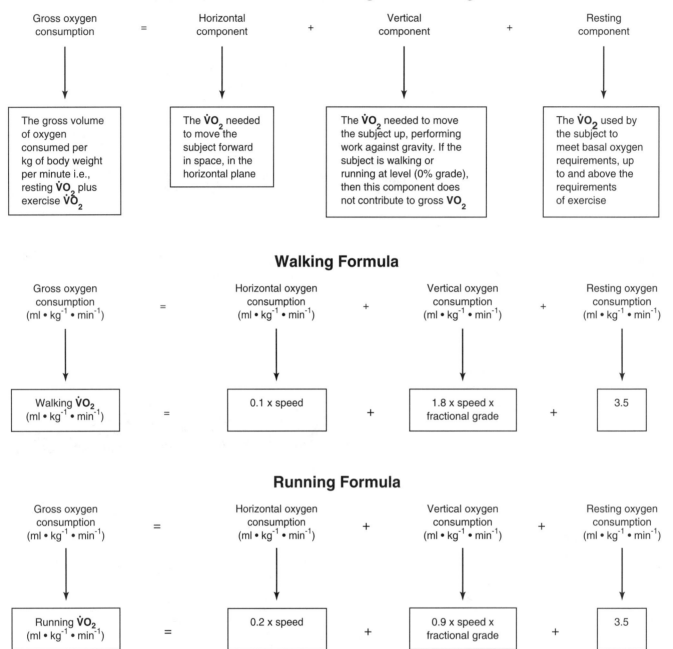

FIGURE 11-3 General structure of the walking and running formulae.

1. **Walking formula**

   –This formula applies to speeds of 50 to 100 m · min^{-1} (1.9 to 3.7 mph).

   a. **Gross $\dot{V}O_2$** is calculated in **relative terms** (ml · kg^{-1} · min^{-1}).

   b. The **horizontal component** is the product of the speed of the treadmill, in meters per minute (m · min^{-1}), multiplied by 0.1 (the O_2 cost of walking). The product, the $\dot{V}O_2$ of walking forward, is in ml · kg^{-1} · min^{-1}.

   c. The **vertical component** is the product of the grade of the treadmill multiplied by the speed of the treadmill (m · min^{-1})

   multiplied by 1.8 (the O_2 cost of walking uphill). The product, the $\dot{V}O_2$ of walking uphill, is in ml · kg^{-1} · min^{-1}. (Do not confuse the percent grade of the treadmill with the degree angle of inclination. **Percent grade of the treadmill** is the amount of vertical rise for 100 units of belt travel. For example, a patient walking on a treadmill at a 5% grade travels 5 meters vertically for every 100 meters of belt travel.)

   d. The **resting component** is 3.5 ml · kg^{-1} · min^{-1}.

General Structure: ACSM Leg and Arm Ergonometry Formulae

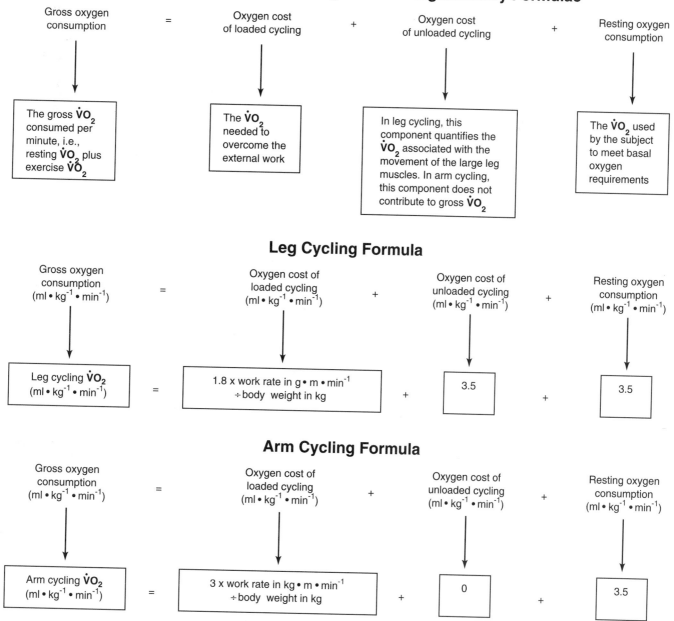

FIGURE 11-4 General structure of the leg and arm ergonometry formulae.

2. **Running formula**

   –This formula applies to running speeds exceeding 134 m · min⁻¹ (5.0 mph) and for true jogging speeds above 80.4 m · min⁻¹ (3.0 mph).

   –This formula may also be used for off-the-treadmill level running, but not for running on a graded track.

   a. **Gross $\dot{V}O_2$** is calculated in **relative terms** (ml · kg⁻¹ · min⁻¹).

   b. The **horizontal component** is the product of the speed of the treadmill (in m · min⁻¹) multiplied by 0.2 (the O_2 cost of running). The product, the $\dot{V}O_2$ of running forward, is in ml · kg⁻¹ · min⁻¹.

   c. The **vertical component** is the product of the grade (elevation) of the treadmill multiplied by the speed of the treadmill (in m · min⁻¹) multiplied by 0.9 (the O_2 cost of running uphill). The product, the $\dot{V}O_2$ of running uphill, is in ml · kg⁻¹ · min⁻¹.

   d. The **resting component** is 3.5 ml · kg⁻¹ · min⁻¹.

B. **LEG AND ARM ERGOMETRY FORMULAE** (Figure 11-4)

   1. **Leg cycling**

      –This formula applies to work rates between 300 and 1200 kg · m · min⁻¹, or 50 to 200 watts (50–200 W).

a. **Gross O$_2$ consumption** is calculated in relative terms (ml · kg^{-1} · min^{-1}).

b. **Oxygen cost of loaded leg cycling.** This is the product of the cost of cycling (1.8) multiplied by the work rate (kg · m · min^{-1}) divided by body weight (kg). The O$_2$ cost of cycling may also be calculated using the following expression:

10.8 · work rate (in watts) ÷ body weight (in kg)

Exam Note: Work Rate

The work rate may be provided to you in the question. You may also be expected to derive it from the cadence of the cycle ergometer and the resistance set on the flywheel.

• Work rate, also known as the **power output** or **workload,** is the product of the resistance set on the flywheel and the speed of cycling (velocity):

Work rate = force (resistance set on the flywheel in kg) · velocity (in m · min^{-1})

The units for the resistance set on the flywheel, **kilogram-force (kgf) and kilopond (kp), can be used interchangeably:** 1 kgf = 1 kp.

• **Calculate velocity from revolutions per minute (RPM)** by multiplying the RPM value by 6 for a Monark cycle ergometer, or by 3 for either a Tunturi or a BodyGuard. For example, an individual cycling at 50 RPM on a Monark leg ergometer is pedaling at a velocity of 300 m · min^{-1}. If the same individual works against a resistance of 2 kp, then the work rate will be 2 · 50 · 6 = 600 kg · m · min^{-1}.

• Work rate can also be expressed in watts:

1 watt = 6.0 kg · m · min^{-1}

---

c. **Oxygen cost of unloaded leg cycling.** Leg cycling incurs a small oxygen cost for the movement of the legs in space.

d. The **resting O$_2$ component** is 3.5 ml · kg^{-1} · min^{-1}.

2. **Arm cycling**

   –This formula applies to work rates between 150 and 750 kg · m · min^{-1} (25 to 125 W).

   a. **Gross O$_2$ consumption** is calculated in relative terms (ml · kg^{-1} · min^{-1}).

   b. **Oxygen cost of loaded arm cycling.** This is the product of the cost of cycling (3) multiplied by the work rate (kg · m · min^{-1}) divided by body weight (kg). The O$_2$ cost of cycling may also be calculated using the following expression:

18 · work rate (in watts) ÷ body weight (in kg)

Exam Note: Work Rate

The work rate may be provided to you in the question. You may also be expected to derive it from the cadence of the cycle ergometer and the resistance set on the flywheel.

• Work rate, also known as the power output or workload, is the product of the resistance set on the flywheel and the speed of cycling (velocity):

work rate = force (resistance set on the flywheel in kg) · velocity (in m · min^{-1})

• Calculate velocity from RPM by multiplying the RPM value by 2.4 for a Monark arm ergometer. The units for the resistance set on the flywheel, kilogram-force (kgf) and kilopond (kp), can be used interchangeably:

1 kgf = 1 kp

For example, an individual arm cycling at 50 RPM on a Monark arm ergometer is pedaling at a velocity of 120 m · min^{-1}. If the same individual works against a resistance of 2 kp, then the work rate will be 2 · 50 · 2.4 = 240 kg · m · min^{-1}.

• Work rate can also be expressed in watts:

1 W = 6.0 kg · m · min^{-1}

---

c. **Oxygen cost of unloaded arm cycling.** Arm cycling does not incur an oxygen cost of unloaded cycling.

d. The **resting component is 3.5 ml · kg^{-1} · min^{-1}.**

C. **STEPPING FORMULA** (Figure 11-5)

–This formula applies to stepping performed on a step box, a bleacher, or a similar stepping object where both concentric (moving up against gravity) and eccentric (moving down with gravity) contractions are involved.

–The formula is appropriate for stepping rates between 12 and 30 steps · min^{-1}, and heights between 0.04 and 0.4 m (1.6 to 15.7 inches).

1. **Gross O$_2$ consumption** is calculated in relative terms (ml · kg^{-1} · min^{-1}).

2. **Horizontal component.** This is the product of the rate of stepping per minute multiplied by 0.2. The product is O$_2$ consumption in ml · kg^{-1} · min^{-1}.

3. **Vertical component.** This the product of the height of each step (in meters) multiplied by the rate of stepping per minute multiplied by 1.33 multiplied by 1.8. The product is O$_2$ consumption in ml · kg^{-1} · min^{-1}.

4. **Resting component** is 3.5 ml · kg^{-1} · min^{-1}.

ACSM Stepping Formula

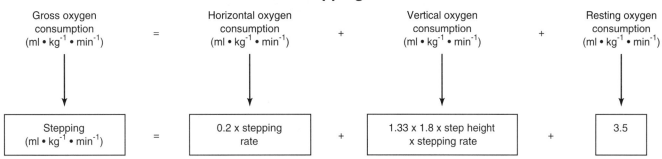

FIGURE 11-5 ACSM stepping formula.

III. SOLVING THE ACSM METABOLIC FORMULAE

A. USING A SYSTEMATIC APPROACH

–The task of solving the ACSM formulae is made easier using a systematic approach, which will help you avoid small but costly mistakes.

1. Read each question carefully and do not proceed until you know what you are asked to calculate. Remember that some questions may be solved without the use of a metabolic formula.

2. Extract only the required information. Do not be misled with extraneous information. If, for example, a question wants you to calculate the $\dot{V}O_2$ for walking on a treadmill, volunteered data about the height, age, or the gender of the subject are irrelevant.

3. Select the correct metabolic equation. A common error committed by many candidates is choosing the wrong formula.

4. Write down each step. *Do not take shortcuts.* Going through all the steps once is faster than two shortcut attempts!

5. On the top left corner of a clean sheet of paper, write the known values and indicate what is the unknown.

6. Where needed, convert all values to the appropriate units (see Table 11-2).
   a. Convert the treadmill speed or cycling cadence to meters per minute (m · min⁻¹).
   b. Convert body weight to kilograms (kg).
   c. Convert step height to meters (m).
   d. Convert work rate to kg · m · min⁻¹.

7. Write down the formula and plug in the known values and constants. Write clearly and place units after all variables.

8. Solve for the unknown. If the unknown is on the left side of the equation (i.e., the $\dot{V}O_2$ value), simply calculate the sum of the three components of the appropriate equation. If the unknown is on the right side of the equation, substitute and solve for the unknown. More on solving for the unknown later.

9. Examine the answer. Is the answer logical? Does it fall within expected "normal" values and human abilities?

10. Examine the choices. Make sure that the answer is in the same units as the answer on the examination, especially if a question does not specify what energy expression is needed (i.e., relative or absolute $\dot{V}O_2$, METs, kcal).

B. SOLVING LINEAR EQUATIONS

–The ACSM metabolic formulae are simple linear regression equations.

–The process of arriving at an answer to a metabolic calculation question is greatly simplified if the unknown is the $\dot{V}O_2$ value.

–In instances where the $\dot{V}O_2$ value is known, you might be expected to calculate an unknown value on the right side of the equation, such as the resistance on the cycle ergometer, the speed of the treadmill, the height of the step bench, etc.

> To solve an equation with an unknown on the right side of the equation, you must simplify the expression so that the unknown stands by itself on one side of the equation and all the known numbers on the other.

1. **Example 1**

   –Solve for χ in the following equation:

   $$\chi - 4 = 10$$

   Solution: Add 4 to both sides of the equation:

   $$\chi - 4 + 4 = 10 + 4$$
   $$\chi = 14$$

2. **Example 2**

   –Solve for α in the following equation:

   $$2\alpha + 7 = 3$$

   Solution: Subtract 7 from both sides of the equation:

   $$2\alpha = -4$$

   Divide both sides by 2:

   $$\alpha = -2$$

3. **Example 3**

   –Solve for β in the following equation:

   $$4\beta - {}^3\!/_4 = {}^7\!/_9$$

   Solution: Add ¾ to both sides of the equation:

   $$4\beta = {}^{55}\!/_{36}$$

   Divide both sides by 4:

   $$\beta = {}^{55}\!/_{144}$$

C. **HELPFUL HINT:** Substitute your answer for the unknown value in the original equation. If the left side equals the right side after the substitution, your answer is correct. For example, in the previous problem, plugging in ${}^{55}\!/_{144}$ in the place of β yields ⅞. Hence, ${}^{55}\!/_{144}$ is the correct answer.

⊚ PRACTICE QUESTIONS: SOLVING LINEAR EQUATIONS

1. What is the gross oxygen cost of walking on a treadmill at 3.5 mph and a 10% grade?

2. A 176-lb patient set the treadmill at 3.0 mph and 2% grade. While exercising, his heart rate was 140 beats · min^{-1} and his blood pressure was 160/80 mm Hg. What was his estimated oxygen consumption in relative terms?

3. What resistance should you set a Monark cycle ergometer at to elicit a $\dot{V}O_2$ value of 2750 ml · min^{-1} while cycling at 50 RPM? The subject is 65 inches tall and weighs 110 pounds.

SOLUTIONS

1. Choose the walking equation.

   a. On the top left corner of a clean sheet of paper, write down your knowns and convert all numbers to the appropriate units:

   Speed in m · min^{-1} = 3.5 mph · 26.8 = 93.8 m · min^{-1}

   b. Write down the ACSM walking formula:

   Walking (ml · kg^{-1} · min^{-1}) = 0.1 · speed +1.8 · speed · fractional grade+3.5 ml · kg^{-1} · min^{-1}

   c. Substitute the variable name with the known values:

   *Walking (ml · kg^{-1} · min^{-1}) = 0.1 · **93.8** m · min^{-1}+1.8 · **93.8** m · min^{-1} · **0.1**+3.5 ml · kg^{-1} · min^{-1}*

   d. Multiply values:

   Walking (ml · kg^{-1} · min^{-1}) = 9.38 ml · kg^{-1} · min^{-1} + 16.88 ml · kg^{-1} · min^{-1}+3.5 ml · kg^{-1} · min^{-1}

   e. Then add numbers:

   *Gross walking $\dot{V}O_2$ = **29.76 ml · kg^{-1} · min^{-1}***

2. The question is clearly asking for $\dot{V}O_2$ in relative terms (ml · kg^{-1} · min^{-1}).

   a. Extract the information you need (speed and elevation of the treadmill) and ignore extraneous information (HR and BP).

   b. Select the walking equation:

   Walking (ml · kg^{-1} · min^{-1}) = Speed (m · min^{-1}) · 0.1+Grade (fraction) · speed (m · min^{-1}) · 1.8+3.5 (ml · kg^{-1} · min^{-1})

   c. On the top left corner of a clean sheet of paper, write down the knowns and convert all numbers to the appropriate units:

   Weight = 176 lb ÷ 2.2 = 80.0 kg

   Speed = 3.0 mph · 26.8 = 80.4 m · min^{-1}

   Treadmill elevation = 2% grade = 2/100 = 0.02

   d. Plug the knowns into the formula and calculate the answer:

   Walking (ml · kg^{-1} · min^{-1}) = Speed (m · min^{-1}) · 0.1+Grade (fraction) · speed (m · min^{-1}) · 1.8 + 3.5 (ml · kg^{-1} · min^{-1})

   *Walking (ml · kg^{-1} · min^{-1}) = **80.4** (m · min^{-1}) · 0.1 + **0.02** · **80.4** (m · min^{-1}) · 1.8 + 3.5 (ml · kg^{-1} · min^{-1})*

Math Reminder

Multiply and divide numbers **before** *adding or subtracting.* For example, in the following expression:

$$Y = 5 + 2 · 5 + 7 · 2$$

Multiply the 2 by the 5 (=10), the 7 by the 2 (=14), and then add the 10, the 14, and the 5 together. The correct answer is Y = 29, not 84.

Walking (ml · kg⁻¹ · min⁻¹) = 8.04 ml · kg⁻¹ · min⁻¹ + 2.89 ml · kg⁻¹ · min⁻¹ + 3.5 ml · kg⁻¹ · min⁻¹

14.43 (ml · kg⁻¹ · min⁻¹) = 8.04 ml · kg⁻¹ · min⁻¹ + 2.89 ml · kg⁻¹ · min⁻¹ + 3.5 ml · kg⁻¹ · min⁻¹

*Relative $\dot{V}O_2$ = **14.43 ml · kg⁻¹ · min⁻¹***

3. Read the question carefully so that you will know what the question is asking for. The question is providing you with the oxygen consumption (2750 ml · min⁻¹), but expects you to calculate the resistance (F) to be set on the cycle ergometer.

   a. Extract the information you need. Only the weight of the subject and the speed of the cycle are needed.

   b. Convert the known units:

      110 pounds = 50.0 kg

   c. Select the leg ergometer equation.

   d. Calculate the gross relative $\dot{V}O_2$ from the given information:

      $\dot{V}O_2$ ml · kg⁻¹ · min⁻¹ = 2750 ml · min⁻¹ ÷ 50.0 kg
      = 55.0 ml · kg⁻¹ · min⁻¹

*Gross oxygen consumption **(ml · kg⁻¹ · min⁻¹)** = Oxygen cost of loaded cycling **(ml · kg⁻¹ · min⁻¹)** + Oxygen cost of unloaded cycling **(ml · kg⁻¹ · min⁻¹)** + Resting oxygen consumption **(ml · kg⁻¹ · min⁻¹)***

*Leg cycling **(ml · kg⁻¹ · min⁻¹)** = **1.8 · work rate ÷ body weight** +3.5 (ml · kg⁻¹ · min⁻¹)+ 3.5 (ml · kg⁻¹ · min⁻¹)*

   e. Note that the unknown (resistance in kg) is part of the work rate. Write out the work rate as force (in kg) · speed (in m · min⁻¹):

55 ml · kg⁻¹ · min⁻¹ = 1.8 · F · speed ÷ body weight + 3.5 (ml · kg⁻¹ · min⁻¹)+3.5 (ml · kg⁻¹ · min⁻¹)

   f. From the given information, we also know that the speed of cycling is 300 m · min⁻¹ (50 RPM · 6). Plug all the knowns into the equation:

55 ml · kg⁻¹ · min⁻¹ = 1.8 · F · 300 m · min⁻¹ ÷ 50 kg + 3.5 (ml · kg⁻¹ · min⁻¹)+3.5 (ml · kg⁻¹ · min⁻¹)

   g. Move the unknown F to one side of the equation, all the knowns to the other side, and calculate for the unknown:

55 ml · kg⁻¹ · min⁻¹ = 1.8 · F · 300 m · min⁻¹ ÷ 50 kg + 3.5 (ml · kg⁻¹ · min⁻¹) + 3.5 (ml · kg⁻¹ · min⁻¹)

55 ml · kg⁻¹ · min⁻¹ – 3.5 ml · kg⁻¹ · min⁻¹ – 3.5 ml · kg⁻¹ · min⁻¹ = 1.8 × F × 300 m/min ÷ 50 kg

48 ml · kg⁻¹ · min⁻¹ = 1.8 · F · 300 m/min · 50 kg

$$\frac{48 \times 50}{1.8 \times 300} = F$$

4.44 kp = F

REVIEW TEST

DIRECTIONS: Carefully read all questions and select the BEST single answer.

1. What is the relative oxygen consumption of walking on a treadmill at 3.5 mph and 0% grade?
   (A) 9.38 ml · kg^{-1} · min^{-1}
   (B) 12.88 ml · kg^{-1} · min^{-1}
   (C) 18.76 ml · kg^{-1} · min^{-1}
   (D) 22.26 ml · kg^{-1} · min^{-1}

2. A patient is walking on a treadmill at 3.4 mph up a 5% grade. What is her $\dot{V}O_2$ in relative terms?
   (A) 9.11 ml · kg^{-1} · min^{-1}
   (B) 11.9 ml · kg^{-1} · min^{-1}
   (C) 24 ml · kg^{-1} · min^{-1}
   (D) 20.81 ml · kg^{-1} · min^{-1}

3. A 70-kg patient is running on a treadmill at 5 mph set at a 5% grade. What is his caloric expenditure rate?
   (A) 12.7 kcal · min^{-1}
   (B) 1.271 kcal · min^{-1}
   (C) 3.633 kcal · min^{-1}
   (D) 36.33 kcal · min^{-1}

4. What is the MET equivalent to level walking on a treadmill at 3.0 mph?
   (A) 5.59 METS
   (B) 3.30 METs
   (C) 2.30 METS
   (D) 3.02 METS

5. What is the relative oxygen consumption of running on a treadmill at 6.5 mph and 0% grade?
   (A) 34.84 ml · kg^{-1} · min^{-1}
   (B) 34.48 ml · kg^{-1} · min^{-1}
   (C) 38.34 ml · kg^{-1} · min^{-1}
   (D) 43.83 ml · kg^{-1} · min^{-1}

6. What is the relative oxygen consumption of running on a treadmill at 5.5 mph and 12% grade?
   (A) 29.48 ml · kg^{-1} · min^{-1}
   (B) 45.4 ml · kg^{-1} · min^{-1}
   (C) 47.2 ml · kg^{-1} · min^{-1}
   (D) 48.9 ml · kg^{-1} · min^{-1}

7. A 150-pound male sets the treadmill speed at 5.0 mph and a 5.2% grade. Calculate his MET value.
   (A) 36.57 METs
   (B) 10.45 METs
   (C) 12.25 METs
   (D) Not enough information to answer the question

8. What is a patient's work rate in watts if he pedals on a Monark cycle ergometer at 50 RPM at a resistance of 2.0 kiloponds?
   (A) 50 watts
   (B) 100 watts
   (C) 200 watts
   (D) 300 watts

9. A 110-pound female pedals a Monark cycle ergometer at 50 RPM against a resistance of 2.5 kiloponds. Calculate her absolute oxygen consumption.
   (A) 300 ml · min^{-1}
   (B) 750 ml · min^{-1}
   (C) 1.25 L · min^{-1}
   (D) 1.7 L · min^{-1}

10. A 55-kilogram phase III cardiac rehabilitation patient trains on a cycle ergometer by pedaling at 60 RPM against a resistance of 1.5 kiloponds. What is her absolute oxygen consumption?
    (A) 1.36 L · min^{-1}
    (B) 2.47 L · min^{-1}
    (C) 3.62 L · min^{-1}
    (D) 3600 ml · min^{-1}

11. The same 55-kilogram patient also trains on a Monark arm ergometer at 60 RPM against a resistance of 1.5 kiloponds. What is her absolute oxygen consumption?
    (A) 1.52 L · min^{-1}
    (B) 773.0 ml · min^{-1}
    (C) 0.840 L · min^{-1}
    (D) 0.774 L · min^{-1}

12. If a 70-kilogram man runs on a treadmill at 8 mph and 0% grade for 45 minutes, what is his caloric expenditure?
    (A) 1067.07 calories
    (B) 392.18 calories
    (C) 730.48 calories
    (D) Not enough information to answer the question

13. Part of your patient's exercise prescription calls for bench stepping. What is the relative oxygen cost of bench stepping if he steps at a rate of 24 steps per minute up a 10-inch stepping box? Your patient weighs 140 pounds.
    (A) 12.91 ml · kg^{-1} · min^{-1}
    (B) 14.61 ml · kg^{-1} · min^{-1}
    (C) 16.41 ml · kg^{-1} · min^{-1}
    (D) 18.11 ml · kg^{-1} · min^{-1}

14. What stepping rate should a patient use if she wishes to exercise at 5 METs? The step box is 6 inches high and she weighs 50 kilograms.
    (A) 12 steps per minute
    (B) 32 steps per minute
    (C) 35 steps per minute
    (D) 96 steps per minute

15. A 143-pound patient regularly exercises on a treadmill at a speed of 5.5 mph and a 2% elevation. What is her caloric expenditure?
    (A) 6.78 kcal · min⁻¹
    (B) 11.58 kcal · min⁻¹
    (C) 20.85 kcal · min⁻¹
    (D) 25.47 kcal · min⁻¹

16. How much weight should your patient expect to lose on a weekly basis if she exercises regularly on a treadmill at a speed of 5.5 mph and a 2% elevation? Her exercise prescription calls for a 45-minute training session at a frequency of 3 sessions per week.
    (A) 1.5 kilograms
    (B) 2.12 kilograms
    (C) 0.25 pounds
    (D) 0.45 pounds

17. What resistance would you set a cycle ergometer at if you want your 80-kilogram patient to train at 6 METs? Assume a 50 RPM cycling cadence.
    (A) 1.5 kilograms
    (B) 2.12 kilograms
    (C) 0.25 pounds
    (D) 0.45 pounds

18. What running speed would you set a level treadmill at to elicit an oxygen consumption of 40 ml · kg⁻¹ · min⁻¹?
    (A) 5.0 mph
    (B) 6.8 mph
    (C) 18.25 m · min⁻¹
    (D) 18.25 mph

19. A 35-year-old client reduced her caloric intake by 1200 kcal per week. How much weight will she lose in 26 weeks?
    (A) 8.9 pounds
    (B) 12.0 pounds
    (C) 26.0 pounds
    (D) 34.3 pounds

20. From question 22, how much weight will she lose in 26 weeks if she integrated a one-mile walk three times per week into her weight loss program?
    (A) 3 pounds
    (B) 6 pounds
    (C) 11 pounds
    (D) 15 pounds

ANSWERS AND EXPLANATIONS

1–B. The steps are as follows:
   a. Choose the ACSM walking formula.
   b. Write down your knowns and convert the values to the appropriate units:
      Knowns: 3.5 mph · 26.8 m · min⁻¹ = 93.8 m · min⁻¹
      0% grade = 0.0
   c. Write down the ACSM walking formula:

Walking = (0.1 · speed) + (1.8 · speed · fractional grade) + (3.5 ml · kg⁻¹ · min⁻¹)

   d. Substitute the known values for the variable name:

$ml · kg^{-1} · min^{-1} = (0.1 · 93.8) + (1.8 · 93.8 · 0) + (3.5)$
$ml · kg^{-1} · min^{-1} = (9.38) + (0) + (3.5)$

   e. Solve for the unknown:

$ml · kg^{-1} · min^{-1} = (9.38) + (3.5)$
Gross walking $\dot{V}O_2$ = 12.88 ml · kg⁻¹ · min⁻¹

2–D. The steps are as follows:
   a. Choose the ACSM walking formula.
   b. Write down your knowns and convert the values to the appropriate units:
      Knowns: 3.4 mph · 26.8 m · min⁻¹
      = 91.12 m · min⁻¹
      5% grade = 0.05
   c. Write down the ACSM walking formula:

Walking = (0.1 · speed) + (1.8 · speed · fractional grade) + (3.5)(ml · kg⁻¹ · min⁻¹)

   d. Substitute the known values for the variable name:

$ml · kg^{-1} · min^{-1} = (0.1 · 91.12) + (1.8 · 91.12 · .05) + (3.5)$
$ml · kg^{-1} · min^{-1} = (9.112) + (8.2008) + (3.5)$

   e. Solve for the unknown:

$ml · kg^{-1} · min^{-1} = (9.112) + (8.2008) + (3.5)$
Gross walking $\dot{V}O_2$ = 20.81 ml · kg⁻¹ · min⁻¹

3–A. The steps are as follows:
   a. Choose the ACSM running formula.
   b. Write down your knowns and convert the values to the appropriate units:
      Knowns: 5 mph · 26.8 = 134 m · min⁻¹
      5% grade = 0.05
   c. Write down the ACSM running formula:

Running = (0.2 · speed) + (0.9 · speed · fractional grade) + (3.5)(ml · kg⁻¹ · min⁻¹)

   d. Substitute the known values for the variable name:

$ml · kg^{-1} · min^{-1} = (0.2 · 134) + (0.9 · 134 · .05) + (3.5)$
$ml · kg^{-1} · min^{-1} = (26.8) + (6.03) + (3.5)$

   e. Solve for the unknown:

$ml · kg^{-1} · min^{-1} = (26.8) + (6.03) + (3.5)$
Gross running $\dot{V}O_2$ = 36.33 ml · kg⁻¹ · min⁻¹

f. The question is asking you to find the patient's caloric expenditure rate, which means that you need to first determine his O_2 consumption in absolute terms:

$$Absolute\ \dot{V}O_2\ (ml \cdot min^{-1}) = relative\ \dot{V}O_2\ (ml \cdot kg^{-1} \cdot min^{-1}) \cdot body\ weight\ in\ kg$$

$$ml \cdot min^{-1} = 36.33\ ml \cdot kg^{-1} \cdot min^{-1} \cdot 70\ kg$$

$$Absolute\ \dot{V}O_2\ (ml \cdot min^{-1}) = 2543.1\ ml \cdot min^{-1}$$

Now, divide by 1000 to get $L \div min^{-1}$:

$$2543.1 \div 1000 = 2.54\ L \cdot min^{-1}$$

g. Multiply absolute $\dot{V}O_2$ by 5.0 to determine his caloric expenditure rate:

$$2.54\ L \cdot min^{-1} \cdot 5.0 = 12.7\ kcal \cdot min^{-1}$$

4–B. The steps are as follows:
   a. Choose the ACSM walking formula.
   b. Write down your knowns and convert the values to the appropriate units:
   Knowns: 3.0 mph · (26.8) = 80.4 m · min^{-1}
   0% grade (level walking) = 0.0
   c. Write down the ACSM walking formula:

$$Walking\ (ml \cdot kg^{-1} \cdot min^{-1}) = (0.1 \cdot speed) + (1.8 \cdot speed \cdot fractional\ grade) + (3.5)$$

   d. Substitute the known values for the variable name:

$$ml \cdot kg^{-1} \cdot min^{-1} = (0.1 \cdot 80.4) + (1.8 \cdot 80.4 \cdot 0) + (3.5)$$

   e. Solve for the unknown:

$$ml \cdot kg^{-1} \cdot min^{-1} = (8.04) + (0) + (3.5)$$

$$Gross\ walking\ \dot{V}O_2 = 11.54\ ml \cdot kg^{-1} \cdot min^{-1}$$

   f. Because this question wants you to find the MET equivalent, we must divide our gross walking $\dot{V}O_2$ by the constant 3.5:

$$METs = relative\ \dot{V}O_2\ (ml \cdot kg^{-1} \cdot min^{-1}) \div 3.5$$

$$METs = 11.54\ ml \cdot kg^{-1} \cdot min^{-1} \div 3.5$$

$$= 3.30\ METs$$

5–C. The steps are as follows:
   a. Choose the ACSM running formula.
   b. Write down your knowns and convert the values to the appropriate units:
   Knowns: 6.5 mph · 26.8 = 174.2 m · min^{-1}
   0% grade = 0.0
   c. Write down the ACSM running formula:

$$Running = (0.2 \cdot speed) + (0.9 \cdot speed \cdot fractional\ grade) + (3.5)(ml \cdot kg^{-1} \cdot min^{-1})$$

   d. Substitute the known values for the variable name:

$$ml \cdot kg^{-1} \cdot min^{-1} = (0.2 \cdot 174.2) + (0.9 \cdot 174.2 \cdot 0) + (3.5)$$

   e. Solve for the unknown:

$$ml \cdot kg^{-1} \cdot min^{-1} = (34.84) + (0) + (3.5)$$

$$Gross\ running\ \dot{V}O_2 = 38.34\ ml \cdot kg^{-1} \cdot min^{-1}$$

6–D. The steps are as follows:
   a. Choose the ACSM running formula.
   b. Write down your knowns and convert the values to the appropriate units:
   Knowns: 5.5 mph · 26.8 = 147.4 m · min^{-1}
   12% grade = 0.12
   c. Write down the ACSM running formula:

$$Running = (0.2 \cdot speed) + (0.9 \cdot speed \cdot fractional\ grade) + (3.5)(ml \cdot kg^{-1} \cdot min^{-1})$$

   d. Substitute the known values for the variable name:

$$ml \cdot kg^{-1} \cdot min^{-1} = (0.2 \cdot 147.4) + (0.9 \cdot 147.4 \cdot 0.12) + (3.5)$$

   e. Solve for the unknown:

$$ml \cdot kg^{-1} \cdot min^{-1} = (29.48) + (15.92) + (3.5)$$

$$Gross\ running\ \dot{V}O_2 = 48.9\ ml \cdot kg^{-1} \cdot min^{-1}$$

7–B. The steps are as follows:
   a. Choose the ACSM running formula.
   b. Write down your knowns and convert the values to the appropriate units:
   Knowns: 5.0 mph · 26.8 = 134 m · min^{-1}
   5.2% grade = 0.052
   c. Write down the ACSM running formula:

$$Running = (0.2 \cdot speed) + (0.9 \cdot speed \cdot fractional\ grade) + (3.5)(ml \cdot kg^{-1} \cdot min^{-1})$$

   d. Substitute the known values for the variable name:

$$ml \cdot kg^{-1} \cdot min^{-1} = (0.2 \cdot 134) + (0.9 \cdot 134 \cdot 0.052) + (3.5)$$

   e. Solve for the unknown:

$$ml \cdot kg^{-1} \cdot min^{-1} = (26.8) + (6.27) + (3.5)$$

$$Gross\ running\ \dot{V}O_2 = 36.57\ ml \cdot kg^{-1} \cdot min^{-1}$$

   f. This question asks us for his MET value so we must divide his gross running $\dot{V}O_2$ (ml · kg^{-1} · min^{-1}) by the constant 3.5 (we can ignore his weight—this is extraneous information):

$$METs = relative\ \dot{V}O_2\ (ml \cdot kg^{-1} \cdot min^{-1}) \div 3.5$$

$$METs = 36.57\ ml \cdot kg^{-1} \cdot min^{-1} \div 3.5$$

$$= 10.45\ METs$$

8–B. This question does not require the use of a metabolic formula because it is asking for the patient's work rate. The steps are as follows:
   a. Write down your knowns and convert the values to the appropriate units:
   Knowns: 50 RPM · 6 meters = 300 m · min^{-1}
   (each revolution on a Monark cycle ergometer = 6 m)
   2.0 kiloponds = 2.0 kilograms
   b. Write down the formula for work rate:

$$work\ rate = force \times distance \div time$$

c. Substitute the known values for the variable name:

$$Work\ rate = 2.0\ kg \cdot 300\ m \cdot min^{-1}$$

$$Work\ rate = 600\ kg \cdot m \cdot min^{-1}$$

d. The question asks for watts, so we must divide the work rate ($kg^{-1} \cdot m \cdot min^{-1}$) by 6:

$$W = kg \cdot m \cdot min^{-1} \div 6\ watts = 600\ kg \cdot m \cdot min^{-1} \div 6$$
$$= 100\ W$$

9–D. The steps are as follows:
  a. Choose the ACSM leg cycling formula.
  b. Write down your knowns and convert the values to the appropriate units:
  Knowns: 110 pounds ÷ 2.2 = 50kg
  50 RPM · 6 meters = 300 m · min⁻¹
  2.5 kp = 2.5 kg
  c. Write down the ACSM leg cycling formula:

$$Leg\ cycling\ (ml \cdot kg^{-1} \cdot min^{-1}) = (1.8 \cdot work\ rate \div body\ weight) + (3.5) + (3.5)$$

  d. Calculate work rate:

$$Work\ rate = kg \cdot m \div min$$
$$= 2.5\ kg \cdot 300\ m \cdot min^{-1}$$
$$= 750\ kg \cdot m \cdot min^{-1}$$

  e. Substitute the known values for the variable name:

$$ml \cdot kg^{-1} \cdot min^{-1} = (1.8 \cdot 750 \div 50) + (3.5) + (3.5)$$

  f. Solve for the unknown:

$$ml \cdot kg^{-1} \cdot min^{-1} = (27) + (3.5) + (3.5)$$

$$Gross\ leg\ cycling\ \dot{V}O_2 = 34\ ml \cdot kg^{-1} \cdot min^{-1}$$

  g. This question is asking for her absolute oxygen consumption, so we must multiply her gross $\dot{V}O_2$ (in relative terms) by her body weight:

$$Absolute\ \dot{V}O_2 = relative\ \dot{V}O_2\ x\ body\ weight$$
$$= 34\ ml \cdot kg^{-1} \cdot min^{-1} \cdot 50\ kg$$
$$= 1700\ ml \cdot min^{-1}$$

  h. To get L · min⁻¹, divide by 1000:

$$1700\ ml \cdot min^{-1} \div 1000 = 1.7\ L\ min^{-1}$$

10–A. The steps are as follows:
  a. Choose the ACSM leg cycling formula.
  b. Write down your knowns and convert the values to the appropriate units:
  Knowns: 55 kg = body weight
  60 RPM · 6 meters = 360 m · min⁻¹
  1.5 kp = 1.5 kg
  c. Write down the ACSM formula:

$$Leg\ cycling\ (ml \cdot kg^{-1} \cdot min^{-1}) = (1.8 \cdot work\ rate \div body\ weight) + (3.5) + (3.5)$$

  d. Calculate work rate:

$$Work\ rate = kg \cdot m \div min = 1.5\ kg \cdot 360\ m \cdot min^{-1}$$
$$= 540\ kg \cdot m \cdot min^{-1}$$

e. Substitute the known values for the variable name:

$$ml \cdot kg^{-1} \cdot min^{-1} = (1.8 \cdot 540 \div 55) + (3.5) + (3.5)$$

  f. Solve for the unknown:

$$ml \cdot kg^{-1} \cdot min^{-1} = (17.67) + (3.5) + (3.5)$$

$$Gross\ leg\ cycling\ \dot{V}O_2 = 24.67\ ml \cdot kg^{-1} \cdot min^{-1}$$

  g. To get her absolute oxygen consumption, multiply by her body weight:

$$Absolute\ \dot{V}O_2 = relative\ \dot{V}O_2 \cdot body\ weight$$
$$= 24.67\ ml \cdot kg^{-1} \cdot min^{-1} \cdot 55\ kg$$
$$= 1356.85\ ml \cdot min^{-1}$$

  h. To get absolute $\dot{V}O_2$ in L · min⁻¹, divide ml · min⁻¹ by 1000:

$$1356.85\ ml \cdot min^{-1} \div 1000 = 1.35685\ L \cdot min^{-1}$$

11–C. The steps are as follows:
  a. Choose the ACSM arm cycling formula.
  b. Write down your knowns and convert the values to the appropriate units:
  Knowns: 55 kg = body weight
  60 RPM · 2.4 meters (each revolution on a Monark arm ergometer = 2.4 m) = 144 m · min⁻¹
  1.5 kp = 1.5 kg
  c. Write down the ACSM formula:

$$Arm\ cycling\ (ml \cdot kg^{-1} \cdot min^{-1}) = (3 \cdot work\ rate \div body\ weight) + (0) + (3.5)\ (ml \cdot kg^{-1} \cdot min^{-1})$$

  d. Calculate work rate:

$$Work\ rate = kg \cdot m \div min$$
$$= 1.5\ kg \cdot 144\ m \cdot min^{-1}$$
$$= 216\ kg \cdot m \cdot min^{-1}$$

  e. Substitute the known values for the variable name:

$$ml \cdot kg^{-1} \cdot min^{-1} = (3 \cdot 216 \div 55) + (0) + (3.5)$$

  f. Solve for the unknown:

$$ml \cdot kg^{-1} \cdot min^{-1} = (11.78) + (0) + (3.5)$$

$$Gross\ arm\ cycling\ \dot{V}O_2 = 15.28\ ml \cdot kg^{-1} \cdot min^{-1}$$

  g. To get her absolute oxygen consumption, multiply her relative oxygen consumption by her body weight:

$$Absolute\ \dot{V}O_2 = relative\ \dot{V}O_2\ x\ body\ weight$$
$$= 15.28\ ml \cdot kg^{-1} \cdot min^{-1} \cdot 55\ kg$$
$$= 840.4\ ml \cdot min^{-1}$$

  h. To get her absolute oxygen consumption in L · min⁻¹, divide ml · min⁻¹ by 1000:

$$840.0\ ml \cdot min^{-1} \div 1000 = 0.8404\ L \cdot min^{-1}$$

12–C. The steps are as follows:
  a. Choose the ACSM running formula.
  b. Write down your knowns and convert the values to the appropriate units:
  Knowns: 8 mph · 26.8 = 214.4 m · min⁻¹
  70 kg = body weight

45 minutes of running
0% grade

c. Write down the ACSM running formula:

Running = (0.2 · speed) + (0.9 · speed · fractional grade) + (3.5) (ml · kg^{-1} · min^{-1})

d. Substitute the known values for the variable name:

ml · kg^{-1} · min^{-1} = (0.2 · 214.4) + (0.9 · 214.4 · 0) + (3.5)

e. Solve for the unknown:

ml · kg^{-1} · min^{-1} = (42.88) + (0) + (3.5)

Gross running $\dot{V}O_2$ = 46.38 ml · kg^{-1} · min^{-1}

f. To find out his total caloric expenditure, we must first put his gross running $\dot{V}O_2$ in absolute terms by multiplying by his body weight:

Absolute $\dot{V}O_2$ = relative $\dot{V}O_2$ x body weight

= 46.38 ml · kg^{-1} · min^{-1} · 70 kg

= 3246.6 ml · min^{-1}

g. Next we must convert ml · min^{-1} to L · min^{-1} by dividing by 1000:

3246.6 ml · min^{-1} ÷ 1000 = 3.2466 L · min^{-1}

h. We must then multiply L · min^{-1} by the constant 5.0 to get kcal · min^{-1}:

3.2466 L · min^{-1} · 5.0 = 16.233 kcal · min^{-1}

i. Finally, we multiply kcal · min^{-1} by the total number of minutes to get total caloric expenditure:

16.233 kcal · min^{-1} x 45 min = 730.48 calories

13–C. The steps are as follows:

a. Choose the ACSM stepping formula.

b. Write down your knowns and convert the values to the appropriate units:
Knowns: Rate = 24 steps per minute
Step height = 10 in x 0.0254 = 0.254 meters
(The body weight is irrelevant in this problem.)

c. Write down the ACSM stepping formula:

Stepping = (0.2 · stepping rate) + (1.33 · step height · stepping rate) + (3.5)(ml · kg^{-1} · min^{-1})

d. Substitute the known values for the variable name:

ml · kg^{-1} · min^{-1} = (0.2 · 24) + (1.33 · 0.254 · 24) + (3.5)

e. Solve for the unknown:

ml · kg^{-1} · min^{-1} = (4.8) + (8.11) + (3.5)

Gross Stepping $\dot{V}O_2$ = 16.41 ml · kg^{-1} · min^{-1}

14–C. The steps are as follows:

a. Choose the ACSM stepping formula.

b. Write down your knowns and convert the values to the appropriate units:
Knowns: 5 METs · 3.5 = 17.5 ml · kg^{-1} · min^{-1}

(This gives us the Relative $\dot{V}O_2$ equivalent, which we will need for the stepping formula)
6 inches · 0.0254 = 0.1524 meters
(Her body weight is irrelevant.)

c. Write down the ACSM stepping formula:

Stepping = (0.2 · stepping rate) + (1.33 · step height · stepping rate) + (3.5)(ml · kg^{-1} · min^{-1})

d. Substitute the known values for the variable name:

17.5 = (0.2 · stepping rate) + (1.33 · 0.1524 · stepping rate) + (3.5)

e. Move all of the knowns on one side of the equation and keep the unknown on the other:

17.5 – 3.5 = (0.2 · stepping rate) + (0.203 · stepping rate)

14 = 0.403 (stepping rate)

f. Divide by 0.403 to get the stepping rate:

34.7 = stepping rate

About 35 steps per minute = stepping rate

15–B. The steps are as follows:

a. Choose the ACSM running formula.

b. Write down your knowns and convert the values to the appropriate units:
Knowns: 143 pounds ÷ 2.2 = 65 kg
5.5 mph = 147.4 m · min^{-1}
2% grade = 0.02

c. Write down the ACSM running formula:

Running (ml · kg^{-1} · min^{-1}) = (0.2 · speed) + (0.9 · speed · fractional grade) + (3.5)

d. Substitute the known values for the variable name:

ml · kg^{-1} · min^{-1} = (0.2 · 147.4) + (0.9 · 147.4 · 0.02) + (3.5)

e. Solve for the unknown:

ml · kg^{-1} · min^{-1} = (29.48) + (2.65) + (3.5)

Gross running $\dot{V}O_2$ = 35.63 ml · kg^{-1} · min^{-1}

f. To find out how many calories per minute she is expending, we must first convert her gross running $\dot{V}O_2$ (in relative terms) to absolute $\dot{V}O_2$ by multiplying by her body weight:

Absolute $\dot{V}O_2$ = relative $\dot{V}O_2$ x body weight

= 35.63 ml · kg^{-1} · min^{-1} · 65 kg

= 2315.95 ml · min^{-1}

g. Convert ml · min^{-1} to L · min^{-1} by dividing by 1000:

2315.95 ml · min^{-1} ÷ 1000 = 2.31595 L · min^{-1}

h. Finally, we can find out how many calories she is expending per minute by multiplying 2.31595 by the constant 5.0:

2.31595 L · min^{-1} · 5.0 = 11.58 kcal · min^{-1}

16–D. This problem expands on problem #15. We established that she is expending 11.58 kcal per minute. The steps are as follows:
  a. Multiply 11.58 kcal per minute by the total number of minutes she exercises (45 minutes × 3 sessions per week = 135 total minutes):

11.58 kcal per minute x 135 total minutes = 1563.3 total calories expended

  b. To find out how many pounds of fat she will lose per week, divide the total calories expended by 3500 (because there are 3500 kcal in one pound of fat):

1563.3 kcal ÷ 3500 = 0.4466 pounds of fat per week of exercise

17–A. The steps are as follows:
  a. Choose the ACSM leg cycling formula.
  b. Write down your knowns and convert the values to the appropriate units:
    Knowns: 6 METs · 3.5 = 21 ml · kg^{-1} · min^{-1}
    80 kg = body weight
  c. Write down the ACSM leg cycling formula:

Leg cycling (ml · kg^{-1} · min^{-1}) = (1.8 · work rate ÷ body weight) + (3.5) + (3.5)

  d. Substitute the known values for the variable name:

21 = (1.8 · work rate ÷ 80) + (3.5) + (3.5)

Assuming he does 50 RPM (or 300 m · min^{-1}):

21 = (1.8 x (F · 300 m · min^{-1} ÷ 80) + (3.5) + (3.5)

  e. Move all of the knowns to one side of the equation, and leave the unknown on the other:

14 = 1.8 · 300 (F) ÷ 80

1120 ÷ 540 = 540 (F) ÷ 540

2.07 = force

About 2.0 kg = force needed

18–B. The steps are as follows:
  a. Choose the ACSM running formula.
  b. Write down your knowns and convert the values to the appropriate units:
    Knowns: 40 ml · kg^{-1} · min^{-1} = relative V̇O$_2$
    Level treadmill = 0% grade

  c. Write down the ACSM running formula:

Running (ml · kg^{-1} · min^{-1}) = (0.2 · speed) + (0.9 · speed · fractional grade) + (3.5)

  d. Substitute the known values for the variable name:

40 = (0.2 · speed) + (0) + (3.5)

  e. Solve for the unknown:

36.5 = 0.2 (speed)

182.5 m · min^{-1} = speed

  f. Convert to m · min^{-1} to mph by dividing m · min^{-1} by 26.8:

182.5 m · min^{-1} ÷ 26.8 = 6.8 mph

19–A. No metabolic formula is needed. The steps are as follows:
  a. Multiply the number of calories per week she is eliminating by the number of weeks:

1200 kcal per week · 26 weeks = 31200 total kcal

  b. Now divide by 3500 to get the total pounds she will lose:

31200 ÷ 3500 total kcal = 8.9 or about 9 pounds over 26 weeks

20–C. No metabolic formula is needed for this question either. The steps are as follows:
  a. One mile of walking or running expends about 100 kcal. Since she walks 1 mile 3 times per week, she expends about 300 kcal per week. Multiply 300 kcal by 26 weeks to determine the total amount of calories she expends by walking:

300 kcal per week · 26 weeks = 7800 kcal

  b. Divide 7800 kcal by 3500 to see how many pounds of fat this represents:

7800 kcal ÷ 3500 = 2.22 pounds or about 2 pounds

So she would lose about 11 pounds over 26 weeks if she incorporated walking into her weight loss program.

CHAPTER 12

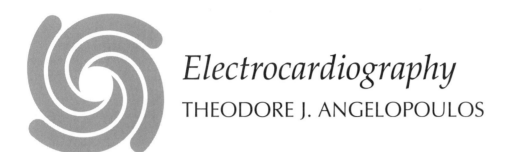

Electrocardiography
THEODORE J. ANGELOPOULOS

I. ELECTRICAL ACTIVITY OF THE HEART AND BASIC ELECTROCARDIOGRAM WAVES

–The electrocardiogram (ECG) records differences in electrical potential (voltage) between two electrodes placed on the skin.

–The electrical conduction system is shown in **Figure 12-1**.

A. PRINCIPLES OF ELECTROPHYSIOLOGY

1. All myocardial cells can be excited in response to external electrical, chemical, and mechanical stimuli.

2. The myocardium comprises ordinary contractile cells located in the atria and

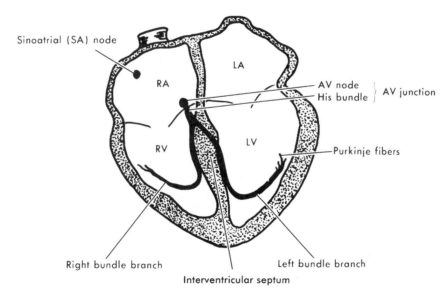

FIGURE 12-1 Conduction system of the heart. Normally the cardiac stimulus is generated in the *sinoatrial (SA) node,* which is located in the *right atrium (RA).* The stimulus then spreads through the *RA* and *left atrium (LA).* Next it spreads through the *atrioventricular (AV) node* and the *bundle of His,* which comprise the *AV junction.* The stimulus then passes into the *left* and *right ventricles (LV and RV)* by way of the *left* and *right bundle branches,* which are continuations of the bundle of His. Finally, the cardiac stimulus spreads to the ventricular muscle cells through the *Purkinje fibers.* (From Goldberger AL: *Clinical Electrocardiography: A Simplified Approach,* 6th ed. St Louis, Mosby, 1999, p 4.)

ventricles, as well as specialized cells that conduct electrical impulses.

3. Cardiac impulses normally arise in the heart's sinoatrial (SA), or sinus, node, located in the right atrium near the opening of the superior vena cava.

4. From the SA node, impulses travel first through the right atrium and then into the left atrium. Thus, the SA node functions as the heart's normal pacemaker.

5. The first phase of cardiac activation involves electrical stimulation of the right and left atria. This in turn signals the atria to contract and to pump blood simultaneously through the tricuspid and mitral valves into the right and left ventricles.

6. The electrical stimulus then spreads to specialized conduction tissues in the atrioventricular (AV) junction (which includes the AV node and the bundle of His) and then into the left and right bundle branches, which transmit the stimulus to the ventricular muscle cells.

7. In the resting period of the myocardial cell, the inside of the cell membrane is negatively charged and the outside of the cell membrane is positively charged. As such, the term "polarized cell" is reserved for the normal resting myocardial cell and describes the presence of electrical potential across the cell membrane due to separation of electrical charges.

8. When an electrical impulse is generated in a particular area in the heart, the outside of the cell in this area becomes negative, and the inside of the cell in the same area becomes positive. This excited state of the cell due to change in polarity is called **depolarization.**

   a. Cardiac impulses originate in the SA node and spread to both atria, causing **atrial depolarization,** represented on the ECG by a P wave.

   b. **Ventricular depolarization** is represented on the ECG by the QRS complex.

9. The return of the stimulated myocardial cells to their resting state is termed **repolarization.**

   a. **Atrial repolarization** is not usually seen on ECG, because it is obscured by ventricular potentials.

   b. **Ventricular repolarization** is represented on the ECG by the ST segment, T wave, and U wave.

B. PRINCIPLES OF ELECTROCARDIOGRAPHY

1. The movement of ions inside and across the membrane of myocardial cells constitutes a flow of electrical charge (ionic current) that is recorded on the ECG.

2. Cardiac electrical potentials are recorded on special ECG graph paper that, under standard conditions, travels at a speed of 25 mm/second.

   a. **Horizontally, the ECG measures duration;** each small square is 0.04 second in duration, and each large square is 0.20 second in duration.

   b. **Vertically, the ECG measures voltages.** Because ECGs are standardized, 1 mV of electrical potential registers a deflection of 10 mm in amplitude.

C. ELEMENTS OF ECG WAVEFORMS (Figure 12-2)

1. The **P wave** is a small positive (or negative) deflection preceding the QRS complex.

2. A **QRS complex** may be composed of a Q wave, an R wave, and an S wave.

   a. A **Q wave** is a negative deflection of the QRS complex preceding an R wave.

   b. An **R wave** is the first positive deflection of the QRS complex.

   c. An **S wave** is a negative deflection of the QRS complex following an R wave.

3. The **ST segment** is that portion of the ECG from the point where the S wave of the QRS ends (**J point**) to the beginning of the T wave.

   –The ST segment should be isoelectric.

   –The ST segment is considered a sensitive indicator of myocardial ischemia or infarction.

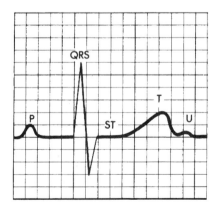

FIGURE 12-2 Basic ECG complexes. The P wave represents atrial depolarization. The PR interval is the time from initial stimulation of the atria to initial stimulation of the ventricles. The QRS represents ventricular depolarization. The ST segment, T wave, and U wave are produced by ventricular repolarization. (From Goldberger AL: *Clinical Electrocardiography: A Simplified Approach,* 6th ed. St Louis, Mosby, 1999, p 8.)

4. The **PR interval** is measured from the beginning of the P wave to the beginning of the QRS complex, and reflects the time needed for the impulse to spread through the atria and to pass through the atrioventricular (AV) junction.

   –The normal PR interval is 0.12–0.20 second.

   –A PR interval prolonged for > 0.20 second with all P waves being conducted and all PR intervals the same indicates first-degree AV block.

5. The **QRS interval** is measured from the beginning of the first wave of the QRS complex to the end of the last wave of the QRS complex.

   –The normal range is 0.04–0.11 second.

6. The **QT interval** is measured from the beginning of the QRS complex to the end of the T wave.

   –Normal QT intervals depend on HR.

   –Factors such as certain drugs, electrolyte disturbances, and myocardial ischemia and infarction may prolong the QT interval.

   –The QT interval may be shortened as result of drug therapy or electrolyte imbalance.

7. The **T wave** represents ventricular repolarization.

   –Normal T waves lack symmetry.

   –Prominent peaked T waves may indicate myocardial infarction or hyperkalemia.

   –Deep, symmetrically inverted T waves suggest myocardial ischemia.

8. The **U wave** represents the last phase of ventricular repolarization.

   –The U wave is frequently hard to detect in a normal ECG. When present, it appears as a small deflection after the T wave.

   –U waves are prominent in hypokalemia and left ventricular hypertrophy.

   –Inverted U waves suggest ischemia.

D. **THE 12-LEAD ECG**

   –represents 12 electrically different views of the heart recorded on special ECG paper.

   1. The 12 leads can be subdivided into three groups (**Figure 12-3**):

      a. **Bipolar standard leads I, II, and III**

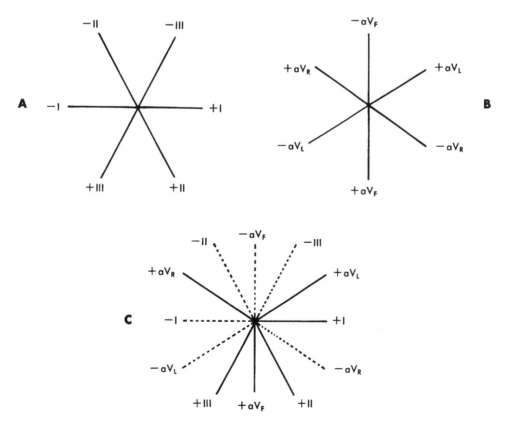

FIGURE 12-3 Derivation of hexaxial lead diagram. **(A)** Triaxial diagram of the bipolar leads (I, II, and III). **(B)** Triaxial diagram of the unipolar leads (aV$_R$, aV$_L$, and aV$_F$). **(C)** The two triaxial diagrams can be combined into a hexaxial diagram that shows the relationship of all six extremity leads. The negative pole of each lead is now indicated by a dashed line. (From Goldberger AL: *Clinical Electrocardiography: A Simplified Approach,* 6th ed. St Louis, Mosby, 1999, p 26.)

b. **Unipolar augmented leads aVR, aVL, and aVF**

c. **Unipolar precordial leads V$_1$–V$_6$**

2. Leads I, II, III, aVR, aVL, and aVF are collectively called **limb leads** because they record potential differences through electrodes placed on limbs.

    a. **Lead I** records the difference in electrical potential between the left arm (positive) and right arm (negative) electrodes.

    b. **Lead II** records the difference in electrical potential between the left leg (positive) and right arm (negative) electrodes.

    c. **Lead III** records the difference in electrical potential between the left leg (positive) and left arm (negative) electrodes.

    d. The **augmented unipolar leads** record electrical potentials at one site relative to zero potential. Electrical potentials are augmented electronically by the ECG.

        (1) For **lead aVR,** the positive electrode is placed on the right arm.

        (2) For **lead aVL,** the positive electrode is placed on the left arm.

        (3) For **lead aVF,** the positive electrode is placed on the left foot.

3. The six **unipolar precordial leads** view the heart's electrical activity in the horizontal plane. An electrode is placed on six different positions on the chest.

    a. **V$_1$:** at the fourth intercostal space on the right sternal border

    b. **V$_2$:** at the fourth intercostal space on the left sternal border

    c. **V$_3$:** at the midpoint of a straight line between leads V$_2$ and V$_4$

    d. **V$_4$:** at the fifth intercostal space, on the left midclavicular line

    e. **V$_5$:** on the anterior axillary line and horizontal to lead V$_4$

    f. **V$_6$:** on the midaxillary line and horizontal to leads V$_4$ and V$_5$

4. The **mean QRS axis** represents the average direction of depolarization as it travels through the ventricles, resulting in excitation and contraction of myocardial fibers.

    –The mean QRS axis can be calculated by simply inspecting leads I, II, III, aVR, aVL, and aVF and applying the following general rules:

    a. The mean QRS axis is directed midway between two leads that register tall R waves of equal amplitude.

    b. The mean QRS axis is directed at right angles (90°) to any extremity lead that registers a biphasic isoelectric complex; for example, in **Figure 12-4**, the mean QRS axis is +90°.

        (1) Axes between -30° and +100° are normal.

        (2) An axis more negative than –30° is considered **left axis deviation** (LAD).

        (3) An axis more positive than +100° is considered **right axis deviation** (RAD).

5. **Heart rate** (HR) is the number of times that the myocardium depolarizes and contracts (beats) in 1 minute.

    –Several techniques are available for determining HR.

    a. If the HR is regular, then the constant 300 is divided by number of large boxes between two consecutive QRS complexes.

    b. If HR is irregular, then the number of cardiac cycles (cardiac cycle: unit between two consecutive R waves) over a 6-second period is multiplied by 10. For example, in **Figure 12-5**, the HR is 100 beats/minute.

II. ARRHYTHMIAS AND CONDUCTION DISTURBANCES

A. SINUS ARRHYTHMIAS (Figure 12-6)

1. **Sinus bradycardia** is characterized by a normal sinus rhythm but with an HR < 60 beats/minute.

2. **Sinus tachycardia** is characterized by a normal sinus rhythm but with an HR of 100–180 beats/minute.

3. Under certain circumstances, the SA node does not maintain a regular sinus rate from beat to beat. This condition is called **sinus arrhythmia** (i.e., respiratory arrhythmia).

4. **Sinus pause (sinus arrest).** The SA node may fail to depolarize the atria for pathological

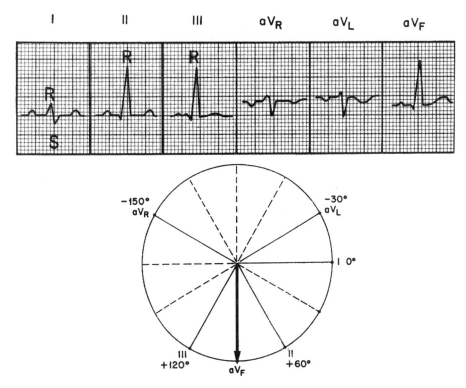

FIGURE 12-4 Mean QRS axis of +90°. (From Goldberger AL: *Clinical Electrocardiography: A Simplified Approach*, 6th ed. St Louis, Mosby, 1999, p 46.)

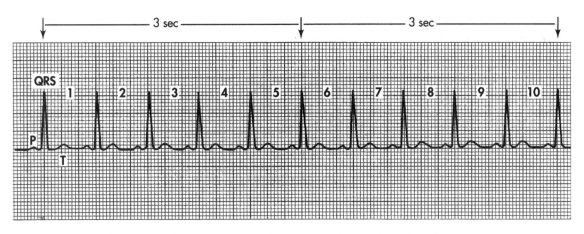

FIGURE 12-5 Measurement of heart rate (beats per minute) by counting the number of cardiac cycles in a 6-second interval and multiplying this number by 10. In this example, 10 cardiac cycles occur in 6 seconds. Therefore the heart rate is 10 × 10 = 100 beats/min. The arrows point to 3-second markers. (From Goldberger AL: *Clinical Electrocardiography: A Simplified Approach*, 6th ed. St Louis, Mosby, 1999, p 16.)

reasons. This condition, differentiated by the absence of P wave or QRS complex, is termed **sinus pause,** or **sinus arrest.** This condition may lead to cardiac arrest unless the AV node or some other focus assumes the role as pacemaker.

B. ATRIAL ARRHYTHMIAS

1. Atrial flutter and atrial fibrillation (Figure 12-7)

–In these arrhythmias, the atria are stimulated not from the SA node, but rather from some ectopic focus or foci.

–The rate of atrial contraction varies from 250–350 beats/minute for atrial flutter and from 400–600 beats/minute for atrial fibrillation.

–With either atrial flutter or atrial fibrillation, the rate of ventricular depolarization depends

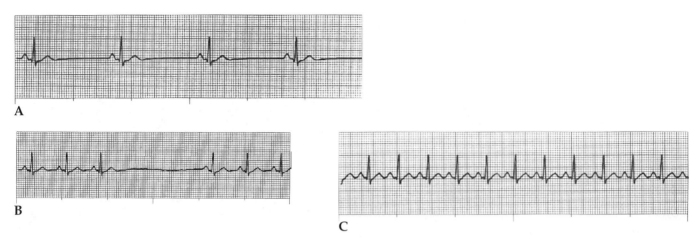

FIGURE 12-6 **(A)** Sinus bradycardia. **(B)** Sinus arrest. **(C)** Sinus Tachycardia. (From Aehlert B: *ECGs Made Easy Pocket Reference.* St Louis, Mosby, 1995, p 25, 29, 26.)

carotid massage begins

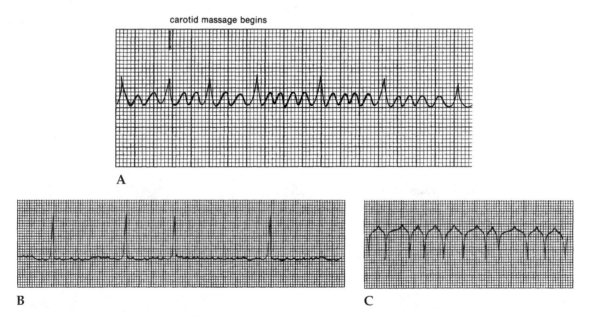

FIGURE 12-7 **(A)** Atrial flutter. Carotid massage increases the block from 3:1 to 5:1. **(B)** Atrial fibrillation with a slow, irregular ventricular rate. **(C)** Another example of atrial fibrillation. In the absence of a clearly fibrillating baseline, the only clue that this rhythm is atrial fibrillation is the irregularly irregular appearance of the QRS complex. (From Thaler MS: *The Only EKG Book You'll Ever Need,* 3rd ed. Philadelphia, Lippincott Williams & Wilkins, 1999, pp 125–126.)

on the rate at which the AV node conducts the supraventricular stimuli.

–The presence of characteristic "sawtooth" waves differentiates atrial flutter, and the absence of P waves and irregular ventricular response characterize atrial fibrillation.

–Atrial flutter and atrial fibrillation can occur in otherwise healthy people as well as in those with heart disease.

2. Supraventricular tachycardia (SVT)
(Figure 12-8)

–is a supraventricular ectopic rhythm with an HR of 140–250 beats/minute.

–Distinguishing features include a regular HR, ectopic P waves, a PR interval that may be normal, and a QRS complex that is typically normal.

C. JUNCTIONAL ARRHYTHMIA (Figure 12-9)

–is a supraventricular ectopic rhythm that results from a focus of automaticity located in the bundle of His.

–ECG waveform characteristics include a regular rhythm, HR of 100–140 beats/minute, normal QRS interval, and P waves (when present) possibly appearing upright or retrograde.

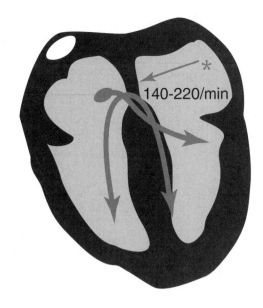

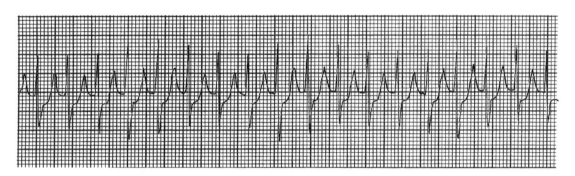

FIGURE 12-8 Atrial tachycardia. (From Davis D: *Quick and Accurate 12-Lead ECG Interpretation,* 3rd ed. Philadelphia, Lippincott Williams & Wilkins, 2001, p 412.)

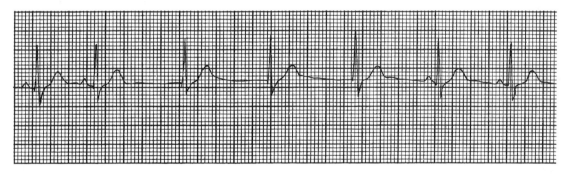

FIGURE 12-9 Sinus rhythm with three junctional escape beats. (From Davis D: *Quick and Accurate 12-Lead ECG Interpretation,* 3rd ed. Philadelphia, Lippincott Williams & Wilkins, 2001, p 408.)

D. VENTRICULAR ARRHYTHMIAS

1. Premature ventricular complexes (PVCs)

–are premature ventricular depolarizations that occur in one of the ventricles and spread to the other ventricle with some delay due to slow conduction through the ventricular myocardial fibers. The ventricles are not depolarized simultaneously, and the duration of the QRS is ≥ 0.12 second.

–PVCs are common in normal individuals and also in patients with organic heart disease. Common causes include emotional stress, electrolyte abnormalities, drug therapy, and myocardial ischemia and/or infarction.

–PVCs linked to acute myocardial infarction are sometimes the forerunners of ventricular tachycardia and ventricular fibrillation.

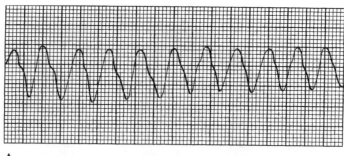

A

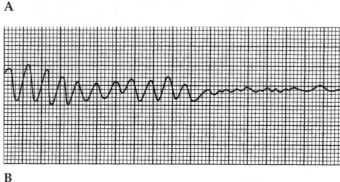

B

FIGURE 12-10 (A) Ventricular tachycardia. The rate is about 200 beats per minute. **(B)** Ventricular tachycardia degenerates into ventricular fibrillation. (From Thaler MS: *The Only EKG Book You'll Ever Need,* 3rd ed. Philadelphia, Lippincott Williams & Wilkins, 1999, p 132,133.)

–PVCs may occur with varying frequency:

   a. Two PVCs occurring in a row is referred to as a **ventricular couplet.**

   b. Three or more PVCs in a row constitute **ventricular tachycardia (Figure 12-10).**

   c. The repetitive pattern of one normal beat and one PVC is called **ventricular bigeminy.**

   d. The repetitive pattern of two normal beats and a PVC is called **ventricular trigeminy.**

2. Ventricular escape

   –is late in relation to the normal R–R cycle, and the QRS is wide.

3. Ventricular fibrillation

   –is often triggered by the simultaneous conduction of ischemic ventricular cells with enhanced automaticity in multiple locations of the ventricles.

   –Distinguishing features include a regular rhythm, a ventricular rate of 150–500 beats/minute, fibrillatory waves, and the absence of a distinct QRS complex.

   –Ventricular fibrillation may occur spontaneously in patients with organic heart disease and is considered the most common cause of sudden cardiac death in patients during an acute myocardial infarction.

   –Ventricular fibrillation necessitates defibrillation.

E. ATRIOVENTRICULAR (AV) BLOCKS (Figure 12-11)

–result when supraventricular impulses are delayed or blocked in the AV node or intraventricular conduction system.

1. First-degree AV block

   –is characterized by a delay in the conduction of the impulse through the AV junction to the ventricles.

   –does not impair cardiac function.

   –The PR interval is > 0.20 seconds.

   –Causes include hyperkalemia, quinidine, digitalis, and ischemic heart disease.

2. Second-degree AV block

   –is subdivided into two types: Mobitz I and Mobitz II.

   a. Mobitz I (Wenckebach AV) block

      –Impulse conduction through the AV junction becomes increasingly more difficult, causing a progressively longer PR interval until a P wave is not conducted. As such, the ECG shows a P wave not followed by a QRS complex, which indicates that the AV junction failed to conduct the impulse from the atria to the ventricles. However, this pause allows the AV node to recover, and the following P wave is conducted with a normal or slightly shorter PR interval.

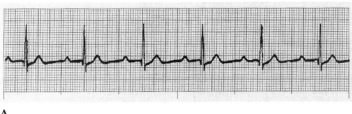

A

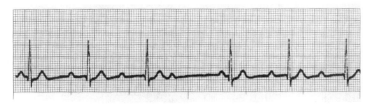

B

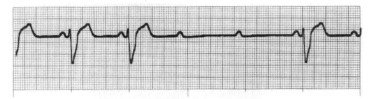

C

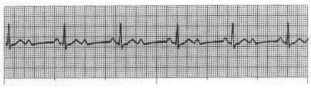

D

FIGURE 12-11 **(A)** Sinus rhythm (borderline sinus bradycardia) at 60 beats per minute with a first-degree AV block. **(B)** Second-degree AV block type I. **(C)** Second-degree AV block type II. **(D)** Second-degree AV block, 2:1 conduction, probably type I. (From Aehlert B: *ECGs Made Easy Pocket Reference.* St Louis, Mosby, 1995, p 61, 62, 63, 64.)

–Causes include certain drugs (digitalis, calcium-channel blockers), ischemic heart disease, and inferior wall myocardial infarction.

b. **Mobitz II block**

–is a delay in AV conduction at the level of the bundle branches.

–is characterized by fixed, normal PR intervals, broad QRS complexes, and nonconducted P waves (dropped beats).

–Causes include anterior wall myocardial infarction and severe conduction system disease.

–Patients with Mobitz II are often considered candidates for a pacemaker.

3. **Third-degree AV block**

–is also called **complete heart block,** because there is no conduction of impulses from the atria to the ventricles.

–Because there is no relationship between the P waves and the QRS complexes, the PR interval changes continually.

–The atria are usually under the control of the sinus node, so that P waves are present with a normal atrial rate.

–The ventricles are paced by a pacemaker located below the point of blockage in the AV junction, so that QRS complexes are seen with a ventricular rate of 30–60 beats/minute. These QRS complexes are of normal or prolonged duration, depending on the pacemaker location.

–Third-degree AV block may occur because of advanced age, digitalis intoxication, or myocardial infarction.

–Patients with third-degree AV block that is not transient (i.e., due to digitalis intoxication) are good candidates for pacemaker implantation.

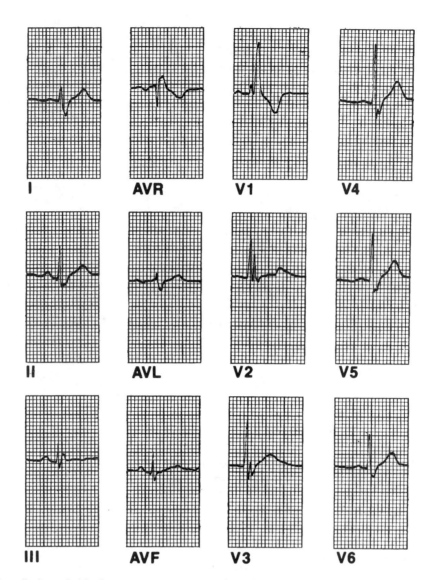

FIGURE 12-12 Right bundle branch block. (From Davis D: *Quick and Accurate 12-Lead ECG Interpretation,* 3rd ed. Philadelphia, Lippincott Williams & Wilkins, 2001, p 155.)

4. **Bundle branch blocks**
   a. **Right bundle branch block (RBBB)**

   –represents a delay in impulse conduction through the right bundle branch (**Figure 12-12**).

   –As a result of delayed depolarization of the right ventricle, the QRS complex is widened (> 0.12 second).

   –Lead V_1 shows an rSR' with a wide R wave, a characteristic ECG change associated with RBBB.

   –Although RBBB may be due to heart disease, it can be present in the absence of organic heart disease.

   b. **Left bundle branch block (LBBB)**

   –represents a delay in impulse conduction through the left bundle branch (**Figure 12-13**).

   –The impulse travels through the right bundle branch and then across the septum, and depolarizes the left ventricle.

   –As a result of delayed depolarization of the left ventricle, the QRS complex is widened (> 0.12 second).

   –Inspection of leads V_1 and V_6 confirms LBBB. A wide negative deflection (QS) is present in lead V_1; lead V_6 shows a wide and tall R wave.

   –LBBB is commonly associated with organic heart disease (e.g., coronary artery disease, hypertension, cardiomyopathy, left ventricular hypertrophy).

5. **Hemiblocks**

   –are blocks involving the anterior or posterior fascicle of the main left bundle branch of the bundle of His.

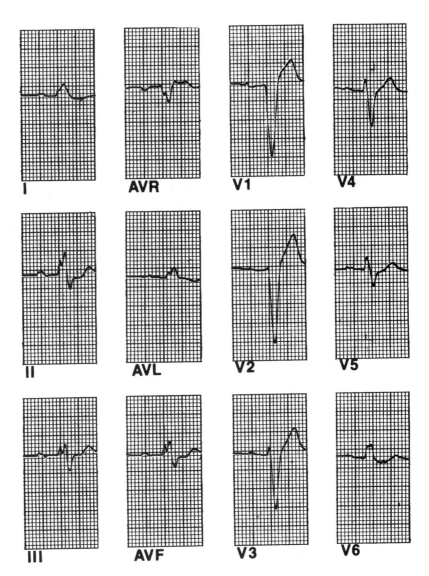

FIGURE 12-13   Left bundle branch block. (From Davis D: *Quick and Accurate 12-Lead ECG Interpretation*, 3rd ed. Philadelphia, Lippincott Williams & Wilkins, 2001, p 159.)

a. Left anterior fascicular block

–is a block in impulse conduction through the anterior fascicle of the main left bundle branch so that the impulse continues down the posterior fascicle.

–A mean QRS axis of > -45° coupled with a QRS duration of < 0.12 second suggests left anterior hemiblock.

b. Left posterior fascicular block

–is a block in impulse conduction through the posterior fascicle of the main left bundle branch, so that the impulse continues to travel down the posterior fascicle of the main left bundle branch.

–A mean QRS axis of > +120° coupled with a QRS duration of < 0.12 second suggest left posterior hemiblock.

III. ECG PATTERNS IN SELECTED DISORDERS

A. CORONARY ARTERY DISEASE (CAD)

–In exercise ECG, usually performed on a treadmill or cycle ergometer, a horizontal or down-sloping ST depression of at least 1 mm lasting for 0.08 second is considered an abnormal test finding and may signify CAD. T wave abnormalities also may be seen in patients with CAD.

B. MYOCARDIAL ISCHEMIA AND INFARCTION

–Myocardial ischemia may occur transiently and may be limited to the inner heart layer (subendocardial ischemia) or may affect the entire thickness of the ventricular wall (transmural ischemia).

–If the myocardial oxygen supply remains inadequate, injury (necrosis) will occur. **Myocardial infarction (MI)** is myocardial injury due to severe ischemia.

–**Table 12-1** summarizes the ECG leads associated with various areas of myocardial injury. **Figures 12-14 and 12-15** illustrate anterior and inferior infarction.

1. **Transmural ischemia with MI**

    –Transmural MI causes changes in both the QRS and ST-T complexes.

    a. ST elevation, or tall, upright T waves, is the earliest sign of transmural MI.

    b. ST elevations may persist for a few hours to a few days. Over this period, Q waves will be formed in those leads showing ST segment elevations.

    c. During the evolving phase, ST segment elevations may return to baseline, and T waves may become inverted.

    d. The Q waves may persist for years following a transmural MI; however, their amplitude decreases and in some cases they may disappear.

    e. In most cases, inverted T waves persist indefinitely over the infarcted area following a transmural MI.

    –Transmural MIs are localized to a specific portion of the left ventricular wall supplied by one of the coronary arteries: left anterior descending artery (LAD), right coronary artery (RCA), and left circumflex (LCx).

    –A transmural MI can be diagnosed by the presence of abnormal Q waves (> 0.04 second and at least 25% of the height of the R wave).

    –Q waves in leads V_1 and V_2 should be examined carefully, because they can be a normal variant or may signify anterior septal MI.

    –An infarction can be determined and localized by careful inspection of certain ECG leads; for example, tall R waves in leads V_1 and V_2 may suggest posterior wall MI or right ventricular hypertrophy.

2. **Subendocardial ischemia and infarction**

    –Subendocardial ischemia usually produces ST segment depression in anterior leads, inferior leads, or both, commonly during attacks of typical angina pectoris.

    –A horizontal or downsloping ST depression of 1 mm lasting 0.08 second is considered an abnormal response during exercise ECG and constitutes a positive exercise test response.

    –Severe subendocardial ischemia may lead to **subendocardial infarction,** marked by persistent ST depression, possible T wave inversion, and usually normal Q waves.

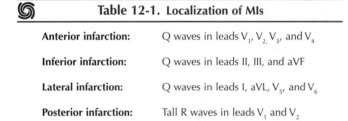

Table 12-1. Localization of MIs

Anterior infarction:	Q waves in leads V_1, V_2, V_3, and V_4
Inferior infarction:	Q waves in leads II, III, and aVF
Lateral infarction:	Q waves in leads I, aVL, V_5, and V_6
Posterior infarction:	Tall R waves in leads V_1 and V_2

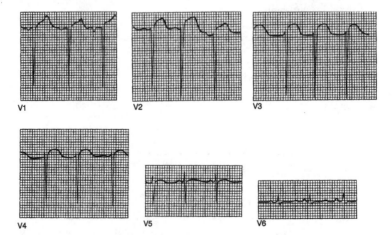

FIGURE 12-14 An anterior infarction with poor R wave progression across the precordium. (From Thaler MS: *The Only EKG Book You'll Ever Need,* 3rd ed. Philadelphia, Lippincott Williams & Wilkins, 1999, p 221.)

C. ATRIAL ENLARGEMENT

1. **Left atrial enlargement** is best demonstrated in lead V_1.

   –A wide P wave of ≥ 0.12 second is seen (**Figure 12-16 B**).

–P wave voltage is normal or slightly increased.

–Sometimes the terminal portion of the P wave, which represents left atrial depolarization, shows a distinct wide negative deflection. As such, lead V_1 may show a biphasic P wave.

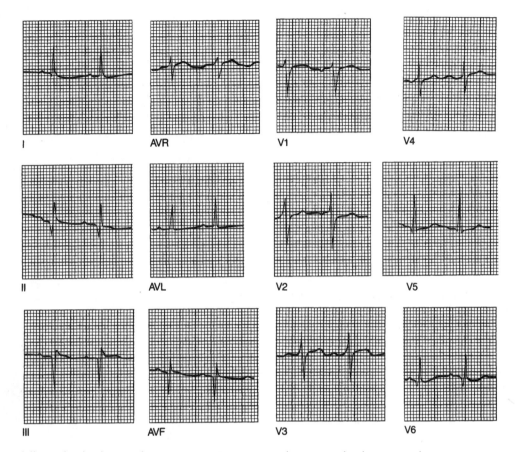

FIGURE 12-15 A fully evolved inferior infarction. Deep Q waves can be seen in leads II, III, and AVF. (From Thaler MS: *The Only EKG Book You'll Ever Need,* 3rd ed. Philadelphia, Lippincott Williams & Wilkins, 1999, p 219.)

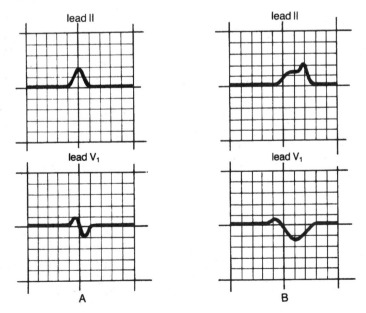

FIGURE 12-16 **(A)** The normal P wave in leads II and V_1. **(B)** Left atrial enlargement. Note the increased amplitude and duration of the terminal, left atrial component of the P wave. (From Thaler MS: *The Only EKG Book You'll Ever Need,* 3rd ed. Philadelphia, Lippincott Williams & Wilkins, 1999, p 80.)

–Wide P waves are often referred to as **P mitrale,** because they are often seen in patients with rheumatic mitral valve disease.

2. **Right atrial enlargement** is best detected in lead II (**Figure 12-17B**).

–P wave amplitude may be increased to > 2.5 mm.

–P wave duration may be normal.

–The tall P wave seen in right atrial enlargement is called **P pulmonale,** because it is common in patients with pulmonary disease.

D. VENTRICULAR HYPERTROPHY

–An increase in the size of either ventricular wall may produce high voltages in the leads over the hypertrophied area.

1. **Left ventricular hypertrophy (LVH)** (**Figure 12-18**)

–typically produces abnormally tall R waves in the left chest leads and abnormally deep S waves in the right chest leads.

–Voltage criteria for the diagnosis of LVH are S wave in lead V_1 + R wave in lead V_5 or V_6 > 35 mm, or R wave in lead aVL > 11 mm.

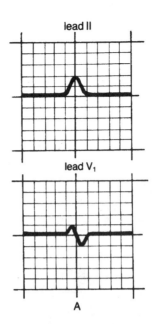
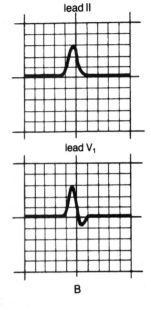

FIGURE 12-17 **(A)** The normal P wave in leads II and V_1. **(B)** Right atrial enlargement. Note the increased amplitude of the early, right atrial component of the P wave. The terminal left atrial component, and hence the overall duration of the P wave, is essentially unchanged. (From Thaler MS: *The Only EKG Book You'll Ever Need,* 3rd ed. Philadelphia, Lippincott Williams & Wilkins, 1999, p 79.)

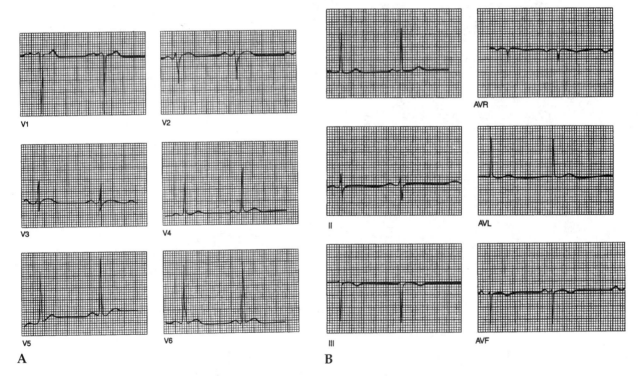

FIGURE 12-18 **(A)** Left ventricular hypertrophy in the precordial leads. Three of the four criteria are met: the R wave amplitude in V_5 plus the S wave amplitude in V_1 exceeds 35 mm, the R wave amplitude in V_6 exceeds 18 mm, and the R wave amplitude in lead V_6 slightly exceeds the R wave amplitude in lead V_5. The only criterion not met is for the R wave in lead V_5 to exceed 26 mm. **(B)** Left ventricular hypertrophy in the limb leads. Criteria 1, 3 and 4 are met; only criterion 2, regarding the R wave amplitude in lead AVF, is not met. (From Thaler MS: *The Only EKG Book You'll Ever Need,* 3rd ed. Philadelphia, Lippincott Williams & Wilkins, 1999, p 85, 86.)

–ST changes and T wave inversions are usually present in leads showing tall R waves.

–LVH is commonly associated with conditions such as aortic stenosis and systemic hypertension.

2. Right ventricular hypertrophy (RVH)
(Figure 12-19)

–produces high voltages in leads V_1 and V_2 and possibly an R wave greater than the S wave in these leads.

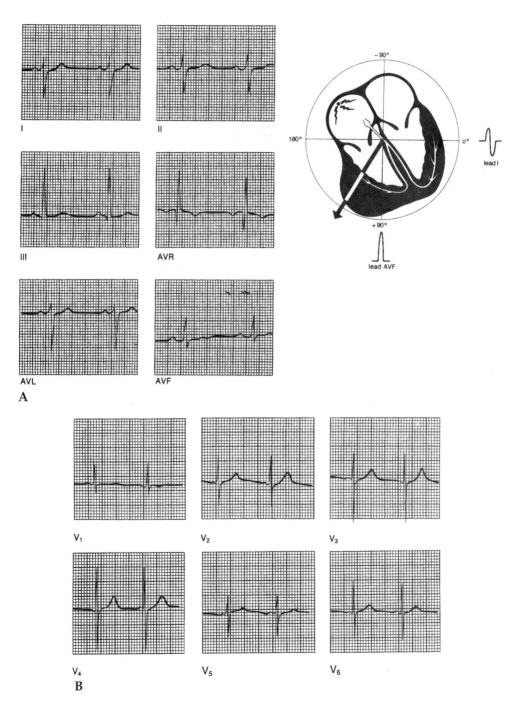

FIGURE 12-19 **(A)** Right ventricular hypertrophy shifts the axis of the QRS complex to the right. The EKG tracings confirm right axis deviation. In addition, the QRS complex in lead I is slightly negative, a criterion that many believe is essential for properly establishing the diagnosis of right ventricular hypertrophy. *(B)* In lead V_1, the R wave is larger than the S wave. In lead V_6, the S wave is larger than the R wave. (From Thaler MS: *The Only EKG Book You'll Ever Need,* 3rd ed. Philadelphia, Lippincott Williams & Wilkins, 1999, p 82, 83.)

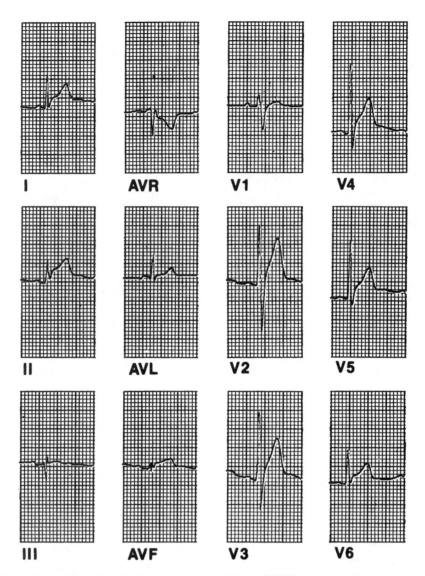

FIGURE 12-20 Pericarditis. (From Davis D: *Quick and Accurate 12-Lead ECG Interpretation,* 3rd ed. Philadelphia, Lippincott Williams & Wilkins, 2001, p 248.)

–RVH also causes right axis deviation and ST changes and T wave inversions in right chest leads.

E. PERICARDITIS

–Acute pericarditis (inflammation of the pericardium) is associated with diffuse ST segment elevation (in contrast to the localized ST segment elevation seen in acute MI), possibly followed by T wave inversion (**Figure 12-20**).

F. PULMONARY DISEASE

–Patients with emphysema (chronic lung disease) often exhibit such ECG changes as low voltage, poor R wave progression in chest leads, and a vertical or rightward QRS axis.

G. HYPERTENSIVE HEART DISEASE

–commonly causes left ventricular hypertrophy that eventually leads to left atrial enlargement.

–Patients with long-standing hypertensive disease often develop LBBB and, in some cases, atrial fibrillation.

H. HYPERVENTILATION

– involves quick, deep breathing for approximately 20 seconds. This procedure is performed before or after a stress test, and any ECG changes are noted. Typical changes include ST segment and T wave abnormalities in all leads (**Figure 12-21**).

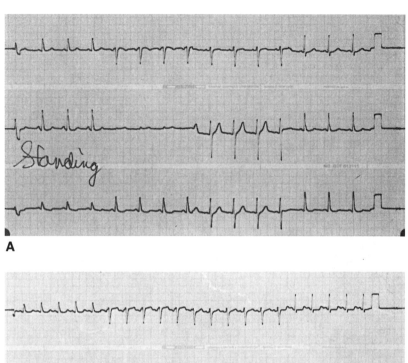

FIGURE 12-21 **(A)** Resting ECG. **(B)** ECG showing results of hyperventilation (i.e., inverted T waves).

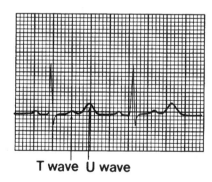

T wave U wave

FIGURE 12-22 Hypokalemia. The U waves are even more prominent than the T waves. (From Thaler MS: *The Only EKG Book You'll Ever Need,* 3rd ed. Philadelphia, Lippincott Williams & Wilkins, 1999, p 247.)

I. ELECTROLYTE ABNORMALITIES

1. **Hypokalemia** produces ST depression with prominent U waves and flattened T waves (**Figure 12-22**).

2. **Hyperkalemia** produces predictable ECG changes depending on severity (**Figure 12-23**).

    a. Mild hyperkalemia causes narrowing and peaking of T waves.

    b. Moderate hyperkalemia is marked by prolonged PR intervals and small or sometimes absent P waves.

    c. Severe hyperkalemia produces wide QRS complexes and asystole.

3. **Hypocalcemia** produces prolonged QT intervals (**Figure 12-24**).

4. **Hypercalcemia** shortens ventricular repolarization and thus shortens the QT interval (see **Figure 12-24**).

J. DRUG THERAPY

1. **Digitalis,** used to treat heart failure and arrhythmias, can produce a shortened QT interval and scooped ST-T complex (**Figure 12-25**). Digitalis toxicity often results in arrhythmias and conduction disturbances.

2. **Quinidine, procainamide,** and **disopyramide,** used to treat arrhythmias, can produce prolonged QT intervals and flattened T waves.

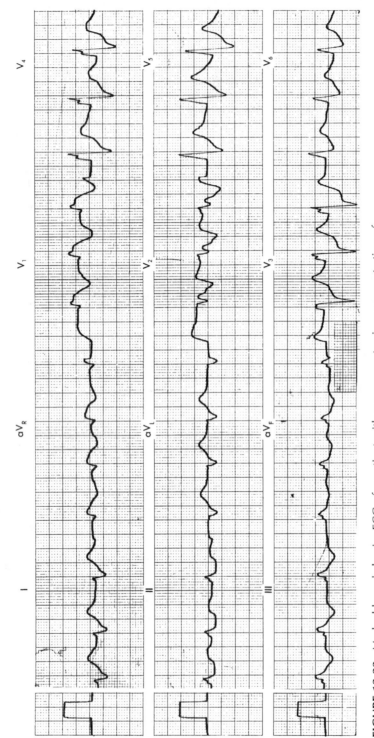

FIGURE 12-23 Marked hyperkalemia: ECG of a patient with a serum potassium concentration of 8.5 mEq/L. Notice the absence of P waves and the presence of bizarre, wide QRS complexes. (From Goldberger AL: *Clinical Electrocardiography: A Simplified Approach*, 6th ed. St Louis, Mosby, 1999, p 118.)

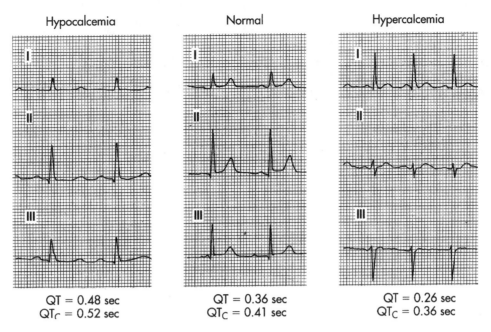

FIGURE 12-24 Hypocalcemia prolongs the QT interval by stretching out the ST segment. Hypercalcemia decreases the QT interval by shortening the ST segment so that the T wave seems to take off directly from the end of the QRS complex. (From Goldberger AL: *Clinical Electrocardiography: A Simplified Approach*, 6th ed. St Louis, Mosby, 1999, p 120.)

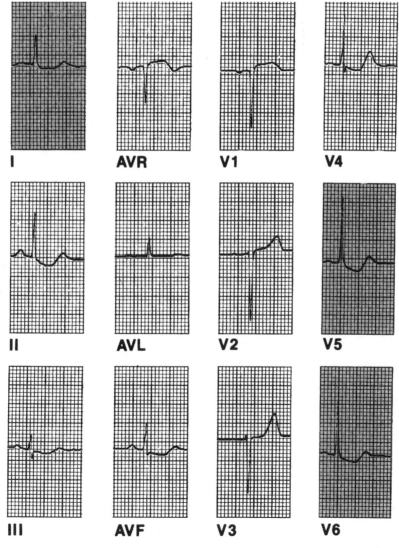

FIGURE 12-25 Digitalis effect. (From Davis D: *Quick and Accurate 12-Lead ECG Interpretation*, 3rd ed. Philadelphia, Lippincott Williams & Wilkins, 2001, p 263.)

REVIEW TEST

DIRECTIONS: Carefully read all questions and select the BEST single answer.

1. Slow conduction in the atrioventricular node is associated with
   (A) prolonged PR interval.
   (B) prolonged QRS interval.
   (C) shortened QT interval.
   (D) elevated ST segment.

2. Examine the six extremity leads shown in the figure below. What is the appropriate mean QRS axis?
   (A) -30°
   (B) 60°
   (C) 90°
   (D) 120°

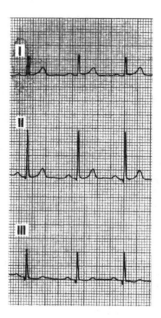
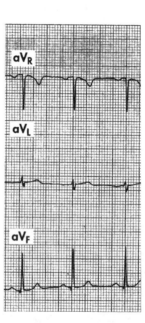

(From Goldberger AL: *Clinical Electrocardiography: A Simplified Approach,* 6th ed. St Louis, Mosby, 1999, p 55.)

3. In the ECG shown following, which of the following conduction abnormalities is indicated?
   (A) Right bundle branch block
   (B) Third-degree atrioventricular block
   (C) First-degree atrioventricular block
   (D) Mobitz I

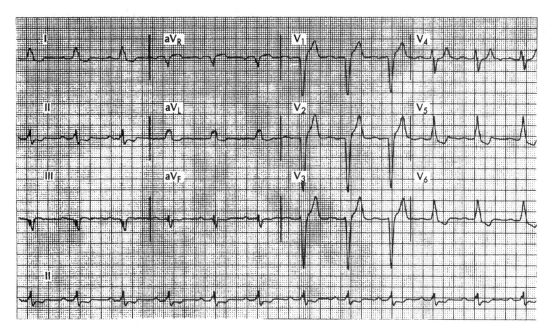

(From Goldberger AL: *Clinical Electrocardiography: A Simplified Approach,* 6th ed. St Louis, Mosby, 1999, p 80.)

4. What condition can cause ST segment elevation?
    (A) Digitalis toxicity
    (B) Hypocalcemia
    (C) Hypokalemia
    (D) Acute pericarditis

5. In the ECG strip shown below, what disorder is indicated?
    (A) Acute pericarditis
    (B) Old inferior myocardial infarction
    (C) Old posterior myocardial infarction
    (D) Anterior myocardial infarction

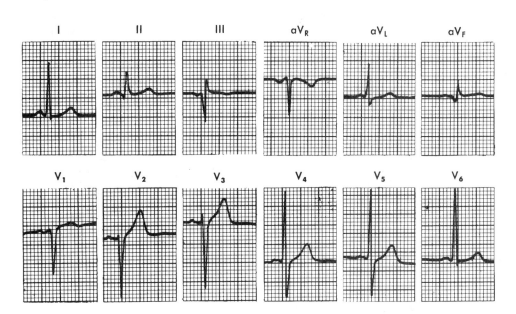

(From Goldberger AL: *Clinical Electrocardiography: A Simplified Approach,* 6th ed. St Louis, Mosby, 1999, p 91.)

6. In the ECG strip shown below, what disorder is indicated?
   (A) Subendocardial ischemia
   (B) Transmural ischemia
   (C) Acute inferior myocardial infarction
   (D) Posterior myocardial infarction

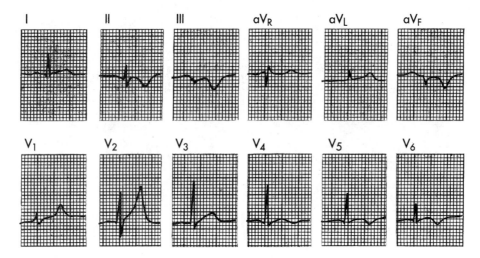

(From Goldberger AL: *Clinical Electrocardiography: A Simplified Approach,* 6th ed. St Louis, Mosby, 1999, p 91.)

7. In the ECG strip shown below, what abnormality is indicated?
   (A) Left bundle branch block
   (B) Posterior wall myocardial infarction
   (C) Right bundle branch block
   (D) Left ventricular hypertrophy

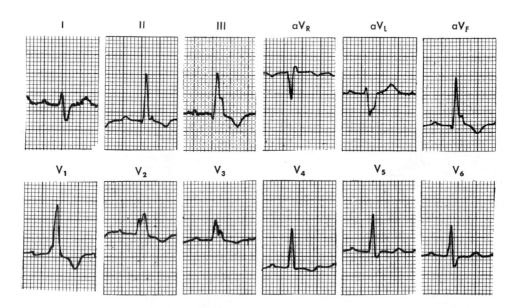

(From Goldberger AL: *Clinical Electrocardiography: A Simplified Approach,* 6th ed. St Louis, Mosby, 1999, p 70.)

8. Subendocardial ischemia usually produces
   (A) ST elevation.
   (B) ST depression.
   (C) Q waves.
   (D) U waves.

9. In the ECG strip shown below, which arrhythmia is present?
    (A) Premature ventricular contractions
    (B) Ventricular tachycardia
    (C) Ventricular trigeminy
    (D) Ventricular bigeminy

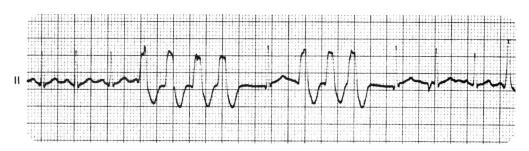

(From Goldberger AL: *Clinical Electrocardiography: A Simplified Approach,* 6th ed. St Louis, Mosby, 1999, p 167.)

10. In the ECG strip shown below, which arrhythmia is indicated?
    (A) Atrial flutter
    (B) Atrial fibrillation
    (C) Premature atrial contractions
    (D) Atrial tachycardia

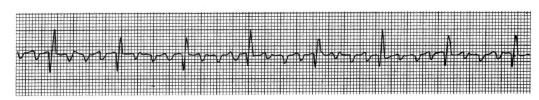

(From Goldberger AL: *Clinical Electrocardiography: A Simplified Approach,* 6th ed. St Louis, Mosby, 1999, p 164.)

11. Abnormally tall and peaked T waves suggest which of the following?
    (A) ~~Hypercalcemia~~ *HyperKalemia*
    (B) Acute pericarditis
    (C) ~~Acute myocardial infarction~~ *Right Bundle Branch Block*
    (D) Hypokalemia

12. Which of the following conditions can prolong the QT interval?
    (A) Hypokalemia and hypercalcemia
    (B) Hyperkalemia and hypercalcemia
    (C) Hypocalcemia and hypokalemia
    (D) Hypocalcemia and hyperkalemia

13. Differentiation between supraventricular and ventricular rhythm is made on the basis of the
    (A) duration (width) of the QRS complex and presence or absence of P waves.
    (B) appearance of the ST segment.
    (C) amplitude of the U wave.
    (D) duration of the PR interval.

14. Which of the following is one cause of a wide QRS complex?
    (A) Hypokalemia
    (B) Defective intraventricular conduction
    (C) Right atrial enlargement
    (D) Abnormal ST segment

15. In response to various stimuli, movements of ions occur, causing the rapid loss of the internal negative potential. This process is known as
    (A) polarization.
    (B) repolarization.
    (C) automaticity.
    (D) depolarization.

16. Digitalis effect refers to
    (A) scooped-out depression of the ST segment produced by digitalis.
    (B) elevation of the PR interval produced by digitalis.
    (C) shortening of the QT interval produced by digitalis.
    (D) prolongation of the QRS complex produced by digitalis.

17. Tall positive T waves may be due to all of the following EXCEPT
    (A) hyperacute phase of myocardial infarction.
    (B) left ventricular hypertrophy.
    (C) acute pericarditis.
    (D) hypocalcemia.

18. In the ECG strip shown below, what abnormalities are indicated?
    (A) Left atrial enlargement and left ventricular hypertrophy
    (B) Right atrial enlargement and right ventricular hypertrophy
    (C) Left anterior fascicular block and left posterior fascicular block
    (D) Subendocardial ischemia and infarction

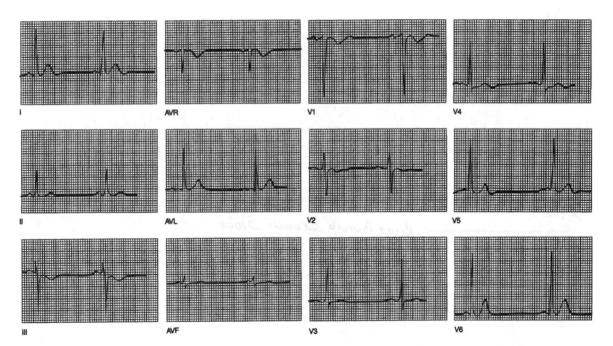

(From Thaler MS: *The Only EKG Book You'll Ever Need,* 3rd ed. Philadelphia, Lippincott Williams & Wilkins, 1999, p 87.)

19. Right axis deviation may be due to
    (A) acute pericarditis.
    (B) right atrial enlargement.
    (C) chronic obstructive pulmonary disease.
    (D) cardiomyopathy.

20. In atrial flutter, the stimulation rate is approximately
    (A) 75 beats/minute.
    (B) 125 beats/minute.
    (C) 200 beats/minute.
    (D) 300 beats/minute.

21. Myocardial cells can be excited in response to all of the following stimuli *except*
    (A) electrical.
    (B) chemical.
    (C) mechanical.
    (D) emotional.

22. The P wave on the electrocardiogram can be
    (A) negative.
    (B) positive.
    (C) isoelectric.
    (D) either positive or negative.

ANSWERS AND EXPLANATIONS

1–A. The PR interval represents the time that it takes for the stimulus to spread through the atria and pass through the atrioventricular (AV) junction. As such, slow conduction in the AV node affects the PR interval. Slow conduction through the AV node is not associated with the duration of the QRS complex or the QT interval.

2–B. The mean QRS axis is 60°. Notice the biphasic QRS complex in lead aVL. As such, the mean QRS axis must point at a right angle to –30°. Obviously, it points at 60°, because leads II, III, and aVF show positive QRS complexes.

3–C. Notice the QS in lead V_1 and the wide R wave in lead V_6. The PR interval is prolonged (> 0.20). As such, first-degree atrioventricular block is present. There is no progressive PR prolongation with a nonconducted P wave; therefore, Mobitz I is not present.

4–D. Acute pericarditis is associated with ST segment elevations. Digitalis produces scooping of the ST-T complex. Hypokalemia produces ST depression, and hypocalcemia prolongs the QT interval.

5–B. Notice the Q waves in leads II, III, and aVF. Posterior infarction produces tall R waves in leads V_1 and V_2. Anterior myocardial infarction results in the loss of R wave progression in the precordial leads and pathologic waves in one or more of the chest leads. Acute pericarditis produces diffuse ST segment elevations.

6–D. Notice the tall R waves in leads V_1 and V_2. Also notice the Q waves in leads III and aVF. Acute

inferior myocardial infarction produces ST segment elevation in leads II, III, and aVF.

7–C. Notice the wide notched R wave in lead V_2 and the secondary T wave inversions in leads V_1, V_2, II, III, and aVF. Left bundle branch block produces a wide QS in lead V_1 and a wide R wave in lead V_6. Posterior wall myocardial infarction produces tall R waves in leads V_1 and V_2 with ST segment depression in the same leads. Left ventricular hypertrophy produces high voltages, marked by tall R waves in lead V_5 or V_6 and deep S waves in lead V_1 or V_2.

8–B. Subendocardial ischemia usually produces ST depression. ST elevations usually appear in transmural ischemia, pericarditis, and acute myocardial infarction (MI). Q waves appear following transmural MI, and U waves are often seen in hypokalemia.

9–B. Ventricular tachycardia is defined as a run of three or more consecutive premature ventricular contractions (PVCs). In ventricular bigeminy, each normal sinus impulse is followed by a PVC. In ventricular trigeminy, a PVC is seen after every two sinus impulses.

10–A. Atrial flutter is characterized by "sawtooth" flutter waves instead of P waves, with a constant or variable ventricular rate. Atrial fibrillation shows fibrillatory waves instead of P waves and an irregular ventricular rate. Atrial tachycardia is defined as three or more consecutive premature atrial beats.

11–C. Hyperkalemia and acute myocardial infarction often show abnormally tall and peaked T waves. Hypokalemia often produces ST depressions with prominent U waves.

12–D. Hypokalemia often produces low-amplitude T waves and sometimes large U waves, which merge, resulting in a prolonged QT interval. Hypocalcemia primarily prolongs the ST segment, resulting in a prolonged QT interval. Hyperkalemia causes narrowed and peaked T waves.

13–A. A narrow QRS complex (< 0.1 second) indicates that the entire ventricular myocardium was depolarized quickly. This can occur only if electrical activation spreads along the ventricular conduction system. A wide QRS complex (> 0.10 second) suggests that electrical activation required considerable time to spread. As such, the impulse did not use the ventricular conduction system to travel. The duration of the PR interval is an indication of the time required for the impulse to travel from the SA node down to the AV node. The ST segment represents the beginning of ventricular repolarization, and U waves are characteristic of hypokalemia or drug therapy.

14–B.   A lesion in the ventricular conduction system will cause a slower spread of activation throughout the ventricles, leading to a wide QRS complex. Hypokalemia does not affect the duration of the QRS complex. Hypokalemia produces ST depressions and prominent U waves. The ST segment represents the beginning of ventricular repolarization and is not related to the duration of the QRS complex.

15–D.   In response to various stimuli, cations (mainly sodium) move inward, causing rapid loss of the internal negative potential. This process is known as depolarization. Polarization refers to the resting state of cardiac muscle cells where the interior of a cell is more negative compared to the exterior. Repolarization is the return of cardiac muscle cells to their resting negative potential. Automaticity refers to the ability of the heart to initiate its own beat.

16–A.   Digitalis effect refers to the characteristic scooped-out depression of the ST segment produced by therapeutic doses of digitalis. A therapeutic dose of digitalis does not produce ST segment elevation. ST segment elevations are often observed in myocardial ischemia or infarction, acute pericarditis, hyperkalemia, and left ventricular hypertrophy. Hypercalcemia is often associated with shortening of the QT interval due to shortening of the ST segment.

17–D.   The hyperacute phase of a myocardial infarction often produces tall positive T waves. Tall positive T waves are also seen in left ventricular

hypertrophy (left precordial leads). Acute pericarditis is occasionally associated with tall T waves.

18–C.   Left atrial enlargement is manifested by P wave duration of > 0.11 second, P wave notching, and a negative P wave deflection in V_1. Left ventricular hypertrophy is demonstrated by large R waves (> 27 mm) in lead V_5 plus deep waves in lead V_1. Left anterior hemiblock is associated with a mean QRS axis of –45° and a QRS width of < 0.12 second.

19–C.   Chronic obstructive pulmonary disease causes right axis deviation because of right ventricular overload. Any cause of right ventricular hypertrophy such as pulmonic stenosis or primary pulmonary hypertension is also associated with right axis deviation. Cardiomyopathy is associated with dilation and usually with diffuse fibrosis.

20–D.   With atrial flutter, the atrial stimulation rate is about 300 beats/minute and the ventricular rate varies depending on the ability of the atrioventricular junction to transmit stimuli from the atria to the ventricles. In atrial flutter, the ventricular rate may not vary.

21–D.   All myocardial cells can be stimulated by external electrical, chemical and mechanical stimuli. The myocardium comprises ordinary contractile cells located in the atria and ventricles as well as specialized cells that conduct the impulses.

22–D.   The P wave on the electrocardiogram can be either positive or negative, depending on the lead. For example, the P wave is always negative in a normal aVR lead, and always positive in a normal V_6 lead.

Recommended Readings

CHAPTER 1–Functional Anatomy and Biomechanics

Cavanagh PR (ed): *Biomechanics of Distance Running.* Champaign, IL, Human Kinetics, 1990.

Cavanagh PR, Kram R: Stride length in distance running: velocity, body dimensions, and added mass effects. *Med Sci Sports Exerc* 21(4):467–479, 1989.

Cavanagh PR, Williams KR: The effects of stride length variation on oxygen uptake during distance running. *Med Sci Sports Exerc* 14(1):30–35, 1982.

Crouch JE: *Functional Human Anatomy,* 3rd ed. Philadelphia, Lea & Febiger, 1978.

Hamill J, Bates BT, Knutzen KM: Ground reaction force symmetry during walking. *Res Quarterly Exerc Sport* 55(3):289–293, 1984.

Hamill J, Knutzen KM: *Biomechanical Basis of Human Movement.* Baltimore, Williams & Wilkins, 1995.

Hogberg P: How do stride length and stride frequency influence the energy-output during running? *Arbeitsphysiologica* 14:437–441, 1952.

Magee DJ: *Orthopedic Physical Assessment,* 3rd ed. Philadelphia, WB Saunders, 1997.

Munro CF, Miller DI, Fuglevand AJ: Ground reaction forces in running: a reexamination. *J Biomech* 20:147–155, 1987.

Nigg B (ed): *Biomechanics of Running Shoes.* Champaign, IL, Human Kinetics, 1986.

Rose J, Gamble JG (eds): *Human Walking,* 2nd ed. Baltimore, Williams & Wilkins, 1994.

Winter DA, Patla AE, Frank JS, et al: Biomechanical walking pattern changes in the fit and healthy elderly. *Phys Ther* 70:340–347, 1990.

CHAPTER 2–Exercise Physiology

American College of Sports Medicine: *ACSM's Guidelines for Exercise Testing and Prescription,* 6th ed. Baltimore, Williams & Wilkins, 2000.

American College of Sports Medicine: *ACSM's Resource Manual for Guidelines for Exercise Testing and Prescription,* 3rd ed. Baltimore, Williams & Wilkins, 1998 (Chapters 14–17, 22, 23, 36, 37, 41, 42, 53, 56 and Appendix).

Astrand P, Rodahl K: *Textbook of Work Physiology.* New York, McGraw Hill, 1977.

Brooks GA, Fahey TD: *Exercise Physiology: Human Bioenergetics and Its Applications.* New York, Macmillan, 1985.

Fletcher GF: *Cardiovascular Response to Exercise: American Heart Association Monograph Series.* Mount Kisco, NY, Futura Publishing, 1994.

MacArdle WD, Katch FI, Katch VL: *Essentials of Exercise Physiology,* 2nd ed. Philadelphia, Lippincott Williams & Wilkins, 1999.

Pashkow FJ, Dafoe WA: *Clinical Cardiac Rehabilitation: A Cardiologist's Guide,* 2nd ed. Baltimore, Williams & Wilkins, 1998.

Pollock ML, Schmidt DH: *Heart Disease and Rehabilitation,* 3rd ed. Champaign, IL, Human Kinetics, 1996.

Pollock ML, Wilmore JH: *Exercise in Health and Disease: Evaluation and Prescription for Prevention and Rehabilitation.* Philadelphia, WB Saunders, 1990.

Powers SK, Howley ET: *Exercise Physiology: Theory and Application to Fitness and Performance.* Dubuque, IA, William C. Brown, 1990.

CHAPTER 3–Human Development and Aging

American College of Sports Medicine, Current Comment: The prevention of sport injuries of children and adolescents. *Med Sci Sports Exerc* 25(8)(suppl):1-7, 1993.

Balady GJ, Chaitman D, Driscoll D, et al: Recommendations for cardiovascular screening, staffing, and emergency policies at health/fitness facilities. Position Statement. *Med Sci Sports Exerc* 30:1009-1018, 1998.

U.S. Department of Health and Human Services: *Physical Activity and Health: A Report of the Surgeon General.* Atlanta, U.S. Department of Health and Human Services, Centers for Disease Control and Prevention, National Center for Chronic Disease Prevention and Health Promotion, 1996.

Krahenbuhl GS, Skinner JS, Kort WM: Developmental aspects of maximal aerobic power in children. *Exerc Sport Sci Rev* 13:503-538, 1985.

Mazzeo RS, Cavanagh P, Evans WJ et al: Exercise and physical activity for older adults. Position Stand. *Med Sci Sports Exerc* 30:992-1008, 1998.

Pollock ML, Gaesser GA, Butcher JD et al: The recommended quantity and quality of exercise for developing and maintaining cardiorespiratory and muscular fitness, and flexibility in healthy adults. Position Stand. *Med Sci Sports Exerc* 30:975-991, 1998.

CHAPTER 4–Pathophysiology/Risk Factors

American College of Sports Medicine: *ACSM's Exercise Management for Persons with Chronic Diseases and Disabilities.* Champaign, IL, Human Kinetics, 1997.

American College of Sports Medicine: *ACSM's Guidelines for Exercise Testing and Prescription,* 5th ed. Baltimore, Williams & Wilkins, 1995.

American College of Sports Medicine: *ACSM's Resource Manual for Guidelines for Exercise Testing and Prescription,* 3rd ed. Baltimore, Williams & Wilkins, 1998.

Lilly LS (Ed): *Pathophysiology of Heart Disease,* 2nd ed. Baltimore, Williams & Wilkins, 1998.

McArdle WD, Katch FI, Katch VL: *Exercise Physiology: Energy, Nutrition, and Human Performance,* 4th ed. Baltimore, Williams & Wilkins, 1996.

West JB: *Pulmonary Pathophysiology: The Essentials,* 5th ed. Baltimore, Williams & Wilkins, 1998.

CHAPTER 5–Human Behavior and Psychology

American Psychiatric Association: *Diagnostic and Statistical Manual of Mental Disorder,* 4th ed. Washington, DC, American Psychiatric Association, 1994.

McKay M, Rogers P, McKay J: *When Anger Hurts.* San Francisco, New Harbinger Publications, 1989.

Williams R, Williams V: *Anger Kills.* New York, Harper, 1993.

Wallston BS, Alagna SW, DeVellis BM et al: Social support and physical health. *Health Psychol* 2:367-391, 1983.

CHAPTER 6–Health Appraisal and Fitness Testing

American College of Sports Medicine: *ACSM's Guidelines for Exercise Testing and Prescription,* 6th ed. Philadelphia, Lippincott Williams & Wilkins, 2000.

American College of Sports Medicine: *ACSM's Resource Manual for Guidelines for Exercise Testing and Prescription,* 3rd ed. Baltimore, Williams & Wilkins, 1998.

American Heart Association Science Advisory: Guide to primary prevention of cardiovascular diseases. A statement for healthcare professionals from the task force on risk reduction. *Circulation* 95:2329-2331, 1997.

Baladay GJ, Caitman B, Driscoll D et al: American College of Sports Medicine and American Heart Association Joint Position Statement: Recommendations for cardiovascular screening, staffing, and emergency policies at health/fitness facilities. *Med Sci Sports Exerc* 30:1009–1018, 1998.

Expert Panel on Detection, Evaluation, and Treatment of High Blood Cholesterol in Adults: Summary of the second report of the National Cholesterol Education Program (NCEP) expert panel on detection, evaluation, and treatment of high blood cholesterol in adults (Adult Treatment Panel II). *JAMA* 269:3015–3023, 1993.

Froelicher V, Marcondes G: *Manual of Exercise Testing.* Chicago, Year Book Medical Publishers, 1989.

Heyward V: *Advanced Fitness Assessment and Exercise Prescription,* 3rd ed. Champaign, IL, Human Kinetics, 1998.

Knight JA, Laubach CA, Butcher RJ et al: Supervision of clinical exercise testing by exercise physiologists. *Am J Cardiol* 75:390-391, 1995.

Kraemer WJ, Fry AC: Strength testing: Development and evaluation of methodology. In *Physiological Assessment of Human Fitness.* Edited by Maud PJ, Foster C. Champaign, IL, Human Kinetics, 1995, pp 115–138.

Ritchie JL, Bateman TM, Bonow RO et al: Guidelines for clinical use of radionuclide imaging. Report of the American College of Cardiology/ American Heart Association Task Force on Assessment of Diagnostic and Therapeutic Cardiovascular Procedures (Subcommittee on Coronary Artery Bypass Graft Surgery). *J Am Coll Cardiol* 17:543–589, 1991.

Ross JG, Pate RR: The national children and youth fitness study II: A summary of the findings. JOPERD 58:51–56, 1987.

US Department of Health and Human Services: *Physical Activity and Health: A report of the Surgeon General.* Atlanta, US Department of Health and Human Services, Centers for Disease Control and Prevention, National Center for Chronic Disease Prevention and Health Promotion, 1996.

CHAPTER 7–Safety, Injury Prevention, and Emergency Care

American College of Sports Medicine: *ACSM's Guidelines for Exercise Testing and Prescription,* 6th ed. Philadelphia, Lippincott Williams & Wilkins, 2000.

American College of Sports Medicine: *ACSM's Resource Manual for Guidelines for Exercise Testing and Prescription,* 3rd ed. Baltimore, Williams & Wilkins, 1998.

Grauer K, Cavallaro D: *ACLS: Rapid Review and Case Scenarios,* 4th ed. St Louis, Mosby, 1996.

Lillegard WA, Rucker KS: *Handbook of Sports Medicine.* Boston, Andover Medical, 1993.

CHAPTER 8–Exercise Programming

Albright A: ACSM Position Stand: Exercise and type 2 diabetes. *MSSE* 32(7), 2000.

American Association of Cardiovascular and Pulmonary Rehabilitation: *AACVPR Guidelines for Cardiac Rehabilitation Programs,* 2nd ed. Champaign, IL, Human Kinetics, 1995.

American Association of Cardiovascular and Pulmonary Rehabilitation: *AACVPR Guidelines for Pulmonary Rehabilitation Programs,* 2nd ed. Champaign, Human Kinetics, 1998.

American College of Sports Medicine: *ACSM's Resource Manual for Guidelines for Exercise Testing and Prescription,* 3rd ed. Baltimore, Williams & Wilkins, 1998.

American College of Sports Medicine: *ACSM Guidelines for Exercise Testing and Prescription,* 6th ed. Philadelphia, Lippincott Williams & Wilkins, 2000.

American College of Sports Medicine: *ACSM's Exercise Management for Persons with Chronic Diseases and Disabilities.* Champaign, IL, Human Kinetics, 1997.

Fletcher GF, Balady GJ et al. Exercise standards: A statement for healthcare professionals from the AHA. *Circulation* 91(2):580, 1995.

Gibbons RJ, Balady GJ et al: ACC/AHA guidelines for exercise testing: A report of the American College of Cardiology/American Heart Association Task Force on Practice Guidelines (Committee on Exercise Testing). *JACC* 30(1):260-315, 1997.

Gordon NF: *Breathing Disorders: Your Complete Exercise Guide.* Champaign, IL, Human Kinetics, 1993.

Gordon NF: *Diabetes: Your Complete Exercise Guide.* Champaign, IL, Human Kinetics, 1993.

Mazzeo RS: ACSM Position Stand: Exercise and physical activity for older adults. *MSSE* 30:992-1008, 1998.

Pate R, Pratt M et al: Physical activity and public health: A recommendation from the Centers for Disease Control and Prevention and ACSM. *JAMA* 273(5): 402-407, 1995.

Pollock ML et al: ACSM Position Stand: The recommended quantity and quality of exercise for developing and maintaining cardiorespiratory and muscular fitness and flexibility in healthy adults. *MSSE* 30:975-991, 1998.

Rejeski J, Kenney E: *Fitness Motivation: Preventing Participant Dropout.* Champaign, IL, Human Kinetics, 1988.

Ruderman N, Devlin JT (eds): *American Diabetes Association: The Health Professional's Guide to Diabetes and Exercise.* Alexandria, American Diabetes Association, 1995.

Squires R: *Exercise Prescription for the High-Risk Cardiac Patient.* Champaign, IL, Human Kinetics, 1998.

Van Norman K: *Exercise Programming for Older Adults.* Champaign, IL, Human Kinetics, 1995.

Wenger N: *Rehabilitation of the Coronary Patient,* 3rd ed. New York, Churchill Livingstone, 1992.

Westcott W, Baechle T: *Strength Training Past 50.* Champaign, IL, Human Kinetics, 1998.

CHAPTER 9–Nutrition and Weight Management

Bennett B, Van Vynckt V: *Dictionary of Healthful Food Terms.* Hauppauge, NY, Barron's Educational Series, 1997.

National Institutes of Health: Health implications of obesity. *NIH Consensus Statement* 5(9):1-7, 1985.

Miller M, Vogel RA: *The Practice of Coronary Disease Prevention.* Baltimore, Williams & Wilkins, 1996.

Position of the American Dietetic Association and The Canadian Dietetic Association: Nutrition for physical fitness and athletic performance for adults. *J Am Diet Assoc* 93(6):691-696, 1993.

Proper and Improper Weight Loss Programs. American College of Sports Medicine Position Stand, 1983.

CHAPTER 10–Program and Administration/Management

American Association of Cardiovascular and Pulmonary Rehabilitation: *Guidelines for Cardiac Rehabilitation and Secondary Prevention Programs,* 3rd ed. Champaign, IL, Human Kinetics, 1999.

American College of Sports Medicine (eds): *Resource Manual for Guidelines for Exercise Testing and Prescription,* 3rd ed. Baltimore, Williams & Wilkins, 1998.

American College of Sports Medicine: *Guidelines for Exercise Testing and Prescription,* 6th ed. Philadelphia, Lippincott Williams & Wilkins, 2000.

American Association of Cardiovascular and Pulmonary Rehabilitation: *Guidelines for Pulmonary Rehabilitation Programs,* 2nd ed. Champaign, IL, Human Kinetics, 1998.

Wenger NK, Froelicher ED, Smith LK et al: *Cardiac Rehabilitation. Clinical Practice Guideline No. 17.* Rockville, MD, U.S. Department of Health and Human Services, Public Health Service, Agency for Health Care Policy and Research and the National Heart, Lung and Blood Institute. AHCPR Publication No. 96-0672. October 1995.

Patton RW, Corry JM, Gettman LR, Graf JS: *Implementing Health/Fitness Programs.* Champaign, IL, Human Kinetics, 1986.

American College of Sports Medicine: *Health/Fitness Facilities Standards and Guidelines,* 2nd ed. Champaign, IL, Human Kinetics, 1997.

Pollock ML, Schmidt DH (eds): *Heart Disease and Rehabilitation,* 3rd ed. Champaign, IL, Human Kinetics, 1995.

Fardy PS, Yanowitz FG: *Cardiac Rehabilitation, Adult Fitness, and Exercise Testing,* 3rd ed. Baltimore, Williams & Wilkins, 1995.

Herbert DL, Herbert WG: *Legal Aspects of Preventative and Rehabilitative Exercise Programs,* 3rd ed. Canton, OH, Professional Reports Corporation, 1993.

CHAPTER 12–Electrocardiography

American College of Sports Medicine: *ACSM's Resource Manual for Guidelines for Exercise Testing and Prescription,* 3rd ed. Philadelphia, Lippincott Williams & Wilkins, 1998.

American College of Sports Medicine: *ACSM's Guidelines for Exercise Testing and Prescription,* 6th ed. Philadelphia, Lippincott Williams & Wilkins, 2000.

Berne RM, Levy MN: *Cardiovascular Physiology,* 7th ed. St Louis, Mosby, 1997.

Goldberger AL: *Clinical Electrocardiography,* 6th ed. St Louis, Mosby, 1999.

COMPREHENSIVE EXAM

DIRECTIONS: Carefully read all questions and select the *best* single answer.

1. Which of the following medications is an endogenous catecholamine that optimizes blood flow to the heart and brain by increasing aortic diastolic pressure, and preferentially shunts blood to the internal carotid artery, thus enhancing cerebral blood flow?
   (A) Lidocaine
   (B) Oxygen
   (C) Atropine
   (D) Epinephrine

2. If a healthy young man exercises at an intensity of 45 ml · kg^{-1} · min^{-1} three times per week for 45 minutes each session, how long would it take him to lose 10 pounds of fat?
   (A) 4 weeks
   (B) 7.14 weeks
   (C) 16.5 weeks
   (D) 19 weeks

3. All of the following techniques are commonly used in the diagnosis of coronary artery disease *except*
   (A) electrocardiography.
   (B) radionuclide imaging.
   (C) echocardiography.
   (D) cardiac spirometry.

4. During mild to moderate exercise, minute ventilation increases primarily through an increase in
   (A) tidal volume.
   (B) respiratory rate.
   (C) forced expiratory volume.
   (D) forced inspiratory volume.

5. Which of the following would be an adequate exercise prescription for a patient who has undergone a heart transplant?
   (A) High intensity, short duration, small muscle groups, high frequency
   (B) High intensity, long duration, small muscle groups, high frequency
   (C) Low to moderate intensity, daily, large muscle groups, moderate duration
   (D) Low intensity, 3 times a week, large muscle groups, moderate duration

6. Recommendations for exercise in patients with diabetes include all of the following *except*
   (A) avoiding injection of insulin into an exercising muscle.
   (B) exercising with a partner.
   (C) exercising only when temperature and humidity are moderate.
   (D) avoiding exercise during peak insulin activity.

7. Which of the following is a reversible pulmonary condition caused by some type of irritant (e.g., dust, pollen) and characterized by obvious narrowing of the bronchial airways, with dyspnea and possibly hypoxia and hypercapnia?
   (A) Emphysema
   (B) Bronchitis
   (C) Asthma
   (D) Pulmonary vascular disease

8. Atrial flutter and atrial fibrillation are examples of
   (A) ventricular arrhythmias.
   (B) supraventricular arrhythmias.
   (C) atrioventricular conduction delays.
   (D) pre-excitation syndromes.

9. Which of the following statements regarding contraindications to graded exercise testing is *not* accurate?
   (A) Some individuals have risk factors that outweigh the potential benefits from exercise testing and the information that may be obtained.
   (B) Absolute contraindications refer to individuals for whom exercise testing should not be performed until the situation or condition has stabilized.
   (C) Relative contraindications include patients who might be tested if the potential benefit from exercise testing outweighs the relative risk.
   (D) All of the above

10. An impulse originating in the sinoatrial node and then spreading to both atria, causing atrial depolarization, appears on the electrocardiogram as a
    (A) P wave.
    (B) QRS complex.
    (C) ST segment.
    (D) T wave.

11. Whole body and segmental movement occurs in three spatial dimensions. Which plane divides the body into symmetrical right and left halves?
    (A) Frontal plane
    (B) Transverse plane
    (C) Sagittal plane
    (D) Medial plane

12. To reduce the risk for certain diseases and to gain health benefits, the recommended weekly caloric expenditure is
    (A) 200–700 kilocalories/week.
    (B) 700–2,000 kilocalories/week.
    (C) 2,000–5,000 kilocalories/week.
    (D) more than 5,000 kilocalories/week.

13. Exercise has been shown to have a beneficial effect on reducing mortality in patients with coronary artery disease. The mechanisms responsible for this include
    (A) its effect on other risk factors.
    (B) reduced myocardial oxygen demand at rest and at submaximal workloads.
    (C) reduced platelet aggregation.
    (D) all of the above.

14. The degradation of carbohydrate to pyruvate or lactate occurs through
    (A) the adenosine triphosphate system.
    (B) anaerobic glycolysis.
    (C) aerobic glycolysis.
    (D) fat metabolism.

15. Which is *least* likely to be an effective means of permanent weight loss?
    (A) Dietary changes
    (B) Increase exercise
    (C) Rapid weight loss
    (D) Diet and exercise

16. Which of the following strategies is most commonly used in patients diagnosed with coronary artery disease who are not responding to other treatments?
    (A) Percutaneous transluminal coronary angioplasty
    (B) Coronary artery stent
    (C) Coronary artery bypass graft surgery
    (D) Pharmacologic therapy

17. Which of the following statements best describes the precautions for exercise taken in patients with an automatic implantable cardioverter defibrillator (AICD)?
    (A) Heart rate must be monitored closely during exercise, to ensure that it does not reach the level of the activation rate and trigger a shock to the patient.
    (B) Most AICDs are set to deliver a shock to the patient only when the heart rate nears 300 beats/minute.
    (C) The patient should avoid exercise-related increases in heart rate.
    (D) The intensity of exercise should be kept very low for this patient.

18. Oxidative phosphorylation uses oxygen as the final acceptor of hydrogen to form adenosine triphosphate and
    (A) phosphocreatine.
    (B) lactate.
    (C) carbon monoxide.
    (D) water.

19. Healthy, untrained subjects have an anaerobic threshold at approximately what percentage of maximal oxygen consumption?
    (A) 25%
    (B) 55%
    (C) 75%
    (D) 95%

20. Which of the following medications reduces myocardial ischemia by lowering myocardial oxygen demand with some increase in oxygen supply, and as a result is used to treat typical and variant angina?
    (A) Beta adrenergic blockers
    (B) Calcium channel blockers
    (C) Aspirin
    (D) Nitrates

21. Which of the following structures is located in the posterior wall of the right atrium, just inferior to the opening of the superior vena cava?
    (A) Sinoatrial node
    (B) Atrioventricular node
    (C) Bundle of His
    (D) Purkinje fibers

22. How many calories will a 110-pound woman expend if she pedals on a Monark cycle ergometer at 50 RPM against a resistance of 2.5 kiloponds for 60 minutes?
    (A) 12.87 calories
    (B) 31.28 calories
    (C 510 calories
    (D 3500 calories

23. Electrocardiographic precordial lead V_4 is placed at the
    (A) fourth intercostal space, left sternal border.
    (B) fourth intercostal space, right sternal border.
    (C) midaxillary line, fifth intercostal space.
    (D) midclavicular line, fifth intercostal space.

24. Which of the following increases curvilinearly with the work rate until it reaches near maximum at a level equivalent to approximately 50% of aerobic capacity and increasing only slightly thereafter?
    (A) Stroke volume
    (B) End-diastolic volume
    (C) Cardiac output
    (D) Oxygen consumption

25. Exposure to which of the following environments causes vasoconstriction (higher blood pressure response), lowering the anginal threshold and possibly provoking angina at rest (variant or Prinzmetal's angina), and can induce asthma, general dehydration, and dryness or burning of the mouth and throat?
    (A) Extreme cold
    (B) Extreme heat
    (C) High altitude
    (D) High humidity

26. What is the equivalent total caloric expenditure of 3 lbs (6.6 kg) of fat?
    (A) 1000
    (B) 5,500
    (C) 10,500
    (D) 15,000

27. Which of the following statements is *not* true about the Continuous Quality Improvement (CQI) process, also known as quality assurance?
    (A) CQI is tied to program certification.
    (B) CQI is a systematic evaluation procedure.
    (C) CQI uses only objective data in its data analytical process.
    (D) The process for CQI should be explained in the policy and procedures manual.

28. Irreversible necrosis of the heart muscle resulting from prolonged ischemia describes
    (A) thrombosis.
    (B) aneurysm.
    (C) infarction.
    (D) thrombolysis.

29. Which of the following medications used to treat heart failure and some arrhythmias can produce electrocardiographic changes of QT interval shortening and ST segment depression (often known as "scooping")?
    (A) Beta-blockers
    (B) Calcium channel blockers
    (C) Potassium
    (D) Digitalis

30. The energy to perform physical work comes from the breakdown of
    (A) testosterone.
    (B) oxygen.
    (C) adenosine triphosphate.
    (D) phosphocreatine.

31. For a patient who has had coronary artery bypass graft surgery or valve replacement surgery, which of the following care measures is *not* indicated?
    (A) The patient should avoid extreme tension on the upper body due to sternal and leg wounds for 2–4 months.
    (B) The clinician should observe for infection or discomfort along the incision.
    (C) The patient should be monitored for chest pain, dizziness and dysrhythmias.
    (D) The patient should avoid high-intensity exercise early in the rehabilitation period.

32. Which of the following is a *modifiable* risk factor for the development of coronary artery disease?
    (A) Increasing age
    (B) Male gender
    (C) Family history
    (D) Tobacco smoking

33. Regular aerobic exercise 5 days/week at 50%–85% $\dot{V}O_2$ for 45 minutes will most favorably affect
    (A) homocysteine levels.
    (B) triglycerides.
    (C) lipoprotein (a).
    (D) low-density lipoprotein cholesterol.

34. Which of the following redistributes blood flow from the trunk to peripheral areas, decreases resistance in the tissues for movement, and increases the tissue temperature and energy production?
    (A) Training effect
    (B) Cool down
    (C) Warm up
    (D) Orthostatic response

35. Regarding risk stratification for exercise testing, individuals who have signs or symptoms suggesting cardiopulmonary or metabolic disease and/or two or more risk factors are considered to be at
    (A) no risk.
    (B) low risk.
    (C) moderate risk.
    (D) high risk.

36. Which of the following conditions is marked by the progressively difficult conduction of an electrical impulse through the atrioventricular junction, producing a progressively longer PR interval until a P wave is not conducted (with the electrocardiogram showing a P wave not followed by a QRS complex)?
    (A) First-degree atrioventricular block
    (B) Second-degree atrioventricular block, Mobitz type I
    (C) Second-degree atrioventricular block, Mobitz type II
    (D) Third-degree atrioventricular block

37. Heart rate increases in a linear fashion with work rate and oxygen uptake during dynamic exercise. The magnitude of the heart rate response is related to
    (A) age.
    (B) body position.
    (C) medication use.
    (D) all of the above.

38. Regular exercise can have a positive effect on all of the following conditions *except*
    (A) obesity.
    (B) dyslipidemia.
    (C) hypertension.
    (D) cirrhosis.

39. On the electrocardiogram, which of the following is considered a sensitive indicator of myocardial ischemia or injury?
    (A) Q waves
    (B) PR interval
    (C) ST segment
    (D) T wave

40. Which of the following evaluation techniques provides the *least* accurate measurement of obesity?
    (A) Body mass index
    (B) Waist to hip ratio
    (C) Body composition analysis
    (D) Height/weight tables

41. A balance between the energy required by the working muscles and the rate of ATP production through aerobic metabolism is referred to as
    (A) oxygen debt.
    (B) oxygen deficit.
    (C) steady-state.
    (D) adaptation.

42. On the electrocardiogram, various combinations of ST segment abnormalities, the presence of Q waves, or the absence of R waves may suggest
    (A) cerebrovascular accident.
    (B) acute myocardial infarction.
    (C) ventricular aneurysm.
    (D) mitral valve prolapse.

43. What is the relative oxygen consumption of walking on a treadmill at 3.5 mph up a 10% grade?
    (A) $181.72 \text{ ml} \cdot \text{kg}^{-1} \cdot \text{min}^{-1}$
    (B) $18.17 \text{ ml} \cdot \text{kg}^{-1} \cdot \text{min}^{-1}$
    (C) $29.76 \text{ ml} \cdot \text{kg}^{-1} \cdot \text{min}^{-1}$
    (D) $27.96 \text{ ml} \cdot \text{kg}^{-1} \cdot \text{min}^{-1}$

44. Which of the following axes lies perpendicular to the frontal plane?
    (A) Longitudinal axis
    (B) Mediolateral axis
    (C) Anteroposterior axis
    (D) Transverse axis

45. Expected benefits of regular exercise in patients with peripheral vascular disease include all of the following *except*
    (A) redistribution and increased blood flow to the legs.
    (B) increased tolerance for walking (improved claudication pain tolerance).
    (C) increased blood viscosity.
    (D) improved muscle cell metabolism.

46. Which of the following patients do *not* need a physician's evaluation prior to initiating a vigorous exercise program?
    (A) Men over age 50 and women over age 50 with fewer than two risk factors for coronary artery disease
    (B) Men under age 40 and women under age 50 with fewer than two risk factors for coronary artery disease
    (C) Men under age 40 and women over age 50 with fewer than two risk factors for coronary artery disease
    (D) Men under age 50 and women under age 50 with fewer than two risk factors for coronary artery disease

47. All of the following are types of intraventricular conduction disturbances *except*
    - (A) left bundle branch block.
    - (B) right bundle branch block.
    - (C) atrioventricular nodal reentrant tachycardia.
    - (D) all of the above.

48. For persons free of absolute contraindications to exercise, the health and medical benefits of exercise clearly outweigh any associated risks. To ensure as safe an environment as possible during exercise testing and training, the clinical exercise specialist must be prepared to do all of the following *except*
    - (A) understand the risks associated with exercise and exercise testing.
    - (B) be able to perform emergency medical procedures.
    - (C) have knowledge of the care of an injury or medical emergency.
    - (D) be able to implement preventive measures.

49. What is defined as a surplus of adipose tissue, resulting from excess energy intake relative to energy expenditure?
    - (A) Overweight
    - (B) Android obesity
    - (C) Obesity
    - (D) Gynoid obesity

50. Although program certification of clinical exercise rehabilitation programs is a relatively new concept, it involves many already established components of the exercise program. Which of the following is *not* a component important to clinical exercise rehabilitation program certification?
    - (A) Staff certification and/or licensure
    - (B) Program outcomes measures
    - (C) The policy and procedures manual
    - (D) Adherence to insurance codes for billing

51. *Preload* of the left ventricle refers to
    - (A) contractility.
    - (B) diastolic filling.
    - (C) ventricular outflow.
    - (D) ejection fraction.

52. A constricting, squeezing, burning, or heavy feeling in the chest area, neck, cheeks, shoulder, or arms, provoked by physical work or stress, are characteristic of
    - (A) angina.
    - (B) asthma.
    - (C) atherosclerosis.
    - (D) arteriosclerosis.

53. Health screening prior to participation in a graded exercise test is indicated for all of the following reasons *except*
    - (A) to determine the presence of disease.
    - (B) to consider contraindications for exercise testing or training.
    - (C) to determine the need for referral to a medically supervised exercise program.
    - (D) to evaluate aerobic capacity.

54. The proper emergency response for a patient who has experienced a cardiac arrest, but who is now breathing and has a palpable pulse, includes
    - (A) continuing the exercise test to determine why the patient had this response.
    - (B) placing the patient in the recovery position with the head to the side to prevent an airway obstruction.
    - (C) placing the patient in a comfortable seated position.
    - (D) beginning Phase I cardiac rehabilitation.

55. A patient weighing 200 pounds (90.01 kg) sets the treadmill speed at 4 miles/hr (107 meters/min) and a 5% grade. During exercise, his blood pressure rises to 150/90 mm Hg, and his heart rate increases to 150 beats/min. What is his estimated energy expenditure in terms of L/min?
    - (A) 1.07 L/min
    - (B) 2.14 L/min
    - (C) 4.28 L/min
    - (D) 8.56 L/min

56. Advancing age brings a progressive decline in bone
    - (A) growth and maturation.
    - (B) mineral density and calcium content.
    - (C) distensibility.
    - (D) fractures.

57. Which of the following procedures provides the *least* sensitivity and specificity in the diagnosis of coronary artery disease?
    - (A) Coronary angiography
    - (B) Echocardiography
    - (C) Radionuclide imaging
    - (D) Electrocardiography

58. When an electrical impulse is generated in a particular area in the heart, the outside of the cells in this area become negatively charged and the inside of the cells become positively charged, in a process known as
    - (A) polarization.
    - (B) repolarization.
    - (C) depolarization.
    - (D) excitation.

59. Cardiac output increases linearly with increased work rate. At exercise intensities up to 50% of maximal oxygen consumption, increased cardiac output is facilitated by an increase in
    (A) heart rate and stroke volume.
    (B) heart rate only.
    (C) stroke volume only.
    (D) neither heart rate nor stroke volume.

60. Which of the following is true of flow-resistive training (a type of breathing retraining for patients with pulmonary disease)?
    (A) It helps coordinate breathing with activities of daily living.
    (B) It increases respiratory muscle strength and endurance.
    (C) It uses a preset inspiratory pressure, usually at a consistent fraction of maximal inspiratory pressure.
    (D) It consists of breathing through a progressively smaller opening.

61. A sustained muscle contraction against a fixed load or resistance with no change in the length of the involved muscle group or joint motion describes
    (A) isometric contraction.
    (B) isotonic contraction.
    (C) muscular weakness.
    (D) muscular strength.

62. Which of the following is a *nonmodifiable* risk factor for the development of coronary artery disease?
    (A) Tobacco smoking
    (B) Dyslipidemia
    (C) Family history
    (D) Hypertension

63. All of the following are examples of capital expenses *except*
    (A) tangible assets.
    (B) staff salaries
    (C) equipment purchases.
    (D) construction.

64. A push or a pull that produces or has the capacity to produce a change in motion of a body is known as
    (A) force.
    (B) torque.
    (C) Newton's law of gravity.
    (D) inertia.

65. The thickest, middle layer of the artery wall, composed predominantly of smooth muscle cells and responsible for vasoconstriction and vasodilation, is the
    (A) endothelium.
    (B) intima.
    (C) media.
    (D) adventitia.

66. What electrocardiographic electrode is positioned at the fourth intercostal space, left sternal border?
    (A) V_1
    (B) V_2
    (C) V_3
    (D) V_6

67. An exercise program for a man weighing 154 lb (70 kg) includes a warm-up at 2.0 METs for 5 minutes, 20 minutes of treadmill running at 9 METs, 20 minutes of leg cycling at 8 METs, and a cool-down of 5 minutes at 2.5 METs. What is this patient's total energy expenditure for an exercise session?
    (A) 162 kcal/session
    (B) 868 kcal/session
    (C) 444 kcal/session
    (D) 1256 kcal/session

68. The "average" cardiac output at maximal exercise is
    (A) 5 L/minute.
    (B) 10 L/minute.
    (C) 20 L/minute.
    (D) 20 ml/minute.

69. For a patient exercising in the heat or in humid environments, the exercise prescription should be altered by
    (A) increasing the intensity and decreasing the duration.
    (B) decreasing the intensity and increasing the duration.
    (C) decreasing the intensity and decreasing the duration.
    (D) increasing the intensity and varying the duration.

70. Which of the following statements regarding an emergency plan is accurate?
    (A) The emergency plan does not need to be written down, as long as everyone understands it.
    (B) As long as everyone knows his or her individual responsibilities during an emergency, a list of each staff member's responsibilities is not needed.
    (C) All emergency situations must be documented with dates, times, actions, people involved, and outcomes.
    (D) There is no need to practice emergencies as long as the staff fully understand their responsibilities.

71. Which of the following is *not* considered to be an orthopedic condition that can lead to limitation of regular exercise (physical conditioning)?
    (A) Osteoarthritis
    (B) Rheumatoid arthritis
    (C) Osteoporosis
    (D) Multiple sclerosis

72. What disorder is characterized by an inflammation and edema of the trachea and bronchial tubes; hypertrophy of the mucous glands, which narrows the airway; arterial hypoxemia, leading to vasoconstriction of smooth muscle in the pulmonary arterioles and venules; and, in the presence of continued vasoconstriction, pulmonary hypertension?
    (A) Emphysema
    (B) Bronchitis
    (C) Atherosclerosis
    (D) Asthma

73. For any high-risk patient, it is prudent to
    (A) skip the warm up and cool down entirely.
    (B) increase the intensity of warm up and decrease the intensity of cool down.
    (C) decrease the intensity of warm up and increase the intensity of cool down.
    (D) prolong both warm up and cool down.

74. Oxygen consumption can be measured by all of the following methods *except*
    (A) direct calorimetry.
    (B) indirect calorimetry.
    (C) estimation from workload.
    (D) chest x-ray.

75. The American College of Sports Medicine (ACSM) recommends that exercise programs for patients with heart disease be under the overall guidance of a(n)
    (A) physician.
    (B) ACSM Program Director$_{SM}$.
    (C) ACSM-certified physician.
    (D) physician and an ACSM Program Director$_{SM}$ or ACSM Exercise Specialist®.

76. The sum of the oxygen cost of physical activity and the resting energy expenditure is known as
    (A) relative oxygen consumption.
    (B) absolute oxygen consumption.
    (C) net oxygen consumption.
    (D) gross oxygen consumption.

77. Ventricular tachycardia is marked by
    (A) two premature ventricular contractions (PVCs) in a row.
    (B) one PVC on every other beat repeatedly.
    (C) two PVCs on every other beat repeatedly.
    (D) three PVCs in a row.

78. In which of the following conditions do necrotic heart muscle fibers degenerate, causing the muscle wall to become very thin and thus increasing the risk of thrombus, arrhythmias, and heart failure?
    (A) Papillary dysfunction
    (B) Ventricular dilation
    (C) Myocardial infarction
    (D) Ventricular aneurysm

79. The exercise prescription for muscular fitness (endurance) when using resistance training is
    (A) 10%–40% of 1 repetition maximum.
    (B) 20%–40% of 1 repetition maximum.
    (C) 40%–60% of 1 repetition maximum.
    (D) 60%–80% of 1 repetition maximum.

80. A slotted stainless-steel tube that acts as a scaffold to hold the walls of a coronary artery open, thereby improving blood flow and relieving the symptoms of coronary artery disease, is known as a
    (A) balloon angioplasty.
    (B) stent.
    (C) lysing device.
    (D) coronary artery graft.

81. Which of the following conditions is indicated by a PR interval prolonged beyond 0.20 seconds, with all P waves conducted and all PR intervals the same?
    (A) First-degree atrioventricular block
    (B) Second-degree atrioventricular block, Mobitz type I
    (C) Second-degree atrioventricular block, Mobitz type II
    (D) Third-degree atrioventricular block

82. Q waves detected by electrocardiogram leads V_1, V_2, V_3, and V_4 are an indication of
    (A) left anterior hemiblock.
    (B) left posterior hemiblock.
    (C) anterior infarction.
    (D) posterior infarction.

83. Atherosclerosis is thought to begin
    (A) at birth.
    (B) during adolescence.
    (C) during middle age.
    (D) only after significant exposure to risk factors.

84. What graded exercise test protocol includes a momentary stoppage while measures are obtained?
    (A) Step test
    (B) Continuous protocol
    (C) Discontinuous protocol
    (D) Field test

85. For patients with congestive heart failure, which of the following statements is accurate?
    (A) Most of the improvement resulting from regular exercise is within the myocardium.
    (B) These patients can never expect improved physical fitness.
    (C) Exercise capacity is improved because of peripheral adaptations.
    (D) Complete bed rest is prescribed for these patients.

86. In which of the following conditions would regular resistance training generally provide the *most* benefit?
    (A) Osteoporosis
    (B) Rheumatoid arthritis
    (C) Stroke
    (D) Hypertension

87. Above 1500 meters (4921 feet) in altitude, what percentage reduction in maximal oxygen consumption can be expected for each subsequent 1000 meters (3280 feet) in altitude?
    (A) 2%
    (B) 10%
    (C) 25%
    (D) 50%

88. The QRS on an electrocardiogram is measured from the beginning of the first wave to the end of the last wave of the QRS complex. A QRS complex duration exceeding 0.20 second may point to
    (A) atrioventricular conduction delay.
    (B) normal cardiac function.
    (C) intraventricular conduction delay.
    (D) acute myocardial infarction.

89. The incidence of cardiac arrest during clinical exercise testing is
    (A) 1 in 10,000.
    (B) 0.4 in 10,000.
    (C) 1.4 in 10,000.
    (D) 1 in 1 million.

90. A regular exercise program will primarily affect which lipid value?
    (A) Total cholesterol level
    (B) Very-low-density and high-density lipoprotein cholesterol levels
    (C) Low density lipoprotein cholesterol level
    (D) Total cholesterol/low density cholesterol ratio

91. In the terminology of the health behavior change model, which of the following refers to early phases of making a change in a health behavior or the intention to make a change?
    (A) Antecedents
    (B) Adoption
    (C) Maintenance
    (D) Instruction

92. An effective strategy in limiting the progression and promoting regression of atherosclerosis is to lower
    (A) low-density lipoprotein cholesterol.
    (B) high-density lipoprotein cholesterol.
    (C) triglycerides.
    (D) glucose.

93. Which of the following is *not* a common type of "field test"?
    (A) Cooper 12-minute test
    (B) 1.5-mile run test
    (C) Rockport walking test
    (D) Treadmill test

94. A transmural myocardial infarction, marked by tissue necrosis in a full-thickness portion of the left ventricular wall, typically produces what changes on the electrocardiogram?
    (A) T wave inversion
    (B) U wave inversion
    (C) ST segment depression
    (D) ST segment elevation

95. Slow, safe activation of the body's responses to exercise and increased range of motion to prepare joints and muscles for vigorous activity occurs during
    (A) stimulus phase.
    (B) cool down.
    (C) warm up.
    (D) resistance training.

96. Which of the following statements is *true*?
    (A) For certain individuals, the risks of testing and exercise outweigh the potential benefits.
    (B) For all patients, the risks of testing and exercise outweigh the benefits.
    (C) Only a small percentage of patients should have undergo exercise testing, because it is too dangerous.
    (D) The potential benefits of testing and exercise always outweigh the risks.

97. Which of the following has a risk ratio in the development of coronary artery disease similar to that of hypertension, hypercholesterolemia, and cigarette smoking?
    (A) Physical inactivity
    (B) Obesity
    (C) Diabetes mellitus
    (D) Psychological stress

98. Which of the following is an example of physical activity requiring anaerobic glycolysis to produce energy in the form of adenosine triphosphate?
    (A) 100-meter sprint
    (B) 400-meter sprint
    (C) 5000-meter run
    (D) Marathon run

99. A mean electrical axis (as measured on the electrocardiogram) of -45 is considered
    (A) normal.
    (B) right axis deviation.
    (C) left axis deviation.
    (D) extreme left axis deviation.

100. Which of the following medications significantly reduces first-year mortality rates in post-myocardial infarction patients by 20%–35%?
    (A) Aspirin
    (B) Calcium channel blockers
    (C) Beta adrenergic blockers
    (D) Nitrates

ANSWERS AND EXPLANATIONS

1–D. Epinephrine is an endogenous catecholamine that optimizes blood flow to the heart and brain by increasing aortic diastolic pressure and preferentially shunting blood to the internal carotid artery. Lidocaine is an antiarrhythmic agent that can decrease automaticity in the ventricular myocardium, as well as raise the fibrillation threshold. Supplemental oxygen ensures adequate arterial oxygen content and greatly enhances tissue oxygenation. Atropine is a parasympathetic blocking agent used to treat bradyarrhythmias.
[Chapter 7]

2–C. The steps are as follows:
   a. Convert relative $\dot{V}O_2$ to absolute $\dot{V}O_2$ by multiplying relative $\dot{V}O_2$ ($ml \cdot kg^{-1} \cdot min^{-1}$) by his body weight. We are not given his body weight so we cannot finish this problem.
   b. Assuming that he is an average 70-kg man:

   $Absolute\ \dot{V}O_2 = relative\ \dot{V}O_2 \times body\ weight$

   $= 45\ ml \cdot kg^{-1} \cdot min^{-1} \times 70\ kg$

   $= 3150\ ml \cdot min^{-1}$

   c. To get $L \cdot min^{-1}$, divide $ml \cdot min^{-1}$ by 1000:

   $3150\ ml \cdot min^{-1} \div 1000 = 3.15\ L \cdot min^{-1}$

   d. Multiply 3.150 $L \cdot min^{-1}$ by the constant 5.0 to get $kcal \cdot min^{-1}$:

   $3.15\ L \cdot min^{-1} \times 5.0 = 15.75\ kcal \cdot min^{-1}$

   e. Multiply 15.75 kcal per minute by the total number of minutes he exercises (45 minutes × 3 times per week = 135 total minutes) to get the total caloric expenditure:

   $15.75\ kcal\ per\ minute \times 135\ minutes$
   $= 2126.25\ total\ kcal\ per\ week$

   f. Divide by 3500 to get pounds of fat:

   $2126.25\ kcal \div 3500 = 0.6075\ pounds\ of\ fat\ per\ week$

   g. Divide 10 pounds by 0.6075 pounds of fat per week to get how many weeks it will take him to lose 10 pounds of fat:

   $10 \div 0.6075 = 16.46\ weeks \approx 16.5\ weeks$
   [Chapter 11]

3–D. In the diagnosis of coronary artery disease, electrocardiography, radionuclide imaging, and echocardiography are commonly used by themselves or with other tests. Other important diagnostic studies for coronary artery disease include coronary angiography.
[Chapter 4]

4–A. During mild to moderate exercise, minute ventilation increases primarily through tidal volume. During vigorous exercise, respiratory rate also increases. The increase in minute ventilation is directly proportional to oxygen consumption and carbon dioxide production during low-intensity exercise.
[Chapter 2]

5–C. Patients who have had heart transplant should exercise at a rating of perceived exertion of between 11 and 16 (moderate) or between 60% and 70% of maximum metabolic capacity (METs) or 40% to 75% of maximal oxygen consumption. Frequency should be 4–6 days/week. Duration should include a prolonged warm up. In addition, resistance training can be used in moderation.
[Chapter 8]

6–C. Recommended precautions for the exercising diabetic patient include wearing the proper footwear, maintaining adequate hydration, monitoring blood glucose level regularly, always wearing a medical identification bracelet or some other form of identification, and avoiding injecting insulin into exercising muscles. There is no reason why a patient with diabetes cannot exercise at any time if proper precautions are followed.
[Chapter 8]

7–C. The only reversible pulmonary disease, asthma is triggered by a mediator (such as dust or pollen) that increases calcium influx into mast cells, resulting in the release of chemical mediators such as histamine. These mediators trigger bronchoconstriction (an increase in smooth muscle contraction of the bronchial tubes) and an inflammatory response. During asthma attacks, the individual becomes dyspneic and is likely to be hypoxic and hypercapnic. Attacks can last for hours or even days if they are not self-reversing or responsive to drug therapy.
[Chapter 4]

8–B. In the presence of atrial flutter and atrial fibrillation, the atria are not stimulated from the sinoatrial node but from some ectopic atrial focus or foci. The rate of atrial depolarization varies between 250 and 350 beats/minute for atrial flutter and between 400 and 600 beats/minute for atrial fibrillation. In either atrial flutter or atrial fibrillation, the rate of ventricular depolarization depends on the rate at which the atrioventricular node conducts the supraventricular stimuli.
[Chapter 12]

9–D. All of the these statements are true regarding contraindications to exercise testing.
[Chapter 6]

10–A. The cardiac impulse originating in the sinoatrial node that spreads to both atria causing atrial depolarization is indicated on the electrocardiogram as a P wave. Atrial repolarization is not usually seen on the electrocardiogram because it is obscured by the other ventricular electrical potentials. Ventricular depolarization is represented on the electrocardiogram by the QRS complex. Ventricular repolarization is represented on the electrocardiogram by the ST-segment, T-wave and at times, the U-wave.
[Chapter 12]

11–C. The sagittal plane divides the body into symmetrical right and left halves. The frontal plane divides the body into front and back halves. The transverse plane divides the body in half superiorly and inferiorly. There is no medial plane.
[Chapter 1]

12–B. The principles of exercise prescription for health and physical fitness dictate that the average caloric expenditure needed to gain health benefits to reduce the risk for certain chronic diseases is between 700 and 2,000 kilocalories weekly.
[Chapter 8]

13–D. The mechanisms responsible for a reduction in deaths from coronary artery disease include its effect on other risk factors, reduced myocardial oxygen demand at rest and at submaximal workloads (resulting in an increased ischemic and angina threshold), and reduced platelet aggregation and improved endothelial-mediated vasomotor tone.
[Chapter 4]

14–B. The degradation of carbohydrate (glucose or glycogen) to pyruvate or lactate occurs in a process termed *anaerobic glycolysis.* Because pyruvate can participate in the aerobic production of adenosine triphosphate (ATP), glycolysis can also be considered the first step in the aerobic degradation of ATP. Anaerobic metabolism results in the accumulation of lactic acid in the blood, which can contribute to fatigue; lactic acid can also be used as a fuel during and following exercise.
[Chapter 2]

15–C. Rapid weight loss is considered to be 3 lb/week for women and 3–5 lb/week for men after the first 2 weeks of the diet. Long-term maintenance is usually a problem with rapid weight loss; one study reported total recidivism within 3–5 years. Modifications in diet and exercise are generally associated with more-permanent weight loss.
[Chapter 9]

16–C. Coronary artery bypass graft surgery is usually reserved for patients who have a poor prognosis for survival or who are unresponsive to pharmacologic treatment, stents, or percutaneous transluminal coronary angioplasty. Such patients include those with angina, left main coronary artery stenosis, multiple vessel disease, and left ventricular dysfunction.
[Chapter 4]

17–A. There are many benefits of chronic exercise for a patient with an automatic implantable cardioverter defibrillator (AICD). However, several precautions need to be taken, including monitoring the heart rate and knowing at what rate the AICD is set to shock the patient. The rate for activation is preset and varies for each patient. Depending, of course, on the exercise prescription, it generally is safe to exercise a patient up to that heart rate.
[Chapter 8]

18–D. The metabolic end products of oxidative phosphorylation include adenosine triphosphate and water. Other byproducts include carbon dioxide. Lactate is the metabolic end product of anaerobic glycolysis.
[Chapter 2]

19–B. A normal, unconditioned person has an anaerobic threshold of approximately 55% of maximal oxygen consumption. A conditioned person can have an anaerobic threshold as high as 70%–90% of maximal oxygen consumption. The onset of metabolic acidosis or anaerobic metabolism can be measured through serial measurements of blood lactate level or by the assessment of expired gases, specifically pulmonary ventilation and carbon dioxide production.
[Chapter 2]

20–D. Nitrates reduce ischemia by reducing myocardial oxygen demand with some increase in oxygen supply and are used in the treatment of typical and variant angina. Beta-adrenergic blockers reduce myocardial ischemia by lowering myocardial oxygen demand; lower blood pressure; control ventricular arrhythmias; and significantly reduce first year mortality rates in post–myocardial infarction patients by 20% to 35%. Calcium channel blockers reduce ischemia by altering the major determinants of myocardial oxygen supply and demand but have not been shown to reduce post–myocardial infarction mortality rates. Aspirin is a platelet-inhibitor.
[Chapter 4]

21–A. Cardiac impulses normally arise in the sinoatrial or sinus node of the heart. The sinoatrial node is located in the right atrium (posterior wall) near the opening of the superior vena cava. From the sinoatrial node, impulses travel to the left atrium and to the atrioventricular node, through the bundle of His and then on to Purkinje fibers in the ventricles.
[Chapter 12]

22–C. The steps are as follows:
   a. Choose the ACSM leg cycling formula.
   b. Write down your knowns and convert the values to the appropriate units:
   Knowns: 110 pounds ÷ 2.2 = 50 kg
   50 RPM × 6 meters = 300 m · min^{-1}
   2.5 kp = 2.5 kg
   60 minutes of cycling
   c. Write down the ACSM formula:

   Leg cycling $(ml \cdot kg^{-1} \cdot min^{-1}) = (1.8 \times work\ rate \div body\ weight) + (3.5) + (3.5)\ (ml \cdot kg^{-1} \cdot min^{-1})$

   d. Calculate work rate:

   Work rate $= kg \cdot m/min = 2.5\ kg \cdot 300\ m \cdot min^{-1}$
   $= 750\ kg^{-1} \cdot m \cdot min^{-1}$

   e. Substitute the known values for the variable name:

   $ml \cdot kg^{-1} \cdot min^{-1} = (1.8 \times 750 \div 50) + (3.5) + (3.5)$

   f. Solve for the unknown:

   $ml \cdot kg^{-1} \cdot min^{-1} = (27) + (3.5) + (3.5)$
   Gross leg cycling $\dot{V}O_2 = 34\ ml \cdot kg^{-1} \cdot min^{-1}$

   g. To find out how many calories she expends, we must first convert her oxygen consumption to absolute terms:

   Absolute $\dot{V}O_2 = relative\ \dot{V}O_2 \times body\ weight$
   $= 34\ ml \cdot kg^{-1} \cdot min^{-1} \times 50\ kg$
   $= 1700\ ml \cdot min^{-1}$

   h. Convert ml · min^{-1} to L · min^{-1} by dividing by 1000:

   $1700\ ml \cdot min^{-1} \div 1000 = 1.7\ L \cdot min^{-1}$

   i. Next we must see how many calories she expends in one minute by multiplying her absolute $\dot{V}O_2$ (in L · min^{-1}) by the constant 5.0:

   $1.7\ L \cdot min^{-1} \times 5.0 = 8.5\ kcal \cdot min^{-1}$

   j. Finally, multiply the number of calories she expends in one minute by the number of minutes she cycles:

   $8.5\ kcal \cdot min^{-1} \times 60\ min = 510\ total\ calories$
   [Chapter 11]

23–D. The proper anatomical location of V_4 is the midclavicular line, fifth intercostal space. Precordial leads V_1 and V_2 are located at the fourth intercostal space, right and left sternal borders. There is no precordial lead site at the midaxillary line, fifth intercostal space.
[Chapter 1]

24–A. During exercise, stroke volume increases curvilinearly with the work rate until it reaches near maximum at a level equivalent to approximately 50% of aerobic capacity and increasing only slightly thereafter. The left ventricle is able to contract with greater force during exercise because of a greater end-diastolic volume and enhanced mechanical ability of muscle fibers to produce force.
[Chapter 2]

25–A. Exposure to the cold causes vasoconstriction (higher blood pressure response), lowers the anginal threshold in patients with angina, can provoke angina at rest (variant or Prinzmetal's angina), and can induce asthma, general dehydration, and dryness or burning of the mouth and throat.
[Chapter 4]

26–C. To convert from pounds of fat to total kcal, multiply the fat weight (in pounds) by 3,500. The correct answer is 3 × 3,500 = 10,500 kcal.
[Chapter 8]

27–C. CQI can and should be both objective and subjective in its approach and data analysis. Subjective data, such as participant opinions on program offerings, as well as objective program attendance data are important.
[Chapter 10]

28–C. A thrombosis is a specific clot that may cause a myocardial infarction. An aneurysm is a condition caused by necrotic muscle fibers of the heart that degenerate, causing the myocardial wall to become very thin. During systole, these nonfunctional muscle fibers do not contract but rather bulge outward, increasing the risk of thrombus, ventricular arrhythmia, and heart failure. Thrombolysis (thrombolytic therapy) uses a specific clot-dissolving agent administered during acute myocardial infarction to restore blood flow and limit myocardial necrosis. Myocardial infarction is irreversible necrosis of the heart muscle resulting from prolonged ischemia.
[Chapter 4]

29–D. Digitalis is used to treat heart failure and certain arrhythmias. Shortening of the QT interval and a "scooping" of the ST–T complex characterize the effects of digitalis on the electrocardiogram.
[Chapter 12]

30–C. The energy to perform physical work comes from the breakdown of adenosine triphosphate (ATP). The amount of directly available ATP is small, with action lasting only 5–10 seconds; thus, ATP must be resynthesized constantly.
[Chapter 2]

31–A. Avoiding tension on the upper body is typically recommended for 4–8 weeks, not 2–4 months. All of the other precautions are accurate.
[Chapter 8]

32–D. Aging, the male gender, and family history of coronary artery disease are risk factors that cannot be controlled. Tobacco smoking, on the other hand, can be modified or eliminated.
[Chapter 4]

33–B. Triglycerides are the only substance listed that has been proven to be directly affected by exercise. Homocysteine and lipoprotein (a) have not been shown to change favorably with exercise. Low-density lipoprotein cholesterol is affected by diet and may be lowered indirectly from weight loss associated with exercise.
[Chapter 9]

34–C. Warm-up exercises tend to redistribute blood flow from the trunk to peripheral areas, decrease resistance in the tissues for movement, and increase tissue temperature and energy production. Cool down has an opposite effect.
[Chapter 2]

35–C. No-risk or low-risk individuals are those who are apparently healthy and asymptomatic and have no more than one coronary risk factor. Moderate-risk individuals are those who have signs or symptoms suggesting possible cardiopulmonary or metabolic disease and/or two or more risk factors. High-risk individuals are those with known cardiac, pulmonary, or metabolic disease.
[Chapter 6]

36–B. Second degree AV block is subdivided into two types: Mobitz Type I and Mobitz Type II. Mobitz Type I is also known as the Wenckebach phenomenon. In this condition, the conduction of the impulse through the AV junction becomes increasingly more difficult, resulting in a progressively longer PR interval until a QRS complex is dropped following a P-wave. This indicates that the AV junction failed to conduct the impulse from the atria to the ventricles. This pause allows the AV node to recover, and the following P-wave is conducted with a normal or slightly shorter PR interval.
[Chapter 12]

37–D. The magnitude of heart rate response is related to age, body position, fitness, type of activity, the presence of heart disease, medications, blood volume, and the environment. In unconditioned persons, a proportionally greater increase in heart rate is observed at any fixed submaximal work rate than is seen in conditioned persons.
[Chapter 2]

38–D. Regular exercise has been shown to increase caloric expenditure in an effort to reduce body weight for those who are obese; increase the activity of lipoprotein lipase, which alters blood fats such as triglycerides; and lower blood pressure. In addition to helping reduce these risk factors for the development of coronary artery disease, exercise also can have positive benefits for those with diabetes mellitus, peripheral arterial disease, osteoporosis, and pulmonary disease.
[Chapter 4]

39–C. ST segments are considered to be sensitive indicators of myocardial ischemia or injury. A Q wave is a negative deflection of a QRS complex preceding an R wave. A "pathological" Q wave is an indication of a old transmural myocardial infarction. The PR interval is the time it takes for the initiation of an electrical impulse in the

sinoatrial node to the initiation of electrical activity in the ventricles. The T wave indicates ventricular repolarization.
[Chapter 12]

40–D. The identification and classification of obesity has been somewhat discretionary with a multitude of techniques available. It appears that height/weight tables provide the least accurate technique, because they do not include any variance for body composition (i.e., amount of fat versus amount of lean tissue).
[Chapter 8]

41–C. A steady-state condition occurs when there is a balance between the energy required by the working muscles and the rate of ATP production through aerobic metabolism. Oxygen debt is the oxygen consumption in excess of the resting oxygen consumption at the end of an exercise session. Oxygen deficit is the difference between total oxygen actually consumed and the amount that would have been consumed in a steady state. Adaptation is a result of long-term sustained exercise training.
[Chapter 2]

42–B. The electrocardiogram is an excellent tool for detecting rhythm and conduction abnormalities, chamber enlargements, ischemia, and infarction. ST segment elevation is a sign of acute myocardial infarction with resulting loss of R waves replaced by Q waves.
[Chapter 4]

43–C. The steps are as follows:
  a. Choose the ACSM walking formula.
  b. Write down your knowns and convert the values to the appropriate units:
    Knowns: 3.5 mph × (26.8) = 93.8 m · min^{-1}
    10% grade = 0.10
  c. Write down the ACSM walking formula:
Walking = (0.1 × speed) + (1.8 × speed × fractional grade) + (3.5)(ml · kg^{-1} · min^{-1})
  d. Substitute the known values for the variable name:
ml · kg^{-1} · min^{-1} = (0.1 × 93.8) + (1.8 × 93.8 × 0.1) + (3.5)
ml · kg^{-1} · min^{-1} = (9.38) + (16.884) + (3.5)
  e. Solve for the unknown:
ml · kg^{-1} · min^{-1} = (9.38) + (16.884) + (3.5)
Gross walking $\dot{V}O_2$ = 29.76 ml · kg^{-1} · min^{-1}
[Chapter 11]

44–D. Segmental movements occur around an axis and in a plane. Each of the planes has an associated axis perpendicular to it. The mediolateral axis is perpendicular to the sagittal plane, and the

anteroposterior axis is perpendicular to the frontal plane. There is no transverse axis.
[Chapter 1]

45–C. The benefits of regular (endurance) exercise for patients diagnosed with peripheral vascular disease include redistribution of and increased blood flow to the legs, increased tolerance for walking and improved claudication pain tolerance, *decreased* blood viscosity, and improved muscle cell metabolism.
[Chapter 8]

46–B. The purpose of health screening prior to engaging in vigorous exercise is to identify clients who require additional medical testing to determine the presence of disease, contraindications for exercise testing or training, or referral to a medically supervised exercise program. Men under age 40 and women under age 50 with fewer than two coronary artery disease risk factors do not require a physician's evaluation prior to initiating vigorous exercise (defined as greater than 60% of maximal oxygen consumption).
[Chapter 6]

47–D. An intraventricular conduction disturbance is an abnormal conduction of an electrical impulse below the Bundle of His. Intraventricular conduction disturbances include right and left bundle branch block, and right and left anterior hemiblock.
[Chapter 12]

48–B. Emergency plans must be created, practiced, and implemented in the event of a medical emergency. Clinical personnel must understand the risks associated with exercise and exercise testing, be able to implement preventive measures, and have knowledge of the care of an injury or medical emergency.
[Chapter 7]

49–C. Obesity is defined as a surplus of adipose tissue, resulting from excess energy intake relative to energy expenditure. Overweight is a deviation in body weight from some standard or "ideal" weight related to height. Android obesity describes fat accumulation over the chest and arms rather than the lower trunk, which is gynoid obesity.
[Chapter 9]

50–D. Program certification of clinical exercise rehabilitation programs, while a new concept, involves many components already established as part of the exercise program, such as a clearly articulated mission statement; a defined

organizational chart; a method of measuring client outcomes; a well-used policy and procedures manual; and so forth. Certification of a program is about the *quality* of the program, not about the financial operations of a program such as billing practices and the use of insurance codes.
[Chapter 10]

51–B. Preload refers to diastolic filling (i.e., the amount of blood in the left ventricular prior to ejection). Contractility is the vigor of contraction and may be influenced by ventricular outflow (afterload). Ejection fraction is the ratio of stroke volume to end-diastolic volume.
[Chapter 2]

52–A. Angina pectoris is the pain associated with myocardial ischemia. The pain is often felt in the chest, neck, cheeks, shoulder, or arms; can be brought on by physical or psychological stress; and is relieved when the stressor is removed. Angina can be either classic (typical) or vasospastic (variant or Prinzmetal's).
[Chapter 4]

53–D. The overall goal of health screening before participation in a graded exercise testing or an exercise program is to obtain essential information that will ensure the safety of the participant. Thus, health screening helps to determine the presence of disease, enables one to consider possible contraindications for exercise testing and training, and helps determine whether referral to a medically supervised exercise program is needed.
[Chapter 6]

54–B. The proper response for a patient who has experienced a cardiac arrest yet is breathing and has a pulse is to place an immediate call to the emergency medical system, place the patient in the recovery position with the head to the side to avoid an airway obstruction, and then stay with the patient and continue to monitor vital signs.
[Chapter 7]

55–B. Use the walking metabolic equation to determine the relative oxygen consumption [(0.1 × speed) + (1.8 × speed × grade) + 3.5]; then convert ml/kg/min to L/min; then L/min to kcal/min.

$$\dot{V}O_2 = (0.1 \times 107) + (1.8 \times 107 \times 0.05) + 3.5$$

$$\dot{V}O_2 = 23.83 \ ml/kg/min$$

$$\dot{V}O_2 = 2.14 \ L/min \ (23.83 \ ml/kg/min \times 90.01 \ kg)/1,000$$

[Chapter 8]

56–B. Advancing age brings a progressive decline in bone mineral density and calcium content. This loss accelerates in women immediately after menopause. As a result, older women are at increased risk for bone fractures, a significant cause of morbidity and mortality in the elderly. Hip fractures are the most common and account for a large share of the disability, death, and high medical costs associated with falls.
[Chapter 3]

57–D. Electrocardiography is the least sensitive and least specific of all these tests. Directly visualizing the coronary arteries by using coronary angiography provides the highest sensitivity and specificity. Radionuclide imaging and echocardiography have about the same sensitivity and specificity.
[Chapter 4]

58–C. In the resting period of the myocardial cell, the inside of the cell membrane is negatively charged and the outside of the cell membrane is positively charged. As such, the term "polarized" cell is reserved for the normal "resting myocardial cell" and describes the presence of electrical potential across the cell membrane due to separation of electrical charges. When an electrical impulse is generated in a particular area in the heart, the outside of the cell in this area becomes negative, whereas the inside of the cell in the same area becomes positive. This state of cell excitation (due to a change in polarity) is called depolarization. The simulated myocardial cells return to their resting state in a process called repolarization.
[Chapter 12]

59–A. At exercise intensities up to 50% of maximal oxygen consumption, the increase in cardiac output is facilitated by increases in heart rate and stroke volume. Thereafter, the increase results almost solely from the continued rise in heart rate.
[Chapter 2]

60–D. Flow-resistive training involves breathing through a progressively smaller opening. Paced breathing helps coordinate breathing with activities of daily living. Respiratory muscle training increases respiratory muscle strength and endurance. A preset inspiratory pressure, usually at the same fraction of maximal inspiratory pressure, is known as threshold loading training.
[Chapter 8]

61–A. Isometric contractions occur when the muscle group contracts against a fixed load or resistance with no change in the length of the involved

muscle group or joint motion. In isotonic contractions, the muscle shortens.
[Chapter 2]

62–C.   Family history of coronary artery disease cannot be changed. The others are modifiable risk factors that, with some intervention, can be changed or modified.
[Chapter 4]

63–B.   Staff salaries are not capital expenses; capital expenses are used to procure something tangible for the program. Rather, staff salaries are an example of a variable expense. The purchase of equipment and the cost associated with construction are excellent examples of capital expenses.
[Chapter 10]

64–A.   Torque is the product of a force and the perpendicular distance from the line of action of the force, whereas force can be seen as a push or a pull that produces or has the capacity to produce a change in motion of a body. Multiple forces from multiple directions may act on a body; however, it is the sum of the forces, or the *net force*, that determines the resulting change in motion. Newton's Law describes the relationship between forces, torques, and the resulting movements.
[Chapter 1]

65–C.   The endothelium comprises a single layer of cells that form a tight barrier between blood and the arterial wall to resist thrombosis, promote vasodilation, and inhibit smooth muscle cells from migration and proliferation into the intima. The intima is the very thin, innermost layer of the artery wall composed mainly of connective tissue with some smooth muscle cells. The media, the thickest layer, comprises predominantly smooth muscle cells. It is responsible for arterial vasoconstriction and vasodilation. The adventitia is the outermost layer of the artery wall and provides the media and intima with oxygen and other nutrients.
[Chapter 4]

66–B.   The electrode position for V_1 is the right sternal border, fourth intercostal space. V_2 is located in the fourth intercostal space, left sternal border. The position of V_3 is at the midpoint of a straight line between V_2 and V_4, and V_6 is located on the midaxillary line and horizontal to V_4 and V_5.
[Chapter 12]

67–C.   The energy expenditure for the warm up is 2.0 METs × 5 minutes = 10 METs.

The energy expenditure for the treadmill is 9.0 METs × 20 minutes = 180 METs.

The energy expenditure for the cycle is 8.0 METs × 20 minutes = 160 METs.

The energy expenditure for the cool down is 2.50 METs × 5 minutes = 12.5 METs.

The total energy expenditure is 10 + 180 + 160 + 12.5 = 362.5 METs. Multipy 362.5 METs by 3.5 (because 1 MET = 3.5 ml/kg/min) which equals 1,268.75 ml/kg. Multiply 1,268.75 ml/kg by body weight (70 kg), which equals 88,812.5 ml. Divide that number by 1,000 (because 1,000 mL equals 1 L), which equals 88.81 L. Multiply 88.81 L by 5 (because 5 kcal equals 1 L of oxygen consumed), which equals 444 kcal.
[Chapter 8]

68–C.   Average maximal heart rate is 200 beats/minute, and average maximal stroke volume is 100 ml/stroke; average maximal cardiac output is the product of these two values, or 20 L/minute.
[Chapter 2]

69–C.   High ambient temperature or relative humidity increases the risk of heat-related disorders, including heat cramps, heat syncope, dehydration, heat exhaustion, and heat stroke. Exercise will increase heart rate responses at submaximal workloads and lower oxygen consumption at maximal workloads. In this type of environment, the exercise prescription should be altered by lowering the intensity and also possibly the duration, and, if necessary, by including intermittent rest periods.
[Chapter 4]

70–C.   The emergency plan must be written down and available in all testing and exercise areas. The plan should list the specific responsibilities of each staff member, the required equipment, and pre-determined contacts for an emergency response. All emergencies must be documented with dates, times, actions, people involved, and results. The plan should be practiced with announced and unannounced drills on a quarterly basis. All staff, including non-clinical staff, should be trained in the emergency plan.
[Chapter 7]

71–D.   Osteoarthritis is a degenerative joint disease, generally localized first on an articular cartilage. Rheumatoid arthritis is an inflammatory disease affecting joints and organs as well. Osteoporosis involve loss of bone density. Multiple sclerosis is a neuromuscular disease.
[Chapter 8]

72–B. Classic symptoms of bronchitis include sputum production, chronic cough, and dyspnea associated with the characteristics listed. The clinical symptom of emphysema is dyspnea associated with hypoxia and hypercapnia resulting from hypoventilation of the alveoli; minute ventilation is also very high. Asthma is a reversible condition characterized by an obvious narrowing of the bronchial airways causing dyspnea. Atherosclerosis is a progressive disease of the systemic arterial system.
[Chapter 4]

73–D. Exercise training can counteract the harmful physiological effects of inactivity often associated with chronic diseases. There are a number of precautions and contraindications to exercise, however; one such precaution is to ensure adequate warm up and cool down periods.
[Chapter 8]

74–D. Direct measurement of oxygen consumption requires an extensive laboratory and specialized equipment. It can be measured in the laboratory using techniques of direct and indirect calorimetry or can be estimated from the workload.
[Chapter 2]

75–D. Supervision and staffing recommendations for various populations are available from a number of professional organizations as well as insurance companies. The ACSM recommends supervision of exercise programs for patients with heart disease be under the overall guidance of a physician and an ACSM Program Director$_{SM}$ or ACSM Exercise Specialist ®.
[Chapter 8]

76–D. Physical activity elevates oxygen consumption above resting levels. This additional oxygen uptake by the body is known as the net oxygen consumption. Total oxygen consumption (resting energy expenditure and the oxygen consumption of physical activity) is the gross energy expenditure (i.e., gross oxygen consumption). Net and gross oxygen consumption can be expressed in relative or absolute terms.
[Chapter 8]

77–D. Two premature ventricular contractions (PVCs) in a row is known as a PVC couplet. Ventricular tachycardia occurs when three PVCs (or more) occur in a row without any normal beats.
[Chapter 12]

78–D. A complication of an extensive myocardial infarction is a ventricular aneurysm. Characteristics of a ventricular aneurysm include a degeneration of the myocardial wall, which becomes very thin and often bulges out during systole. These fibers do not contract during systole.
[Chapter 4]

79–C. The amount of weight or resistance and repetitions will vary for strength versus endurance. Rapid strength gains will be realized at higher resistance or weight (80%–100% of 1 repetition maximum) and lower repetitions (6–8). For muscular endurance, a lower weight is used (40%–60% of one repetition maximum) and higher repetitions (8–15).
[Chapter 8]

80–B. Mounted on a balloon catheter that is inflated or expanded at the site of a coronary artery blockage, a stent is a slotted stainless steel tube that is permanently implanted in the artery, where it acts as a scaffold to hold the walls of a coronary artery open.
[Chapter 4]

81–A. The PR interval is measured from the beginning of the P wave to the beginning of the QRS complex. It represents the time required for the impulse to spread through the atria and to pass through the atrioventricular junction. Normal PR interval is 0.12–0.20 second; a PR interval prolonged beyond 0.20 second with all P waves conducted and all PR intervals the same indicates first-degree atrioventricular block.
[Chapter 12]

82–C. Myocardial infarction can be determined and localized by careful inspection of certain electrocardiographic leads. Pathological Q waves on the anterior leads indicate a transmural myocardial infarction of the anterior wall of the left ventricle.
[Chapter 12]

83–A. Atherosclerosis is thought to begin at an early age—at birth, according to some. The disease process is related to the presence of risk factors. Progression does not necessarily occur in a stable, linear manner; some lesions may develop slowly and are relatively stable, whereas other lesions progress very quickly as a result of frequent plaque rupture, formation of thrombi, and changes in the intima.
[Chapter 4]

84–C. Various graded exercise test protocols are available. Some are continuous (with measurements taken without interruption), and others are discontinuous (involving a momentary stop while measurements are obtained). Some

test protocols are taken during a step test, whereas others are taken in the field.
[Chapter 6]

85–C.   Exercise has various benefits for patients with congestive heart failure. It appears as though most of the physical improvements are peripheral (i.e., within the skeletal muscle) and not central. Other benefits of regular exercise for patients with congestive heart failure are a decrease in symptoms and an enhanced quality of life.
[Chapter 8]

86–A.   Although strength training (resistance training) may be beneficial to all of these special populations, regular resistance training helps conserve bone mass, thus decreasing the progression of osteoporosis.
[Chapter 8]

87–B.   Even after exposure and training, an approximate 10% reduction in maximal oxygen consumption occurs per 1,000 meters of altitude above 1,500 meters. After acclimatization, expect a continued increase in pulmonary ventilation and heart rate response at submaximal workloads but a reduced cardiac output, stroke volume, and heart rate at maximal exercise.
[Chapter 4]

88–C.   A QRS duration exeeding 0.20 second indicates an intraventricular conduction delay. Examples of intraventricular conduction delays include premature ventricular contractions and left bundle branch block.
[Chapter 12]

89–B.   With the physical demands of exercise, emergency situations can occur, especially in a clinical setting where patients with disease are exercising. The incidence of a cardiac arrest during exercise testing is 0.4 in 10,000.
[Chapter 12]

90–B.   Very-low-density lipoprotein cholesterol is composed almost entirely of triglycerides, which are converted to a fuel source by the enzyme lipoprotein lipase (which increases with exercise). High-density lipoprotein cholesterol is also increased by regular exercise: The very-low-density lipoprotein remnants serve as precursors to high density lipoprotein cholesterol.
[Chapter 4]

91–B.   The health behavior change model comprises three phases: antecedents, adoption, and maintenance. *Antecedents* refers to all conditions that exist that can support, initiate, or hinder changes in health behavior, including information, instruction, role

models, and previous experience. *Adoption* is the early phase of making a change in a health behavior or the intention to make a change (often a difficult decision). This phase involves any environmental and physical prerequisites, self-efficiency and outcome efficiency, cues to action, goal setting, and behavioral intention. The *maintenance* phase is one of continued response and includes relapse prevention, reinforcement, monitoring, and contracting.
[Chapter 5]

92–A.   Lowering total cholesterol and low-density lipoprotein cholesterol has proven effective in reducing and even reversing atherosclerosis. The goal is to reduce the availability of lipids to the injured endothelium. In primary prevention trials, lowering total cholesterol and low-density lipoprotein cholesterol has been shown to reduce the incidence and mortality of coronary artery disease.
[Chapter 4]

93–D.   Field tests are those that can be administered with minimal equipment and in varying conditions. In the Cooper 12-minute test, the subject covers the greatest distance possible during the 12-minute test period. Maximal oxygen consumption is estimated from the distance covered in meters. The 1.5-mile test is an estimate of maximal oxygen consumption taken as a result of the time needed to cover the distance. The Rockport walking test is a submaximal test that requires the patient to walk 1 mile as fast as possible; immediate postexercise heart rate is measured and maximal oxygen consumption is predicted based on gender, time, and heart rate. Treadmill testing is a complicated procedure normally performed in a laboratory setting.
[Chapter 6]

94–D.   Transmural myocardial infarction produces changes in both the QRS complex and the ST segment. ST segment elevation or tall upright T waves are the earliest signs associated with transmural myocardial infarction. ST segment elevation may persist for a few hours to a few days.
[Chapter 12]

95–C.   The purpose of the warm up is to slowly and safely activate the body's responses to exercise and to increase the range of motion to prepare joints and muscles for vigorous activity. Beneficial physiological responses include increased heart rate and stroke volume, increased body temperature and muscle temperature, and increased metabolic activity.
[Chapter 8]

96–A. It is essential that clinicians be familiar with contraindications to exercise and exercise testing. For a certain group of patients, the risks of exercise testing and exercise in general outweigh the benefits.
[Chapter 7]

97–A. Physical inactivity (sedentary life style) has been determined to have a similar risk in the development of atherosclerosis as the other major risk factors (smoking, hypertension and elevated cholesterol). Obesity, diabetes mellitus, and stress are important risk factors but are not thought to be as significant as smoking, high blood pressure or high cholesterol.
[Chapter 4]

98–B. The 400-meter sprint is an example of physical activity requiring anaerobic glycolysis to produce energy in the form of adenosine triphosphate (ATP). Shorter sprints rely on ready stores of ATP and phosphocreatine. Longer runs require aerobic metabolism to produce ATP.
[Chapter 2]

99–C. A mean electrical axis between –30° and +100° is considered to be normal. An axis that is more negative than –30° is considered to be left axis deviation; an axis greater than +100° is considered to be right axis deviation until it reaches –180° and then it is considered to be extreme right axis deviation or extreme left axis deviation.
[Chapter 12]

100–C. Beta-adrenergic blockers significantly reduce first-year mortality rates in post-MI patients. Aspirin is a platelet inhibitor. Calcium channel blockers reduce ischemia by altering the major determinants of myocardial oxygen supply and demand but have not been shown to reduce post-myocardial infarction mortality rates. Nitrates reduce ischemia by reducing myocardial oxygen demand with some increase in oxygen supply and are used in the treatment of typical and variant angina.
[Chapter 4]

Index

Note: Page numbers in *italics* indicate illustrations; those followed by t indicate tables. Q and A denote questions and answers.